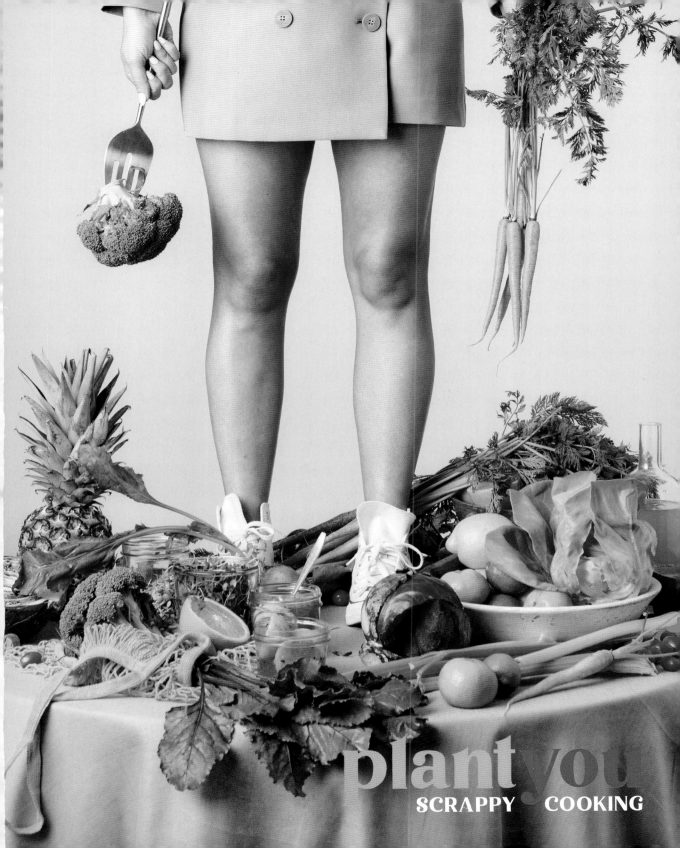

plantyou

SCRAPPY COOKING

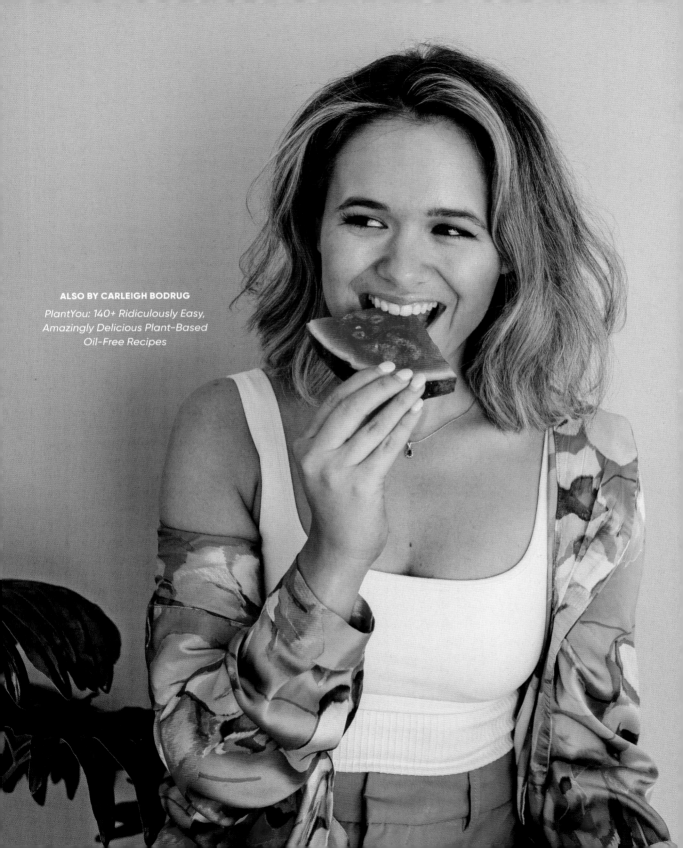

plantyou
SCRAPPY COOKING

140+ Plant-Based Zero-Waste Recipes That Are Good for You, Your Wallet, and the Planet

Carleigh Bodrug

hachette
BOOKS

NEW YORK

Copyright © 2024 by Carleigh Bodrug

Interior photos by Shahad Odah, Foodie's Flare
Jacket photos by Linda Pugliese
Cover design by Amanda Kain
Cover copyright © 2024 by Hachette Book Group, Inc.

Hachette Go, an imprint of Hachette Books
Hachette Book Group
1290 Avenue of the Americas
New York, NY 10104
HachetteGo.com
Facebook.com/HachetteGo
Instagram.com/HachetteGo

First Edition: April 2024

Published by Hachette Go, an imprint of Hachette Book Group, Inc. The Hachette Go name and logo is a trademark of the Hachette Book Group.

The Hachette Speakers Bureau provides a wide range of authors for speaking events. To find out more, go to hachettespeakersbureau.com or email HachetteSpeakers@hbgusa.com.

Hachette Go books may be purchased in bulk for business, educational, or promotional use. For information, please contact your local bookseller or Hachette Book Group Special Markets Department at special.markets@hbgusa.com.

The publisher is not responsible for websites (or their content) that are not owned by the publisher.

Library of Congress Cataloging-in-Publication Data

Names: Bodrug, Carleigh, author.
Title: PlantYou: scrappy cooking: 140+ plant-based zero-waste recipes that are good for you, your wallet, and the planet / Carleigh Bodrug.
Description: New York, NY: Hachette Go, 2024. | Includes index.
Identifiers: LCCN 2023030616 | ISBN 9780306832420 (hardcover) | ISBN 9780306832437 (ebook)
Subjects: LCSH: Vegan cooking. | Cooking (Leftovers) | Food Waste—Prevention. | Waste minimization. | LCGFT: Cookbooks.
Classification: LCC TX837 .B5647 2024 | DDC 641.5/6362—dc23/eng/20230728
LC record available at https://lccn.loc.gov/2023030616

ISBNs: 978-0-306-83242-0 (hardcover); 978-0-306-83243-7 (ebook);
978-0-306-83550-6 (signed edition); 978-0-306-83549-0 (B&N signed edition)

Printed in China

IM

10 9 8 7 6 5 4 3 2

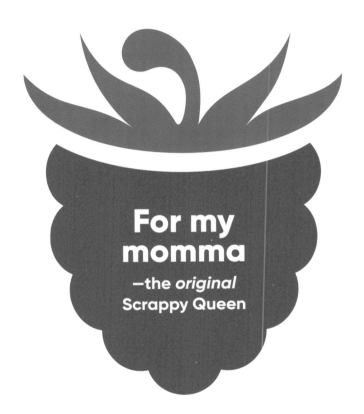

For my
momma
—the *original*
Scrappy Queen

Contents

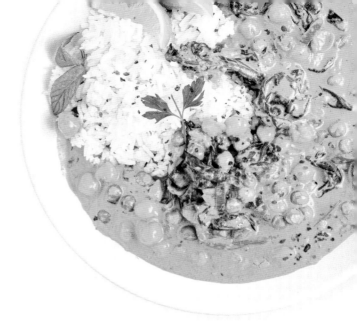

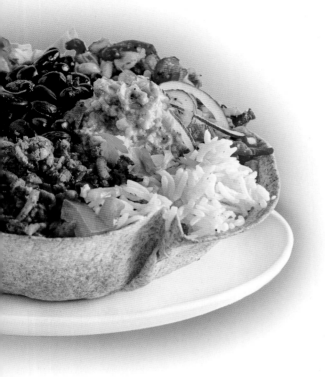

CHAPTER 8
Sustainable Sweets

CHAPTER 6
The Main Bowl

CHAPTER 7
Eco Entrées

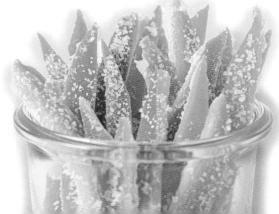

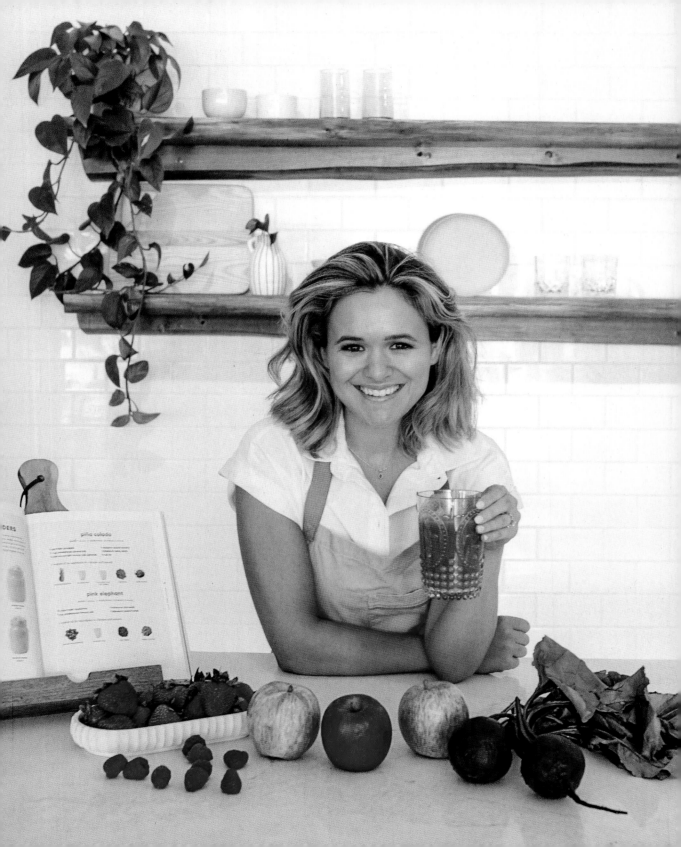

Introduction

Scrappy:

1. made of scraps, consisting of odds and ends

2. spirited, energetic, and resilient
(hey . . . I'm looking at you)

Picture yourself getting home from work after a hectic day. Your stomach is growling, and it's time to cook up a delicious dinner. You open the fridge with anticipation, only to find a vegetable graveyard. Half a bell pepper, a wilted box of spinach, and, of course—a decapitated broccoli stem in the back of the fridge. You think to yourself, *"What the heck can I make with this?!"*

Lucky for you, you're holding the solution in your hands. You see—when I wrote this cookbook, I really didn't want it to be a simple compilation of low-waste hacks to leaf through every so often (although—we've got you covered for those too)! Instead, this is a cookbook you can lean on when you're wondering how to use up anything from radish tops to a can of chickpeas. Inside, you will find over 150 practical, nutritious recipes that help you *use what you already have* for breakfast, lunch, dinner, dessert, and more!

Welcome to the *Scrappy* side, my friend.

This isn't about being perfect. . . . In fact, it's the opposite. This is our little corner of the world where everyone is invited. I officially welcome you to a club that's all about making do with what you've got, learning to improvise, making mistakes, and coming out with something tasty and nourishing in the end.

Come on in, take a seat at my table, and let me teach you how to cook up some delicious food that's good for you, your wallet, and the planet.

Are you ready to get a little weird in the kitchen and embrace your inner *Scrappy*?

Let's do this.

A LITTLE ABOUT ME AND THIS *SCRAPPY* THING

Hey, I'm Carleigh.

Most people know me as the girl behind the food blog and social media brand PlantYou, where I'm cooking up simple and delicious plant-based and low-waste recipes (*OK OK . . . while also posting daily pictures of my cat, King Tut*). Over the years I've been super fortunate to garner an audience of millions of people who are interested in eating more plants, and even wrote a *New York Times* bestselling cookbook called *PlantYou*, teaching people the basics.

Then, a few years back, I learned a statistic about food waste that just about stopped me in my tracks. You might not know this either, but an estimated 30 to 40 percent of the ENTIRE United States food supply ends up in landfills, and a lot of this stems from household waste. We'll dig more into this later, but food waste is a not-so-great thing for our planet (and, obviously, our pocketbooks as well)!

Now, as a vegan food blogger, I already considered myself someone who was pretty conscious about food waste and my environmental impact. Having grown up in Canada, grocery sticker shock is a real thing to me, so in *Scrappy* fashion, I was constantly trying to make the most of the ingredients I bought from the store each week. I threw radish tops into pesto, I chopped broccoli stems into my weekly stir-fry, and of course I kept a reusable bag of scraps in the freezer to make broth each month.

So, one day on Instagram, I decided to post an impromptu video about how to transform orange peels into a delicious candy reminiscent of gummy worms (page 254). As I threw an orange into the air, I yelled, "STOP THROWING OUT THOSE ORANGE PEELS! . . . MAKE ORANGE PEEL CANDY INSTEAD!" I then showed how to make the simple recipe in a quick, thirty-second clip. After posting, I signed off and went about my day, only to return to the app a few hours later to find out the video had been viewed an unexaggerated one *million* times.

I couldn't believe how many people were jazzed about reducing their food waste and eating more plants. This was the perfect opportunity to teach people the years of culinary tips I had learned by experimenting in the kitchen with scraps—and BAM, *Scrappy Cooking* was born.

An estimated 30 to 40 percent of the ENTIRE United States food supply ends up in LANDFILLS.

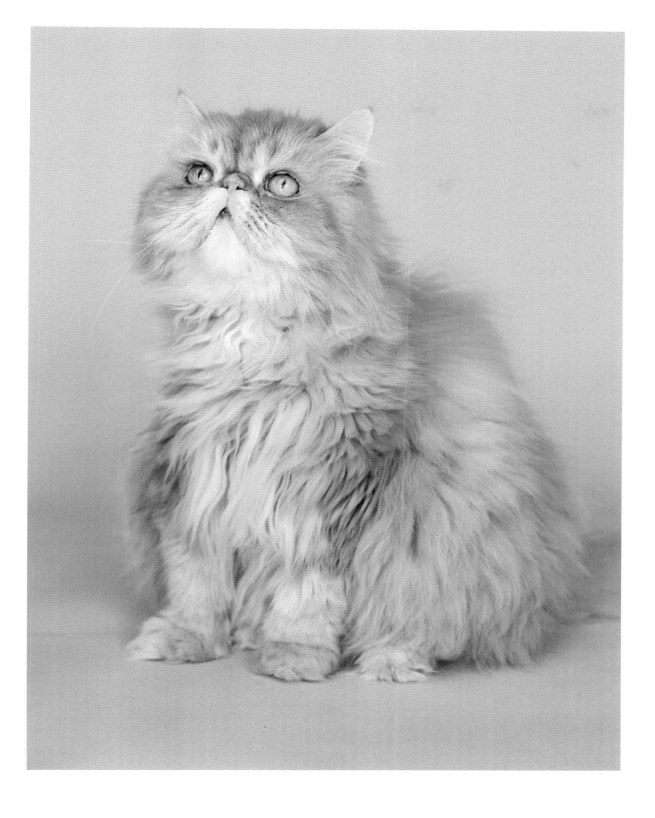

BUT ENOUGH ABOUT ME . . . THIS BOOK IS ABOUT *YOU*

At its core, PlantYou has always been about showing you that cooking nourishing and delicious whole-food, plant-based recipes doesn't have to be time-consuming or complicated.

Scrappy Cooking takes that concept one step further by arming you with the skills to make recipes that are not only great for your health but help you reduce food waste and save money as well.

With this in mind, you'll notice all recipes in this book contain no animal products, with very limited use of any heavily processed food, such as store-bought vegan meat or cheeses (nothing wrong with these, but they're not always accessible). Every single recipe also provides nut-, gluten-, and oil-free substitutions where possible. For your convenience, the macronutrient amounts for each recipe (calories, protein, fat, and carbs) are listed at the back of the book for quick reference.

That's why there are recipes for breakfast, lunch, dinner, and dessert that utilize food we tend to toss—yep, scraps (like how to transform your carrot tops into a life-changing chimichurri, page 272)—but also are, most important, heavily customizable to the ingredients you might have lying around right now. (Recipes earmarked as *Kitchen Raid* are those you can mix and match with any ingredients you have on hand.)

I've also provided a helpful visual index (page 18) that lists some of the most commonly wasted foods—and corresponding recipes for using them up. You can refer to the notes section of every recipe to see what you can do with any leftover scraps, as well as storage instructions. When I say *Scrappy Cooking*, I mean *Scrappy Cooking*!

STAGGERING STATS FOR PERSPECTIVE

Food waste is a bigger problem than most of us realize in North America and beyond. To put this in perspective, the US Department of Agriculture (USDA) estimates 133 billion pounds of food is wasted in the US each year, and costs the average American family $1,800 annually on their groceries. Shockingly, a report by ReFED found that one of the largest sources of food waste in the US is actually *in the household*, which accounts for 43 percent of all food waste after it goes to market, followed by restaurants and food service. This doesn't capture the food that is lost before market, due to post-harvest storage, inedible produce, and transportation.

But food waste doesn't just hurt our wallets, does it? It's bigger than that.

Food that makes it to landfills decomposes and releases methane, a potent greenhouse gas about twenty-eight times more powerful than CO_2 in terms of its warming potential over a hundred-year period.

According to the United States Environmental Protection Agency (EPA), food waste is estimated to make up around 24 percent of the material in landfills, and the largest component of municipal solid waste. This doesn't begin to quantify the energy used to produce, transport, store, and process food that is lost.

While we talk about the environmental impact of the food on our plate, I'd be remiss not to mention again that all recipes in this cookbook, and at PlantYou, are entirely free of animal products, and with good reason. This is important for not only our health but the health of our planet.

Avoiding meat and dairy products is the single biggest way an individual can reduce their environmental impact. A study by Poore and Nemecek[1] showed that meat and dairy provide just 18 percent of calories to feed the world, yet use up to 85 percent of farmland, also contributing 60 percent of agriculture's greenhouse gas emissions.

How's that for perspective?!

I know all that was pretty depressing (and scary), but sometimes we need to have that kind of knowledge before we can change our lifestyle, change our thinking, and, yes, change our cooking. So, in that vein (and with the stats tucked away), let's have some scrappy fun—with a slight detour into understanding the contents of our own kitchens and grocery purchases. Let's talk about what's being wasted and how to achieve tasty streamlining. After all, we can't get *Scrappy* unless we understand where the scraps are hiding!

1   Joseph Poore and Thomas Nemecek, "Reducing Food's Environmental Impacts Through Producers and Consumers," *Science* 360 (2018): 987–992.

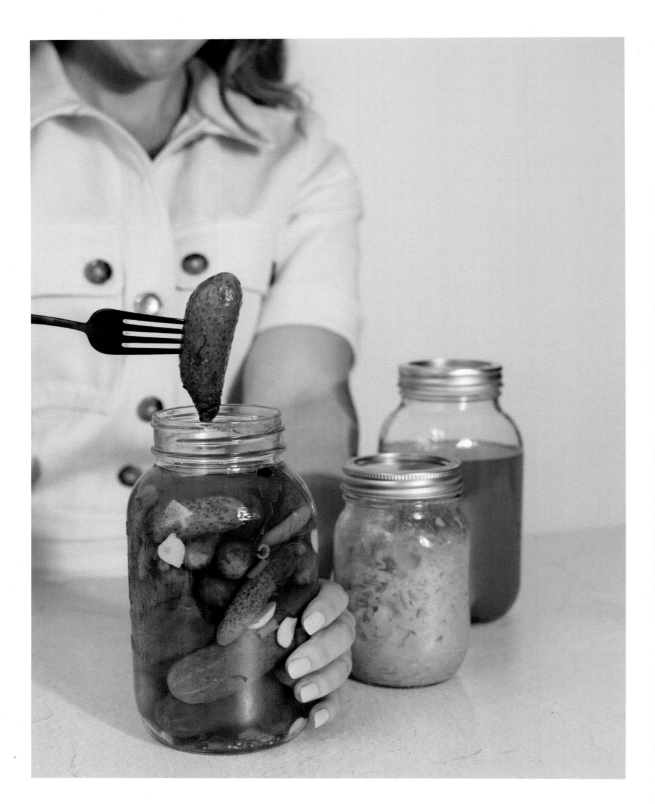

SOOOO . . . LET'S STOP WASTING SO MUCH FOOD—AND MONEY!

Now that we know so much food goes to waste in our homes, let's talk about the problems and, more important, the practical solutions to help us navigate our daily cooking lives.

I want to start by acknowledging that, for many, being able to purchase food is a privilege. In 2021, 10.2 percent of US households were insecure at some point throughout the year, according to the USDA. That number is staggering, and as grocery prices continue to skyrocket, it's more important than ever to figure out ways to save and use up every bit of the food we are purchasing, as well as a grassroots approach to reducing food waste at every stage of the system. Here are some simple adjustments you might be able to make in your home to make the most of what you have.

Problem: Food storage

Unfortunately, a lot of fresh produce spoils because we simply don't know how to store it in the most effective way. I'm going to cover some of the most commonly purchased food items here, and how to store them for longevity.

Solution

LEAFY GREENS AND HERBS—such as spinach, kale, chard, and parsley

- Before storing your greens, wash them thoroughly and dry them completely. You want to remove as much moisture as possible to avoid wilting and spoilage.

- After washing and drying, wrap leafy greens in a clean cloth. The cloth will absorb any excess moisture and keep the leaves crisp and dry.

- Store your wrapped greens in a sealable glass or plastic container in the refrigerator. Avoid storing leafy greens near fruits that produce ethylene gas, such as apples and bananas, as they will speed up the spoiling process.

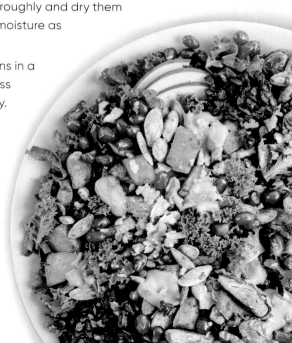

OTHER VEGGIES

- Store other vegetables in a cool, dry place, such as the crisper drawer in your fridge. Be sure not to overload this drawer, as it can prevent air circulation.
- Some vegetables, such as carrots and celery, can be sliced and stored in jars of water in the fridge to keep them fresh and crisp. Just make sure to swap out this water every few days.
- For vegetables with leafy tops, such as carrots, beets, and radishes, it is best to remove the greens and store them separately, as they can draw moisture from the vegetables, causing them to wilt more quickly.

FRUIT

- Most fruit can be stored in the fridge to keep fresh. However, bananas, avocados, and tomatoes should be stored at room temperature until they are ripe, when they can be moved to the fridge to slow down the spoiling process.

BREAD

- Bread and baked goods should be stored in a cool, dry place, such as a bread box or pantry.
- You can also freeze bread to make it last longer. If you purchase a large loaf and know you generally don't get through the whole thing in a week, slice it in half and store it in a sealed container in the freezer to thaw as you need it.

POTATOES

- Potatoes should be stored in a cool, dark, and dry place, ideally between 45°F and 55°F, in a paper bag, if possible. Storing them in a warm or moist environment will cause them to spoil quickly.

NUTS & SEEDS

- Nuts and seeds are subject to mold and can go rancid quickly. To prevent this, store your nuts and seeds in sealed glass containers in the fridge, if possible.
- If the fridge isn't an option, a cool, dry, and dark environment is best.

OTHER DRY GOODS

- Store dry goods, such as pasta, rice, and cereal, in a cold, dry place in your pantry, ideally in airtight containers.

Problem: Overpurchasing

We live in a consumer culture where food is readily available 24/7, a hop, skip, or click away. Which means that it's easy to overbuy—with much food spoiling before it can be eaten.

Solution

It can't be overemphasized. Instead of heading to the grocery store and aimlessly purchasing this and that, plan out your meals for the week so that you are buying food with meticulous *intention*.

This can be as simple as jotting down in the notes app on your phone, breakfast, lunch, and dinner plans and what you will need for each meal.

By doing this simple ritual, you can also "shop" your fridge and pantry to see what you already have in stock, to prevent buying duplicates. You will also save time at the grocery store with a handy list.

Before you go shopping for the week, you can also refer to any of the *Kitchen Raid* meals in this book, which are designed to help you use up the fresh produce you have on hand.

Problem: "Best Before" Dates

Now, I'm not going to tell you to start drinking expired oat milk. BUT . . . "best before" dates can be misleading because they are often misinterpreted as expiration dates. However, they simply indicate at which point a food item will still retain its optimal quality, flavor, and nutritional value—not necessarily when a food is unsafe to eat.

Solution

In most cases, food (particularly whole food) is still safe to eat as long as it has been stored properly and does not show signs of spoilage. Check for any off odor, unusual texture, or signs of mold before consuming or tasting it. Otherwise, let's *not* make it landfill fodder!

Problem: Scraps

In North America in particular, we often misinterpret which part of the food can be eaten, and which should be discarded. This applies to such things as beet greens, broccoli stalks, radish tops, skins, peels, and much more—all of which make wonderful foundations for absolutely delicious and nourishing meals. When we're purchasing these whole foods by weight and throwing part of them away needlessly, we're not only wasting great food but actually throwing money down the drain!

Solution

You've got it in your hands! In this cookbook, I arm you with the knowledge of how to use commonly discarded scraps for delicious recipes, such as Carrot Top Chimichurri (page 272), Broccoli Stem Summer Rolls (page 108), and We-Got-the-Beet Chips (page 62).

Problem: Imperfect Produce

As consumers, we often overlook or reject food that doesn't look shiny and perfect (think about that butternut squash that has a bit of a wonky shape). It might surprise you to learn that individual bananas are bought far less than bunches, and inevitably are often wasted because their perceived value is less. This results in a lot of food being discarded as "waste" by grocery stores.

Solution

I've been very encouraged over the last few years to see many grocery store chains discounting or donating imperfect produce. As consumers, we can also do our part to help waste by going out of our way to purchase the wonky bell pepper or single bananas.

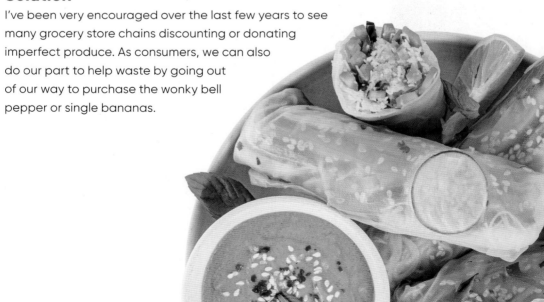

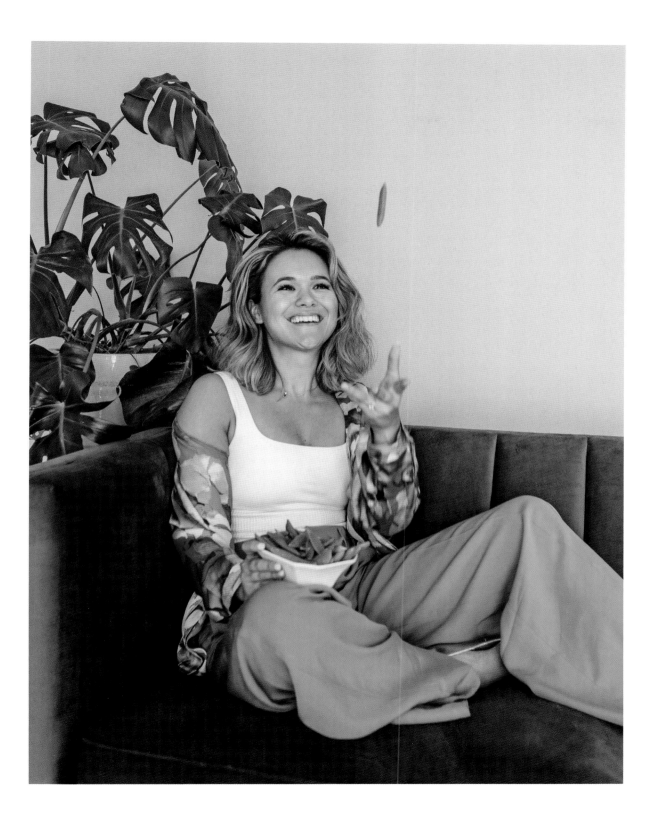

COMPOSTING

Despite my best efforts to use up every bit of the plants I buy, there are still some inevitable scraps that can't be consumed. *C'est la vie!*

Rather than trash the scraps (and let them pile up in our landfills), consider the greenest choice you can make in your scrappy kitchen: regular composting and/or participation in a green bin program. Composting breaks down organic matter, such as food scraps, yard waste, or biodegradable material, into a nutrient-rich soil.

I'm very fortunate to live in a city that has a green bin program that picks up unlimited organic waste every week for compost. A quick Google search should tell you whether your town or city offers the same, and will list what items are acceptable. Some cities even have farmers' markets where you can drop off your compost.

If you do have access to a backyard and make the decision to compost, there are several ways you can approach this—traditional composting, vermicomposting (with worms), or bokashi composting (using fermentation). The best option will depend on your climate, yard space, and preference, so do a little digging (*ha ha*) and determine the best course of action for your household compost.

WHAT ABOUT THE P-WORD?

Yep, plastic. We all know single-use plastic is an enormous issue for our planet, with virtually every single piece of plastic ever made still existing in some form. According to earthday.org, five trillion plastic bags are produced worldwide annually, and each one takes up to a thousand years to disintegrate completely.

Because plastic is so built into our everyday lives, it can feel near impossible to avoid. I always tell myself and others to try our best with the circumstance we're in. The last thing I want with this cookbook is to leave you feeling a bunch of eco-anxiety with every purchase you make! Here are some super-simple ways I've found to reduce single-use plastics.

- Invest in a reusable water bottle and metal or glass straws.
- Bring reusable grocery bags to the store. But in case you forget them, keep a laundry bin in your trunk so you can off-load groceries directly into that instead of using plastic bags.
- Avoid those clingy produce bags at the grocery store by placing fresh fruit and vegetables right in the cart. They need to be washed when you get home anyway.
- If possible, fill up nuts, pastas, rice, and other grains at bulk-bin stores, using glass or reusable plastic containers.
- Purchase such things as nut butters and juice in glass jars as opposed to plastic, when possible.

Once you start implementing these simple swaps into your life, you might notice other areas in your day-to-day where there's unnecessary plastic—and opportunities to adjust accordingly. Again, the *Scrappy* life is about trying your best and having fun doing it!

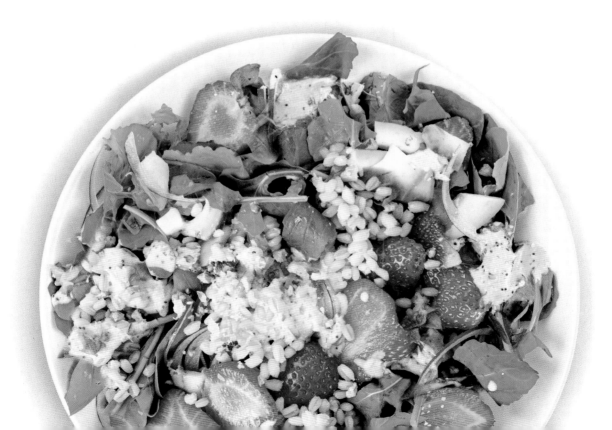

OUTFITTING A *SCRAPPY* KITCHEN

The most zero-waste thing you can do in your sustainable kitchen journey is to use what you already have. As tempting as it is to buy a whole swath of shiny new bamboo kitchen utensils, making sure you've gotten the last life out of your existing plastic kitchen scrubber and containers is essential.

Taking this one step further, it's also valuable to look around at the products you're buying and see where there might be an opportunity to upcycle some of those containers. In any eco-warrior cupboards, you'll find an overflowing shelf of reusable peanut butter, jam, or marinara jars that now serve as storage containers for ferments or a portable breakfast. Thrift stores are also packed with mason jars, reusable containers, and the like.

Now that we've gotten that out of the way, here are a few of my basic cooking essentials that will serve you well on your *Scrappy* cooking journey.

REUSABLES

- Stainless-steel water bottle, in place of plastic
- Cloth bags, in place of plastic, for the grocery store
- Linen napkins or cloths, in place of paper towels
- Stainless-steel straws, in place of paper or plastic

APPLIANCES

- Blender (high-speed, such as Vitamix or Ninja, if possible)
- Food processor
- Oven

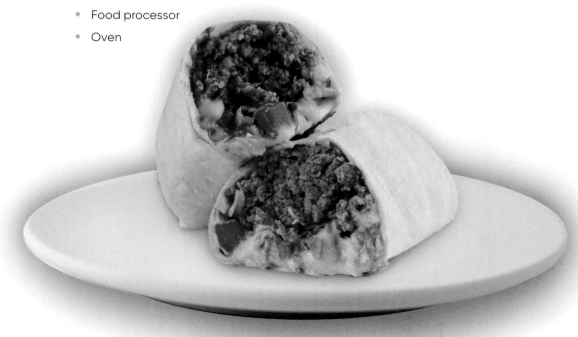

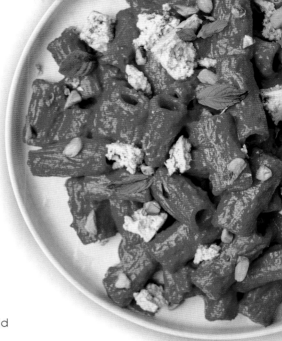

NICE TO HAVE

- Air fryer
- Immersion blender

COOKWARE & BAKEWARE

- Baking sheet (13 x 18-inch recommended)
- Reusable silicone baking mats
- Large stockpot with lid or Dutch oven (5- to 12-quart recommended)
- Medium-size saucepan with lid
- Large nonstick or stainless-steel skillet with lid
- Muffin tin (standard 12-well recommended)

STORAGE CONTAINERS

- Reusable glass containers
- Mason jars (8-ounce for zero-waste powders; 16-ounce for smoothies, juices, and canning; 32-ounce for broths)
- Reusable freezer bags

BASIC UTENSILS

- Cutting board
- Chef's knife
- Paring knife
- Measuring cup
- Measuring spoons
- Mixing bowls
- Slotted spoon
- Spatula
- Tongs

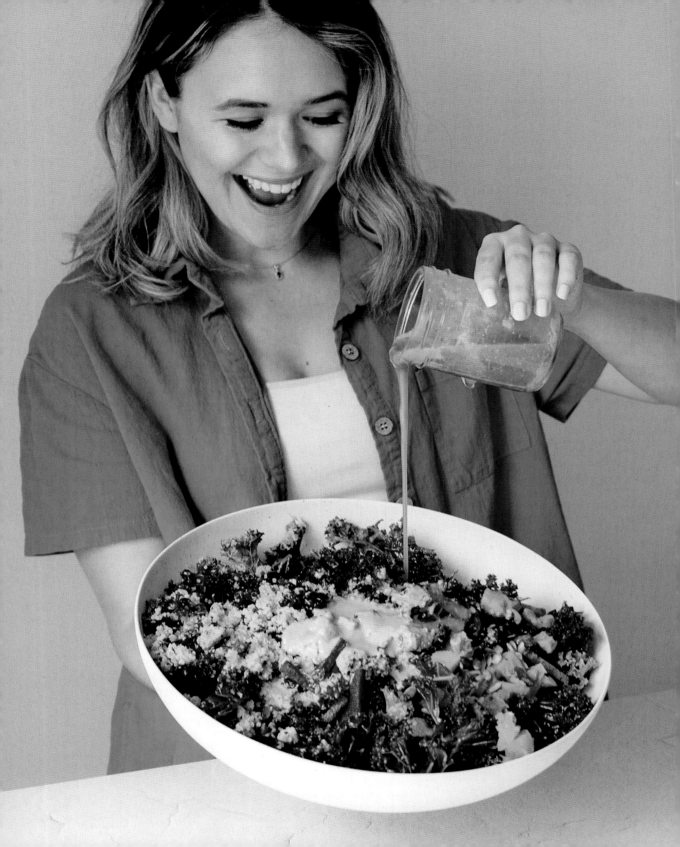

BEANS, GRAINS & STARCHES COOKING CHART

This basic cooking chart might be familiar from *PlantYou*, but it's a really great page to have on hand when you're making just about any grain, bean, or starch. In this book, you will find I often opt for canned beans and lentils. Cans are recyclable, and they're just so convenient. But if you'd rather buy dried beans in bulk, this is a great chart to work from.

How to use this chart: Rinse the grains or legumes in a fine-mesh sieve before cooking to help remove debris. Place in water or vegetable broth and bring to a boil over high heat. Lower the heat to low and simmer for the suggested amount of time.

1 cup (235 ml) grain or legume or starch	Water needed	Cooking time and notes	Cups yielded
BLACK BEANS	4 cups (945 ml)	Soak overnight, drain, and rinse, then simmer for 1¼ hours.	2¼ cups (530 ml)
CHICKPEAS	4 cups (945 ml)	Soak overnight, drain, and rinse, then simmer for 1¼ hours.	2 cups (475 ml)
KIDNEY BEANS	3 cups (710 ml)	Soak overnight, drain, and rinse, then simmer for 1 hour.	2¼ cups (530 ml)
NAVY BEANS	3 cups (710 ml)	Soak overnight, drain, and rinse, then simmer for 1¼ hours.	2¾ cups (650 ml)
PINTO BEANS	3 cups (710 ml)	Soak overnight, drain, and rinse, then simmer for 1¼ hours.	2¾ cups (650 ml)
GREEN OR BROWN LENTILS	2 cups (250 ml)	Rinse. Cook for 30 minutes; drain excess water after cooking.	2½ cups (591 ml)
RED LENTILS	2 cups (250 ml)	Rinse. Cook for 15 to 20 minutes; drain excess water after cooking.	2½ cups (591 ml)
QUINOA	2 cups (475 ml)	Rinse. Cook for 20 minutes, plus 5 minutes of steaming.	2¾ cups (650 ml)
BROWN RICE	2 cups (475 ml)	55 minutes	3 cups (710 ml)
BASMATI RICE	1¾ cups (415 ml)	35 minutes	3 cups (710 ml)
WILD RICE	2½ cups (590 ml)	50 minutes	4 cups (945 ml)

Got This? Make That!

Here's a handy visual index that showcases some of the most common items you might have going to waste in your fridge and pantry, and corresponding recipes to use them up. I couldn't include *everything* here, so I prioritized produce and commonly wasted foods. For a more detailed list, refer to the index at the back of the book.

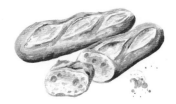

Stale Bread

The world's number one wasted food.

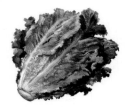

Wilted Greens

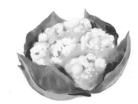

Cauliflower

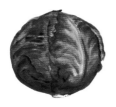

Cabbage

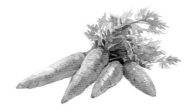

Carrots

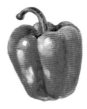

Bell Peppers

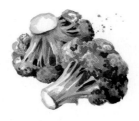

Broccoli Florets & Stems

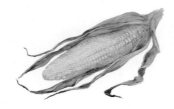

Corn

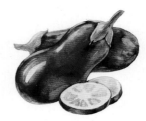

Eggplant

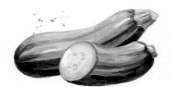

Zucchini

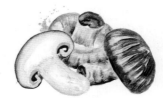

Mushrooms

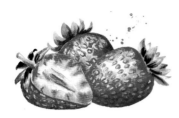

Mushy Berries

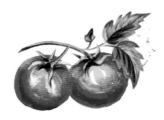

Tomatoes

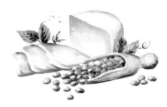

Tofu

For my soy-free friends, check out how to make tofu from beans.

KITCHEN RAID RECIPES

These are a collection of earmarked recipes in which you can use up just about any vegetable, grain, or bean that's starting to overstay its welcome in your fridge or pantry.

THINGS TO KNOW BEFORE YOU START YOUR *SCRAPPY* JOURNEY

A few housekeeping notes for my *Scrappy* chefs:

- **Kitchen Raid!** The recipes marked with a *Kitchen Raid* badge indicate that you can use up a variety of vegetables or items from your pantry based on what you have—not a rigid ingredients list. They are earmarked for your convenience in the visual index (page 18). You can make every single recipe on your own, based on what you have on hand.

- **Use What You Got!** These recipes are designed for simplicity and convenience. In all cases, plant-based milks can be homemade (pages 312 and 314) or purchased; tomatoes can be canned, fresh, hand-crushed, or diced; beans can be canned or cooked ahead of time from scratch and substituted one-for-one according to measurements.

- **Use It All!** You will notice there are a lot of overlapping ingredients used in recipes, such as sunflower seeds (which were chosen because they're an affordable, generally allergy-friendly, sustainable crop), flaxseed or flax meal, sauces, and various grains and vegetables. This is done intentionally, so you can use up ingredients and plan your week to save money and reduce waste. In all instances, you can use store-bought salad dressings, tomato sauces, and such things as vegan mayonnaise and vegan cheese, instead of making the homemade versions.

- **Save 'em and Store 'em.** Storage instructions and uses for scraps are included with each recipe.

- **Au Naturel.** Vegetables are washed and never peeled, unless stated otherwise—in which case I provide a use for the peels in another recipe.

- **Peel Etiquette.** When utilizing the peels for recipes—such as pomegranate peel powder, banana peel bacon, pineapple skin tea, and otherwise—purchase organic produce, if possible, and scrub clean using a vegetable cleaning spray or a mix of water and vinegar (1 part vinegar to 4 parts water).

- **No Gluten? No Oil? No Nuts? No Problem.** Gluten-free, oil-free, and nut-free substitutions for just about every recipe are included in the ingredients list.

- **Macros Index.** Macronutrient information (including the calories, protein, fat, and carbohydrates) is listed at the back of the book for each recipe, so you can access that if you would like, or completely ignore it.

Let's get cooking!

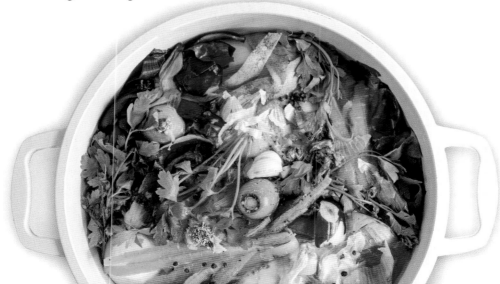

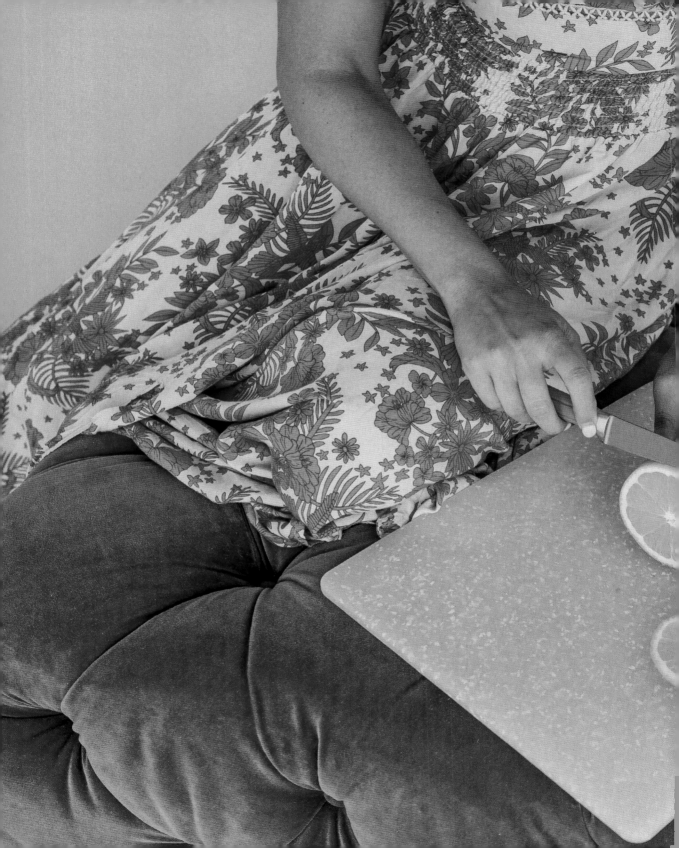

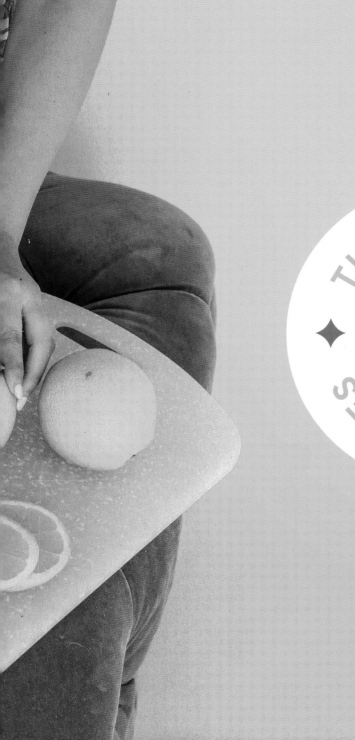

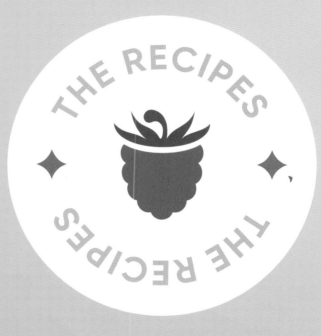

THE RECIPES

THE RECIPES

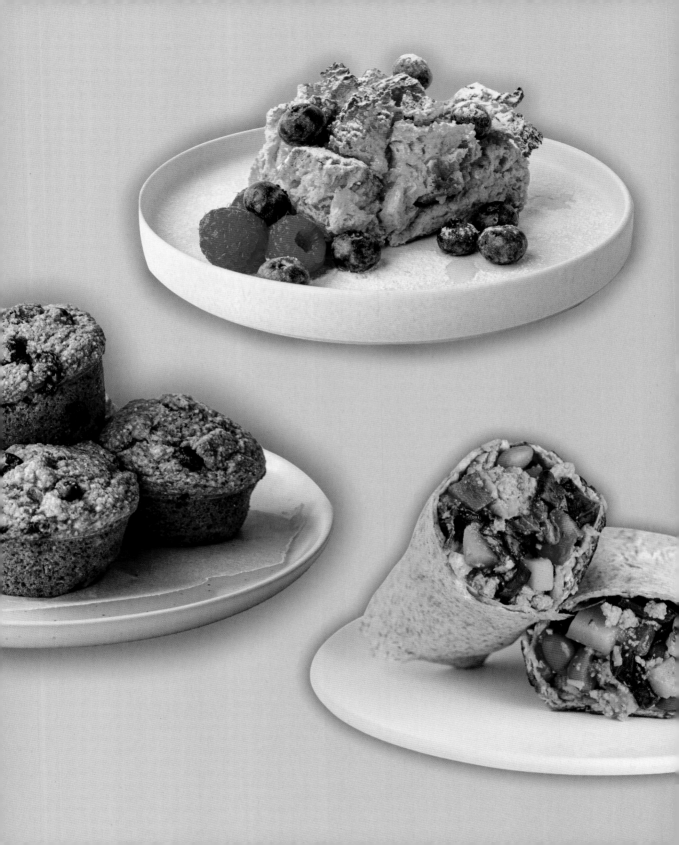

CHAPTER 1

Scrappy Sunrises

Grab that reusable coffee mug, throw on your apron, and get ready to transform your kitchen scraps into a breakfast masterpiece.

Common Ground Granola

Whoa! Stop right there. Don't throw out those spent coffee grounds. Instead, start your morning right with this incredible granola that uses the lofty leftovers from your morning cuppa joe. Packed with fiber and full-bodied flavor, this granola is a true grain changer.

MAKES 12 servings ✦ **START TO FINISH:** 40 minutes

3 cups gluten-free rolled oats

1 cup chopped walnuts, pecans, or pumpkin seeds

2 tablespoons ground flaxseed

¼ cup unsweetened cocoa powder

¼ teaspoon sea salt

⅔ cup pure maple syrup or liquid sweetener

½ cup brewed coffee or tea

3 tablespoons spent coffee grounds or tea leaves

2 tablespoons tahini or nut butter of choice

½ cup vegan dark chocolate chips or cacao nibs

1. Preheat the oven to 350°F, and line a baking sheet with a reusable baking mat or parchment paper.

2. In a bowl, combine the oats, nuts, ground flaxseed, cocoa powder, and salt.

3. In a separate bowl, combine the maple syrup, brewed coffee, coffee grounds, and tahini.

4. Pour the wet mixture into the dry mixture and stir until fully combined. Spread the mixture evenly on the prepared baking sheet.

5. Bake for 30 minutes, tossing it every 10 minutes to ensure the mixture is baked evenly. Remove from the oven and allow to cool completely before stirring in the chocolate chips.

6. Enjoy with plant-based milk or vegan yogurt, or as a topping on morning cereal.

Storage: Store in a sealed container for a few weeks at room temperature, or in the freezer for a month or longer.

Substitution Note: If you're not a coffee drinker, omit the spent coffee grounds and replace the brewed coffee with ½ cup of your favorite brewed tea.

Pro Tip: Spent coffee grounds can be kept in an uncovered bowl in your fridge as a natural deodorizer or utilized as a fertilizer for some plants.

ROLLED OATS

WALNUTS

GROUND FLAXSEED

COCOA POWDER

MAPLE SYRUP

COFFEE

COFFEE GROUNDS

TAHINI

CHOCOLATE CHIPS

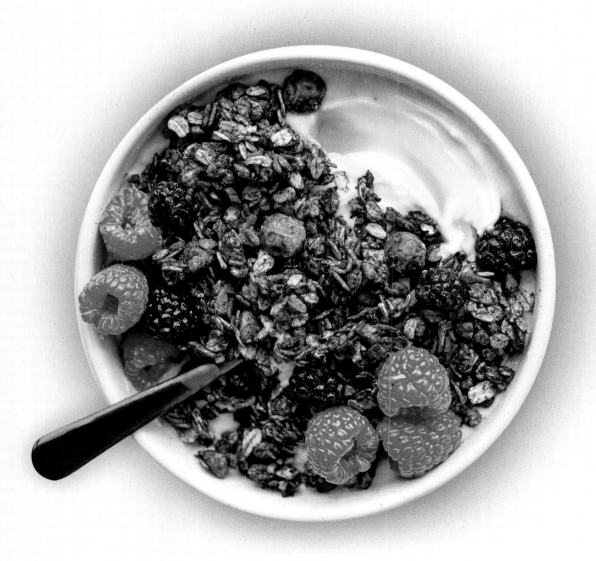

Chia & Overnight Oat Fruity Parfaits

Choose your own adventure! These Chia & Overnight Oat Fruity Parfaits are a breakfast that is easy to make, full of healthy stuff like fiber and omega-3s, and perfect for meal prep. Customize with whichever fruit you have on hand to make a multicolored morning treat.

CHIA PUDDING VERSION

MAKES 2 servings ✦ **START TO FINISH:** 5 minutes

½ cup fruit of choice (mango for yellow, raspberries for pink, blueberries for purple)

¾ cup unsweetened plant-based milk (soy, almond, cashew, or oat)

¼ cup coconut milk

1 teaspoon pure maple syrup

1 teaspoon Homemade Vanilla Extract (page 324) or store-bought pure vanilla extract

3 tablespoons chia seeds

1 cup unsweetened Cultured Vegan Yogurt (page 48) or store-bought coconut or soy yogurt

1. In a blender, combine the fruit, plant-based milk, coconut milk, maple syrup, and vanilla. Transfer the mixture to a sealable container and stir in the chia seeds until evenly dispersed.

2. Cover and allow to set in the fridge for at least 2 hours. Once thickened, transfer to jars with your vegan yogurt of choice on top.

OVERNIGHT OATS VERSION

MAKES 2 servings ✦ **START TO FINISH:** 5 minutes

½ cup fruit of choice (mango for yellow, raspberries for pink, blueberries for purple)

1½ cups unsweetened plant-based milk (soy, almond, cashew, or oat)

1 tablespoon pure maple syrup

1 teaspoon Homemade Vanilla Extract (page 324) or store-bought pure vanilla extract

1½ cups rolled oats, gluten-free if desired

1½ tablespoons chia seeds

1 cup unsweetened Cultured Vegan Yogurt (page 48) or store-bought coconut or soy yogurt

Vegan granola, for serving (optional)

1. In a blender, combine the fruit, plant-based milk, maple syrup, and vanilla. Transfer the mixture to a sealable container and stir in the oats and chia seeds.

2. Cover and allow to set in the fridge for at least 2 hours. Once thickened, transfer to jars with your vegan yogurt of choice on top, and granola if desired.

Storage: Seal and store in the fridge for up to 3 days.

Save the Scraps: Leftover coconut milk in Coo-Coo for Coconut Caramel (page 260) or Firecracker Tofu with Coconut Rice (page 184).

RASPBERRIES
/ MANGO /
BLUEBERRIES

PLANT-BASED
MILK

MAPLE SYRUP

VANILLA
EXTRACT

CHIA SEEDS

YOGURT

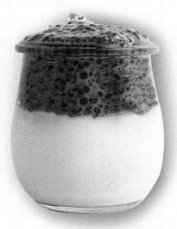
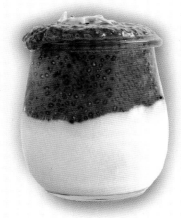
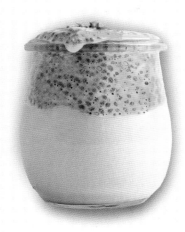

RASPBERRIES
/ MANGO /
BLUEBERRIES

PLANT-BASED
MILK

MAPLE SYRUP

VANILLA
EXTRACT

ROLLED OATS

CHIA SEEDS

YOGURT

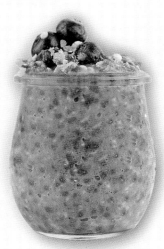
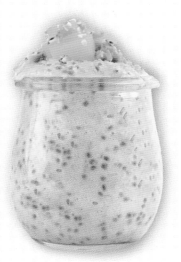
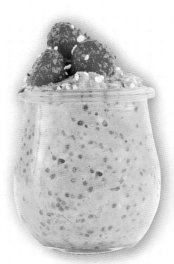

Berry Baked Oatmeal

If you have berries in your fridge that are a little on the mushy side, don't toss them. Transform them into the breakfast of your dreams. The best part about this recipe is that it can be prepped in 15 minutes, and comes together in a single casserole dish for minimal cleanup. After baking, you'll have a healthy breakfast ready for the workweek.

MAKES 6 servings ✦ **START TO FINISH:** 55 minutes

2 tablespoons chia seeds or ground flaxseed

5 tablespoons warm water

2 medium-size bananas

¼ cup (choose your fave) peanut butter, almond butter, sunflower seed butter, or tahini

3 tablespoons pure maple syrup

1½ cups unsweetened Cultured Vegan Yogurt (page 48) or store-bought coconut or soy yogurt

½ cup unsweetened plant-based milk (soy, almond, cashew, or oat)

1 teaspoon Homemade Vanilla Extract (page 324) or store-bought pure vanilla extract

2 cups gluten-free rolled oats

1 tablespoon baking powder

1½ cups mushy berries of choice

1. Preheat the oven to 375°F.

2. First, make a chia seed egg: In a jar or small bowl, mix the chia seeds with the water. Allow to set for 10 minutes, or until a gel is formed.

3. Mash the bananas in the bottom of an 8-inch square pan, then add the chia egg, nut butter, maple syrup, vegan yogurt of choice, plant-based milk, and vanilla. Mix until combined.

4. Add the oats and baking powder, and mix. Fold in 1 cup of the berries, then disperse the remaining ½ cup around the top.

5. Place, uncovered, in the oven and bake for 40 minutes, or until cooked through.

6. Serve warm or enjoy cold, as desired.

Storage: Store in a sealed container in the fridge for up to 5 days, or in a sealed container in the freezer for up to 2 months.

Save the Scraps: Banana peels for Two-Way "Bacon" Street (page 50).

CHIA SEEDS

BANANA

PEANUT BUTTER

MAPLE SYRUP

YOGURT

PLANT-BASED MILK

VANILLA EXTRACT

ROLLED OATS

BAKING POWDER

MUSHY BERRIES

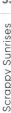
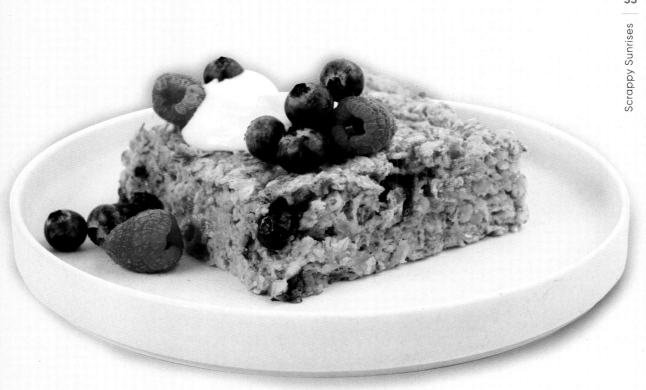

Super Seedy Granola Bars

Skip the packaged granola bars from the store, and make this nutrient-dense homemade version instead. The ingredients come together in less than 20 minutes, and you have a perfect healthy snack or breakfast for the workweek. These bars are gluten-free and vegan, and can be made nut-free by using sunflower seed butter or tahini or another alternative. Seedy can be a *good* thing!

MAKES 12 servings ✦ **START TO FINISH:** 25 minutes

2 cups gluten-free rolled oats

¼ cup ground flaxseed

¼ cup ground hemp hearts

3 tablespoons chia seeds

Pinch of salt

¾ cup (choose your fave) peanut butter, almond butter, sunflower seed butter, or tahini

½ cup pure maple syrup

1 tablespoon plant-based milk

1 teaspoon Homemade Vanilla Extract (page 324) or store-bought pure vanilla extract

½ cup vegan mini dark chocolate chips

1. Preheat the oven to 375°F, and line an 8-inch square baking pan with parchment paper or spray with oil.

2. In a bowl, combine the oats, ground flaxseed, hemp hearts, chia seeds, and salt. In a separate bowl, combine the nut butter (I used almond butter), maple syrup, plant-based milk, and vanilla. If needed, microwave the nut butter mixture for 10 to 15 seconds to make it drippy.

3. Pour the wet mixture into the dry mixture and mix until fully combined. Fold in the chocolate chips. Transfer the mixture to the prepared pan.

4. Using the bottom of a measuring cup, press the granola mixture down into the pan until firmly packed.

5. Bake for 18 minutes, or until set. Remove from the oven and allow to cool for 25 minutes. After cooling, chill in the fridge for 1 hour before slicing.

Storage: Store in an airtight container for up to 5 days at room temperature, or in a sealed container in the freezer for up to 1 month. Slice and place in a reusable bag or wrap in parchment for the perfect grab-and-go snack.

ROLLED OATS

GROUND FLAXSEED

HEMP HEARTS

CHIA SEEDS

PEANUT BUTTER

MAPLE SYRUP

PLANT-BASED MILK

VANILLA EXTRACT

CHOCOLATE CHIPS

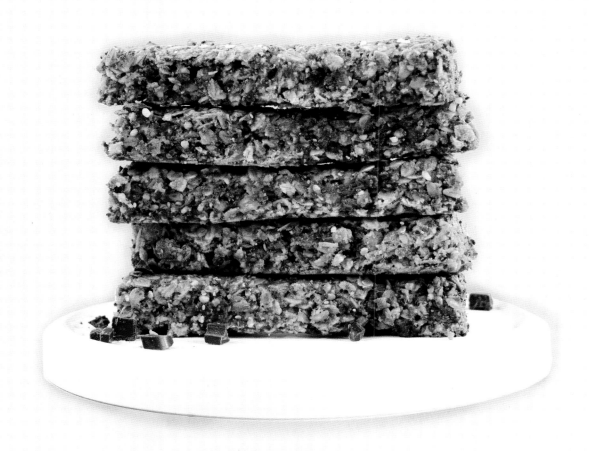

Brown Banana Muffins

Is a bunch of overripe bananas staring at you from your kitchen counter? You're in luck. Whip up a batch of these simple Brown Banana Muffins that taste like they came straight from the bakery. The more bananas ripen, the sweeter they get, providing a perfect base for these fiber-filled breakfast bad boys. If you don't have time to bake today, toss the bananas (with peels on) into the freezer. Take out, thaw, and use as you would fresh. And, oh yeah, you can use those peels separately too (check out Two-Way "Bacon" Street, page 50).

MAKES 12 muffins ✦ **START TO FINISH:** 35 minutes

2 tablespoons ground flaxseed or ground chia seeds

5 tablespoons water

4 medium-size brown bananas, peeled

¼ cup unsweetened plant-based milk (soy, almond, cashew, or oat)

1 teaspoon Apple Scrap Vinegar (page 350) or store-bought apple cider vinegar

½ cup pure maple syrup

1 teaspoon Homemade Vanilla Extract (page 324) or store-bought pure vanilla extract

2 cups gluten-free oat flour or all-purpose flour

1 teaspoon baking soda

2 teaspoons baking powder

2 tablespoons coconut or dark brown sugar

Pinch of salt

½ cup vegan dark chocolate chips

1. In a large bowl, combine the ground flaxseed with the water. Allow to thicken for 10 minutes.

2. Preheat the oven to 415°F, and line a standard twelve-well muffin tin with reusable liners or spray with oil.

3. Add the bananas to the bowl of thickened flaxseed. Mash with a potato masher or the back of a fork, then stir to combine with the "flax egg." Add the plant-based milk, Apple Scrap Vinegar, Apple Scrap Honey, and vanilla, and stir until combined. Allow to sit for an additional 5 minutes.

4. Next, add the oat flour, baking soda, baking powder, coconut sugar, and salt to the bowl. Gently stir until a smooth batter is formed. Fold in the chocolate chips.

5. Divide the batter equally among the prepared muffin wells.

6. Bake for 10 minutes to help the muffins rise, and then lower the heat to 375°F and bake for an additional 7 to 10 minutes to cook through, or until the muffins spring back when lightly pressed in the center.

For Banana Bread: Bake the batter in a loaf pan at 355°F for 55 to 65 minutes until a toothpick inserted in the center comes out clean.

Storage: Store in an airtight container on the counter for up to 5 days, or in a sealed container in the freezer for up to 2 months.

GROUND FLAXSEED

 BANANA

 PLANT-BASED MILK

 APPLE CIDER VINEGAR

 MAPLE SYRUP

 OAT FLOUR

 BAKING SODA

 BAKING POWDER

 COCONUT SUGAR

 CHOCOLATE CHIPS

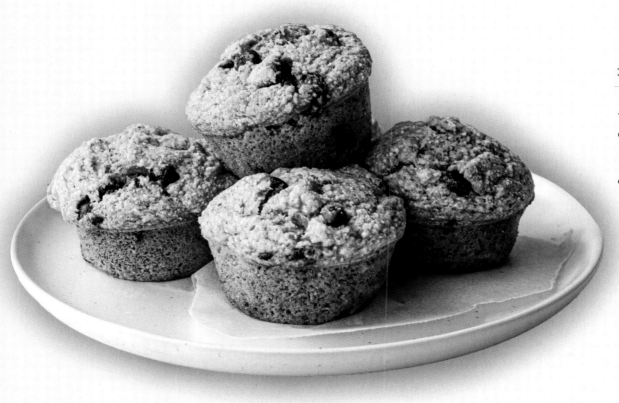

Note: You can make your own oat flour by throwing rolled oats in a blender or food processor, and blitzing until they are finely ground.

Save the Scraps: Banana peels for Two-Way "Bacon" Street (page 50).

"Death by Chocolate" Flapjacks

"Regular" pancakes are great and all. But how might we make them extra delish? Well, obviously, chocolate. But sometimes that's not enough. We want oomph. We want a twist. We want scrappy. *Et voilà*, orange peels. Now we've got fluffy chocolate pancakes with dark chocolate chips dripping with a chocolate syrup on top—all finished off with a sprinkle of Citrus Peel Powder. (No powder? No problem—these are delish without it too!)

MAKES 8 to 10 pancakes ✦ **START TO FINISH:** 20 minutes

PANCAKES

1 cup whole wheat or gluten-free oat flour

1 tablespoon baking powder

½ cup unsweetened cocoa powder

Pinch of salt

1⅓ cups unsweetened plant-based milk (soy, almond, cashew, or oat)

1 teaspoon Homemade Vanilla Extract (page 324) or store-bought pure vanilla extract

3 tablespoons pure maple syrup

¼ cup vegan mini dark chocolate chips

1 tablespoon Citrus Peel Powder (page 332; optional)

CHOCOLATE SAUCE (OPTIONAL)

⅔ cup coconut milk

1 cup vegan dark chocolate chips

1. Make the pancakes: In a bowl, combine the flour, baking powder, cocoa powder, and salt. In a separate bowl, combine the plant-based milk, vanilla, and maple syrup.

2. Fold the wet mixture into the dry mixture, and allow the batter to sit for 5 minutes. Fold in the chocolate chips.

3. Heat a large nonstick skillet over medium heat. If you do not have a really effective nonstick pan, you will want to spray it with a small amount of oil. Put in ⅓ cup of batter per pancake, and cook for 3 to 4 minutes, or until the edges look dry and bubbles have formed. Flip, then cook for an additional 3 minutes, or until browned.

4. Make the chocolate sauce (if using): Place a saucepan over medium heat, pour in the coconut milk, and bring to a boil. Lower the heat and stir in the chocolate chips. Whisk frequently until the chocolate chips are melted into a nice sauce, about 3 minutes.

5. Serve the pancakes immediately with vegan yogurt, pure maple syrup, the chocolate sauce, and/or fruit, with ½ teaspoon of zested orange or more citrus peel powder on top.

Storage: Store the pancakes only in an airtight container in the fridge for up to 3 days, or in the freezer for up to 1 month. When ready to eat, you can pop the pancakes into a toaster to heat until warm.

Save the Scraps: Leftover coconut milk for Coo-Coo for Coconut Caramel (page 260) or Firecracker Tofu with Coconut Rice (page 184).

WHOLE WHEAT FLOUR

BAKING POWDER

COCOA POWDER

PLANT-BASED MILK

VANILLA EXTRACT

MAPLE SYRUP

OPTIONAL: CHOCOLATE CHIPS, COCONUT MILK, CITRUS PEEL POWDER

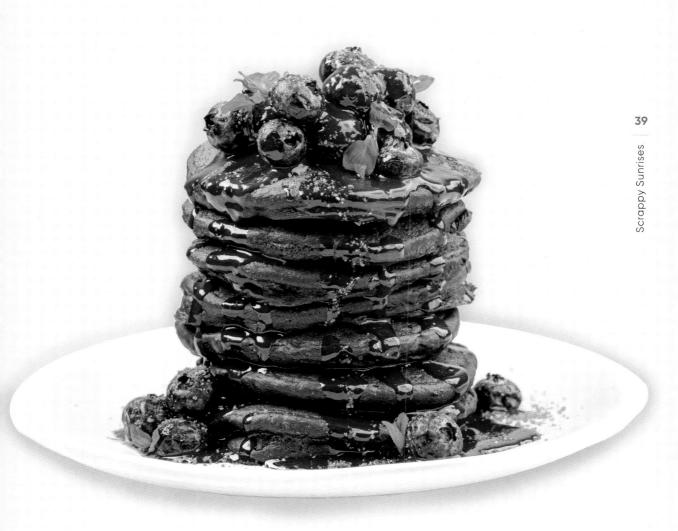

Fritzy Fritters

Take a peek in your fridge. . . . What vegetables are on the fritz? Time to grate them up and make these incredible Fritzy Fritters. (I offer suggestions below, but use whatever you have on hand!) These are the perfect savory snack for when you're on the go, or as the ideal companion to my Eggless Omelet (page 44).

MAKES 8 patties ◆ **START TO FINISH:** 40 minutes

VEGETABLES

1 medium-size zucchini, celeriac, or small squash, grated, about ⅔ cup

2 medium-size Yukon Gold potatoes or potatoes of choice, grated

1 medium-size carrot or parsnip, grated

½ teaspoon salt

BATTER

2 tablespoons ground flaxseed

5 tablespoons warm water

¼ cup vegan kimchi, chopped, or sauerkraut, such as Turmeric Sauerkraut (page 340)

½ cup chickpea flour or all-purpose flour

1 teaspoon garlic powder

1 tablespoon soy sauce or gluten-free tamari

1 tablespoon chili garlic sauce (optional, for spice)

FOR SERVING

Creamy Vegan Tzatziki (page 276)

1. Preheat the oven to 400°F, and line a baking sheet with a reusable baking mat or parchment paper.

2. Prepare the vegetables: In a bowl, combine the grated vegetables. Add the salt, mix well, and let stand for 10 minutes. Transfer the vegetable mixture to a nut milk bag or thin, clean dish towel and squeeze out as much excess water as possible. Discard the excess water.

3. Make the batter: First, make the flax egg. In a small bowl, mix the ground flaxseed with the warm water. Allow to set for 10 minutes, until a gel is formed.

4. In a large bowl, combine the drained vegetables, flax egg, kimchi, chickpea flour, garlic powder, soy sauce, and garlic chili sauce, and mix until a batter is formed.

5. In ¼-cup batches, transfer the mixture, in mounds, to the prepared baking sheet, placing them 2 inches apart. Use the back of a spoon to gently flatten them into 1-inch-thick patties. To get a perfectly round patty, wiggle the top of a glass or mug on the batter in a circular motion.

6. Bake the fritters for about 20 minutes, or until golden brown, flipping halfway through. Enjoy with the tzatziki.

Storage: Store in a sealed container in the fridge for up to 4 days.

Save the Scraps: Carrot tops for Carrot Top Chimichurri (page 272).

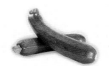

ZUCCHINI

POTATOES

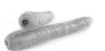

CARROT

GROUND FLAXSEED

KIMCHI

ALL-PURPOSE FLOUR

GARLIC POWDER

SOY SAUCE

CHILI GARLIC SAUCE

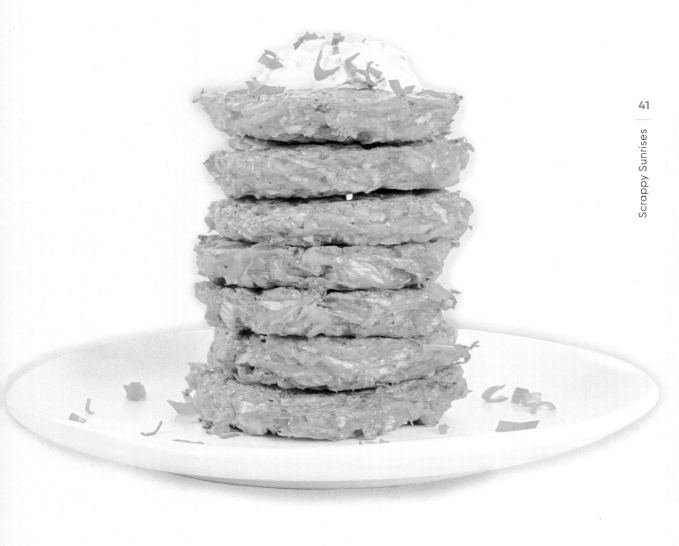

Last Week's Loaf Breakfast Casserole

Bread . . . It's the world's No. 1 most loved and wasted food, with more than 240 million slices ending up in US trash cans each year alone. Stop loafing around, and use up your tired bread in this sinfully delicious French toast–inspired breakfast casserole. This is an amazing meal prep recipe that can also feed a hungry crowd.

MAKES 8 servings ✦ **START TO FINISH:** 60 minutes

CUSTARD

1½ cups unsweetened plant-based milk (soy, almond, cashew, or oat)

¾ cup Cultured Vegan Yogurt (page 48) or store-bought coconut or soy yogurt

¼ cup cornstarch or arrowroot powder

2 tablespoons coconut or light brown sugar

¼ cup pure maple syrup

1 tablespoon ground flaxseed or ground chia seeds

½ teaspoon ground turmeric

1 teaspoon Homemade Vanilla Extract (page 324) or store-bought pure vanilla extract

2 teaspoons ground cinnamon

Juice of ½ lemon

5 cups torn, dry vegan sourdough bread, French loaf, or gluten-free bread of choice (1-inch chunks)

½ cup crushed walnuts, for topping (optional)

FOR SERVING

Berries and more plant-based yogurt and maple syrup (optional)

1. Preheat the oven to 350°F.

2. In a bowl, prepare the custard by combining the plant-based milk, vegan yogurt, cornstarch, coconut sugar, maple syrup, ground flaxseed, turmeric, vanilla, cinnamon, and lemon juice. Mix well, then let stand for 10 minutes, or until slightly thickened.

3. Lightly oil or line a 7 x 11–inch casserole dish with parchment paper. Place the torn bread in an even layer.

4. Pour the custard evenly over the torn bread, and use a spatula to make sure that the bread is covered. Sprinkle the crushed walnuts on top (if using). Allow the bread to soak for 5 minutes.

5. Bake the casserole, uncovered, for 30 minutes, or until the bread is slightly crusty on top and the custard has thickened. Serve warm with berries and more vegan yogurt and maple syrup, if desired.

Storage: Store in an airtight container in the fridge for up to 4 days. Enjoy warm or cold.

Save the Scraps: Lemon peels for Candied Citrus Peels (page 254) or Citrus Peel Powder (page 332).

PLANT-BASED MILK

YOGURT

CORNSTARCH

COCONUT SUGAR

MAPLE SYRUP

GROUND FLAXSEED

TURMERIC

VANILLA EXTRACT

CINNAMON

LEMON

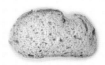

SOURDOUGH BREAD

OPTIONAL: WALNUTS

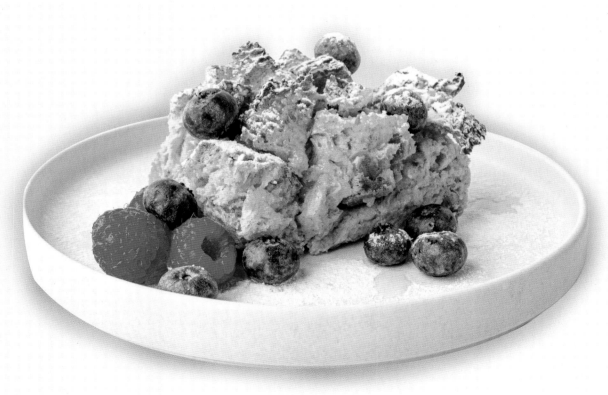

Eggless Omelet

You won't give a cluck about missing the eggs in this vegan breakfast omelet. Chickpea flour provides a silky, egg-like base that's cheap, high in protein, and, yes, delicious. To round out this meal, add any of the vegetables you have hanging out in your crisper. If you can't find chickpea flour in your grocery store, search for gram flour or besan!

MAKES 1 omelet ✦ **START TO FINISH:** 15 minutes

VEGETABLES

1 cup diced vegetables of choice (I used: ¼ red bell pepper, seeded and diced; ¼ red onion, diced; a handful of spinach, chopped; ½ cup cherry tomatoes, sliced in half)

½ teaspoon salt

1 to 2 tablespoons water or extra-virgin olive oil, for pan

OMELET

¼ cup chickpea flour

2 tablespoons nutritional yeast

½ teaspoon garlic powder

½ teaspoon onion powder

½ teaspoon kala namak (black salt) or regular salt

¼ teaspoon ground turmeric

½ teaspoon baking powder

⅓ cup lukewarm water

FOR SERVING

Fresh herbs, hot sauce, ketchup, and freshly ground black pepper

Two-Way "Bacon" Street (page 50; your choice, banana peel or mushroom)

1. Make the vegetables: In a large nonstick skillet over medium heat, combine all the vegetables and salt with the water. Sauté until softened, about 4 minutes.

2. Meanwhile, make the omelet batter: Combine the chickpea flour, nutritional yeast, garlic powder, onion powder, kala namak, turmeric, and baking powder in a bowl and stir well. Slowly pour the water into the mix, whisking to create a smooth, egg-like batter.

3. Once the vegetables are cooked, transfer to a dish and place the pan back on the stove over medium heat. If you do not have a high-quality nonstick skillet, it's essential that you use oil spray or vegan butter to lubricate, or the omelet will fall apart. Alternatively, you can use a spatula to scramble the batter.

4. Pour in the omelet batter and allow it to spread across the entire surface of the pan. Place the lid on the pan and allow the batter to cook until the top of the omelet appears slightly dry, about 3 minutes.

5. Carefully flip the omelet and allow it to cook, covered, for another 1 to 2 minutes, or until dry on top. Add the cooked vegetables to one-half the omelet, and evenly fold over the other half to form a half-moon.

6. Enjoy immediately, garnished with fresh herbs, hot sauce, ketchup, and freshly ground black pepper, as desired. Serve with your choice of Two-Way "Bacon" Street.

1 CUP VEGETABLES OF CHOICE:
RED BELL PEPPER, RED ONION, CHERRY
TOMATOES, SPINACH

CHICKPEA FLOUR

NUTRITIONAL YEAST

GARLIC POWDER

ONION POWDER

KALA NAMAK

TURMERIC

BAKING POWDER

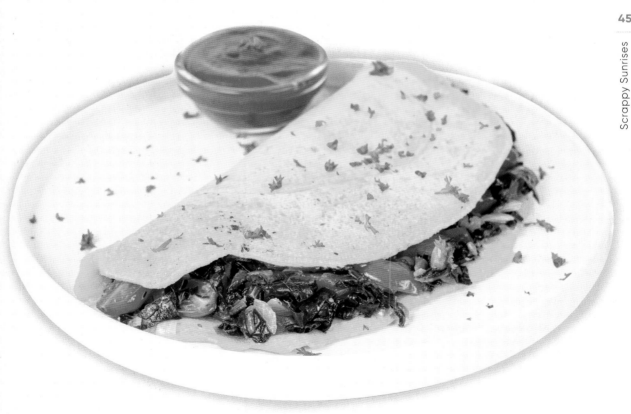

Grab & Glow BurritOH

Skip the drive-thru and all that plastic packaging. Instead, prep a batch of these OH-so-tasty burritos for the week. Protein. Fiber. Flavor. Portable. They'll have you glowing from the inside out. They're also freezer-friendly for grab-and-go (glow?). Now that's a wrap!

MAKES 4 to 6 burritos ✦ **START TO FINISH:** 30 minutes

1 to 2 tablespoons water or extra-virgin olive oil, for pan

1 medium-size yellow onion, diced

2 garlic cloves, minced

1 Yukon Gold potato, diced

1 red bell pepper, seeded and diced

1 (14-ounce) block extra-firm tofu, drained, patted dry, and crushed with the back of a fork

1 (15-ounce) can pinto beans, drained and rinsed

5 slices Two-Way "Bacon" Street (page 50; your choice, banana peel or mushroom), diced (optional)

½ teaspoon ground turmeric

1 teaspoon kala namak (black) or regular salt

¼ cup nutritional yeast

1 tablespoon tomato paste

2 cups spinach, chopped

4 to 6 It's a (Flax) Wrap wraps (page 70) or store-bought vegan whole wheat wraps or gluten-free tortillas

1. Heat the water in a large skillet over medium heat, then add the onion and garlic. Sauté until fragrant, about 3 minutes.

2. Add the potato and bell pepper. Sauté for an additional 5 minutes, or until softened.

3. Add the crushed tofu, pinto beans, "bacon," turmeric, kala namak, nutritional yeast, and tomato paste. Stir until combined. Cook for 5 to 7 more minutes, or until the potatoes are soft, everything is well incorporated, and some of the moisture has evaporated from the mixture. Fold in the spinach.

4. To assemble, place a generous spoonful of the burrito mixture on each tortilla. Then, fold in the side edges of the tortilla and roll. For easier rolling, you can warm the tortillas in a skillet over medium heat for 20 to 30 seconds per side.

Storage: If using these for meal prep, allow the filling to cool for 10 minutes before assembling in the wraps. Store the filling in an airtight container in the fridge for up to 5 days, or in the freezer for up to a month. Reheat in a microwave in 1-minute intervals, or grill in a skillet on the stove top for 3 to 5 minutes.

Save the Scraps: Onion peels for Onion Peel Powder (page 336), Scrappy Broth (page 102), or Bouilliant Bouillon Powder (page 336).

YELLOW ONION

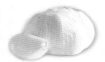

GARLIC

POTATOES

RED BELL PEPPER

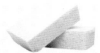

TOFU

PINTO BEANS

TWO-WAY "BACON" STREET

TURMERIC

KALA NAMAK

NUTRITIONAL YEAST

TOMATO PASTE

SPINACH

WHOLE WHEAT
TORTILLAS

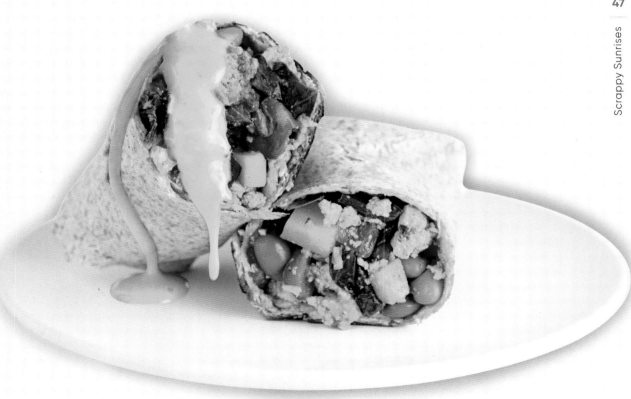

Cultured Vegan Yogurt

Your gut and taste buds will thank you for this homemade probiotic-rich vegan yogurt. Made with a blend of nuts, tofu, and coconut milk, it's the perfect balance of protein, fats, and energy to start your day on the right foot. Serve with cereal, on its own, or as a sweet dessert with leftover fruit.

MAKES 2 to 4 servings ✦ **START TO FINISH:** 1 to 2 days

1 cup raw cashews or sunflower seeds, soaked in water overnight or boiled for 10 minutes

½ cup extra-firm tofu

1 cup canned full-fat coconut milk

¼ to ½ cup water, depending on desired thickness

2 teaspoons Homemade Vanilla Extract (page 324) or store-bought pure vanilla extract, if sweetness is desired

2 tablespoons pure maple syrup, if sweetness is desired

2 vegan probiotic capsules

1. In a blender, combine all the ingredients, except the probiotic capsules, and blend until smooth. Pour into a dry, clean, sterilized glass jar or container. I use a quart-size mason jar.

2. Empty the probiotic capsules into the yogurt, and using a wooden or plastic spoon (not metal, as it can react negatively with the probiotics), stir until fully combined.

3. Cover the jar with a piece of cheesecloth or a clean dish towel and secure with a rubber band. Allow the yogurt to sit for 24 hours in a warm place in your home, about 75°F. If you are in a cooler climate, you can place the yogurt in the oven with the light on.

4. After a full day, taste the yogurt to see whether it has your desired tanginess. It should be thickened and slightly tangy at this point. Enjoy immediately, or place in the fridge to thicken even further.

Storage: Store in a sealed container in the fridge for up to 7 days.

Notes: To sterilize jars, rinse thoroughly with boiling water and then allow to dry completely before adding the ingredients.

To make a new batch of yogurt, you can use 1 tablespoon of this yogurt as a starter, instead of probiotic capsules.

Substitutions: For a nut-free version, use raw sunflower seeds in place of the cashews. For a soy-free version, use an additional ½ cup of nuts in place of the tofu.

Save the Scraps: Use the leftover coconut milk in Coo-Coo for Coconut Caramel (page 260) or Firecracker Tofu with Coconut Rice (page 184).

CASHEWS

TOFU

COCONUT MILK

VANILLA EXTRACT

MAPLE SYRUP

PROBIOTIC CAPSULES

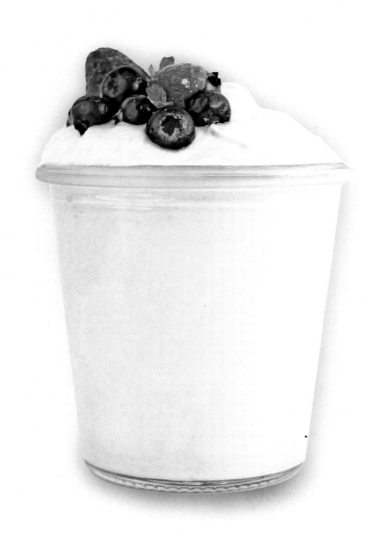

Two-Way "Bacon" Street

Contrary to what many believe, banana peels are perfectly safe to eat and quite nutritious, packed with antioxidants, fiber, and potassium. Scrub them clean with a sponge, then transform them into this unbelievable banana-peel bacon. If you don't ride the banana-peel boat, you can make this same delicious bacon with oyster mushrooms.

MAKES 2 servings ✦ **START TO FINISH:** 60 minutes

1 to 2 organic, ripe banana peels, scrubbed clean

OR

2 to 4 king oyster mushrooms

MARINADE

¼ cup soy sauce or gluten-free tamari

1 tablespoon extra-virgin olive oil or vegetable broth

1 teaspoon Apple Scrap Vinegar (page 350) or store-bought apple cider vinegar

½ teaspoon smoked paprika

½ teaspoon garlic powder

1 tablespoon nutritional yeast

½ teaspoon chopped fresh parsley

1 teaspoon pure maple syrup

Sprinkle of salt

1. If you are using banana peels, use a spoon to scoop out (and discard) any leftover flesh on the inside lining. Slice the banana peels into about four strips per peel or the oyster mushrooms lengthwise, around ³/₈ inch thick.

2. Make the marinade: In a medium-size dish, combine all the marinade ingredients and mix well. Submerge the banana peels or mushroom slices in the marinade and soak for 10 minutes to an hour, as you like.

3. Preheat the oven to 400°F, and line a baking sheet with a reusable baking mat or parchment paper.

4. Transfer the marinated peels or mushroom slices to the prepared baking sheet. Brush with more marinade to coat.

5. Bake for about 15 minutes, until crispy, flipping halfway through. Serve immediately.

Storage: Store in the fridge for up to 3 days.

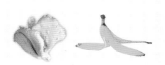

OYSTER MUSHROOM /
BANANA PEEL

SOY SAUCE

OLIVE OIL OR VEGETABLE
BROTH

APPLE CIDER VINEGAR

SMOKED PAPRIKA

GARLIC POWDER

NUTRITIONAL YEAST

PARSLEY

MAPLE SYRUP

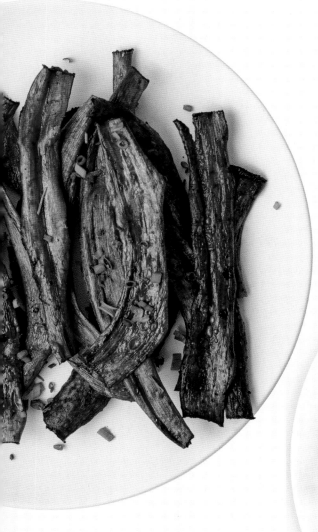

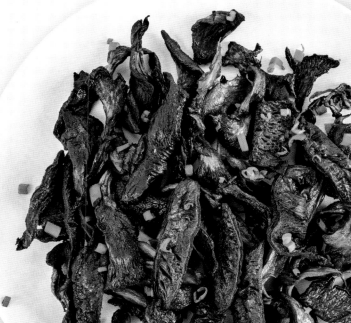

Juicer-Free Green Juice

Nothing makes me feel healthier than starting the day with a big glass of beaming green juice. This feeling shouldn't be exclusive to those with an expensive juicer. You can whip up an amazing vibrant juice in your blender with this nifty recipe—and be sure to save the pulp for some other *Scrappy* recipes noted below!

MAKES 2 to 3 servings ✦ **START TO FINISH:** 5 minutes

1½ cups water

3 cups spinach

2 celery ribs, chopped

1 medium-size cucumber, chopped

1 medium-size orange, peeled and chopped

1 cup fresh parsley, chopped

1. In a blender, combine all the ingredients and blend until smooth.

2. If desired, drain, using a fine-mesh strainer or nut milk bag. This can also be enjoyed as a delicious smoothie.

Storage: Store in a sealed bottle in the fridge for up to 3 days, or freeze for up to 2 months in ice cube trays.

Save the Scraps: Reserve the pulp for the Palak "Paneer" (page 192). Orange peel for Citrus Peel Powder (page 332) or Candied Citrus Peels (page 254). Celery leaves in Celery Leaf "Tabbouleh" (page 106) or Scrappy Broth (page 102).

SPINACH

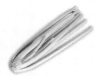
CELERY

CUCUMBER

ORANGE

PARSLEY

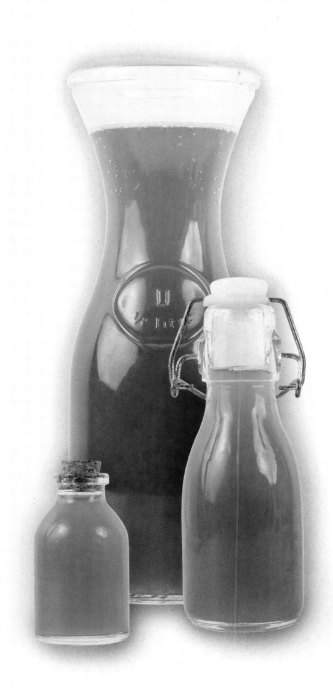

smoothie bombs

Smoothie bombs are your new secret weapon to supercharging any smoothie with nutrition, and using up excess produce (ahem . . . I'm talking about the sad container of spinach hiding at the back of your fridge). Next time you're making a smoothie, add one of the bombs to your blender with your other ingredients of choice. More nutrition and less waste . . . Now we're talking!

EACH MAKES about 32 cubes ✦ **START TO FINISH:** 5 minutes

1. Combine each bomb's listed ingredients, pour into an ice cube tray, and freeze overnight. Once frozen, the smoothie bombs can be transferred to a reusable freezer bag. When ready to make a smoothie, transfer one to three cubes to a blender with 1 cup of plant-based milk plus other ingredients, such as fresh fruit or greens, as desired. Blend until smooth.

2. Alternatively, you can add three or four of the anti-inflammatory, fiber-filled, or berry bombs to 1 cup of plant-based milk, and allow them to melt for an on-the-go premade smoothie.

Storage: Store in the freezer for up to 3 months.

Save the Scraps: Banana peels for Two-Way "Bacon" Street (page 50). Pineapple skin for Pineapple Skin Tea (page 302) or Tangy Tepache (page 304). Date seeds for Date Seed Coffee (page 300).

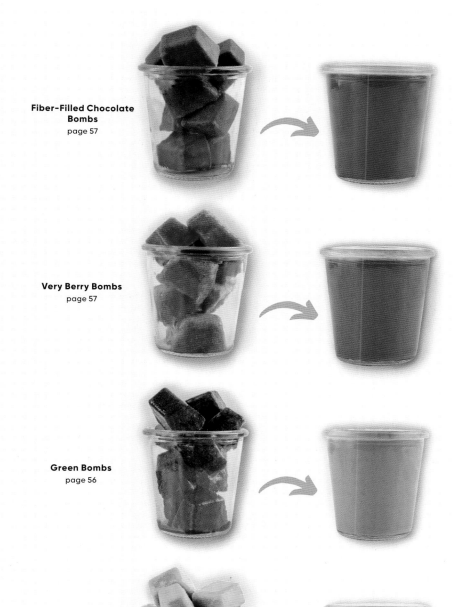

Fiber-Filled Chocolate Bombs
page 57

Very Berry Bombs
page 57

Green Bombs
page 56

Fruity, Spicy Anti-inflammatory Bombs
page 56

Scrappy Sunrises

Greens Bombs

6 to 8 handfuls of spinach, kale, or other greens

1 teaspoon chia seeds

2 to 3 cups coconut water

To make a Digestion Elixir Smoothie with these bombs, add three or four of them to a blender along with a heaping cup of frozen fruit and 1 cup of plant-based milk of choice.

SPINACH

CHIA SEEDS

COCONUT WATER

Fruity, Spicy Anti-inflammatory Bombs

1½ cups cubed pineapple

1½ cups cubed mango

1 teaspoon ground turmeric

1 tablespoon grated fresh ginger

⅛ teaspoon freshly ground black pepper

2 to 3 cups water or unsweetened plant-based milk (soy, almond, cashew, or oat)

To make a Flare Fighter Smoothie with these bombs, add three or four to a blender along with a frozen banana and 1 cup of unsweetened plant-based milk.

PINEAPPLE

MANGO

TURMERIC

GINGER ROOT

BLACK PEPPER

PLANT-BASED MILK

Fiber-Filled Chocolate Bombs

1 cup hemp hearts

¼ cup unsweetened cocoa powder

¼ cup ground flaxseed

¼ cup chia seeds

3 Medjool dates, pitted

2 to 3 cups water or unsweetened plant-based milk (soy, almond, cashew, or oat)

To make a Brownie Batter Smoothie with these bombs, add three or four to a blender along with a frozen banana and 1 cup of unsweetened plant-based milk.

HEMP HEARTS

COCOA POWDER

GROUND FLAXSEED

CHIA SEEDS

MEDJOOL DATES

PLANT-BASED MILK

Very Berry Bombs

2 to 3 cups fresh or frozen berries

1 banana

2 tablespoons ground flaxseed

½ cup Cultured Vegan Yogurt (page 48) or store-bought soy or coconut yogurt

2 to 3 cups water or unsweetened plant-based milk (soy, almond, cashew, or oat)

To make a Berry Powerhouse Smoothie with these bombs, add three or four to a blender along with 1 cup of unsweetened plant-based milk.

RASPBERRIES

BANANA

GROUND FLAXSEED

YOGURT

PLANT-BASED MILK

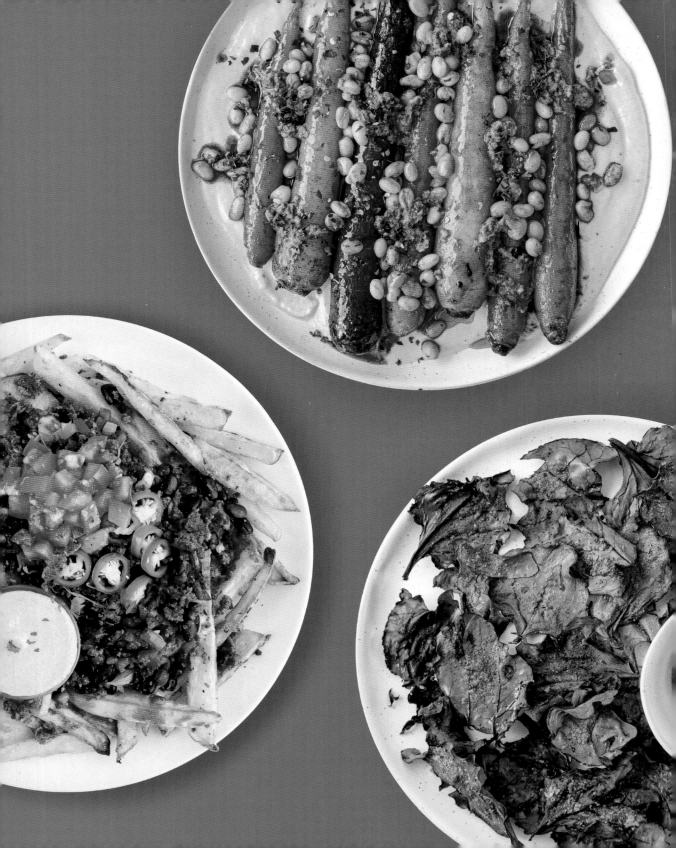

CHAPTER 2

Scrappetizers & Sides

Transform kitchen scraps into party snacks.

Fiesta Fries

Step aside, spuds! Fiesta Fries have arrived to the party. Fresh-cut Yukon Gold potatoes, loaded sky-high with Vegan Ground Beef, black beans, and a creamy sunflower "cheese" sauce—this dish is chock-full of fiber and plant-packed nutrients (*although you'd never know it*).

MAKES 4 servings ✦ **START TO FINISH:** 45 minutes

6 medium-size Yukon Gold potatoes, sliced to desired size, around ½ to ¾ inch recommended

1 tablespoon garlic powder

1 tablespoon salt

2 cups Vegan Ground Beef (page 222) or your favorite vegan ground beef substitute

1 (15-ounce) can black beans, pinto beans, or red kidney beans, drained and rinsed

1 yellow or red onion, diced

1 red bell pepper, seeded and diced

2 garlic cloves, minced

1 teaspoon ground cumin

1 tablespoon chili powder

1 to 2 tablespoons water or extra-virgin olive oil

SUGGESTED TOPPINGS

Load these up with whatever you've got in your fridge

1 tomato, diced

1 jalapeño pepper, seeded and diced

Handful of fresh cilantro (optional)

Juice of 1 lime

½ cup Sunflower Cream Sauce (page 272)

1. Preheat the oven to 375°F, and line a baking sheet with a reusable baking mat or parchment paper.

2. In a bowl, combine the sliced potatoes with the garlic powder and salt and toss until coated.

3. Transfer to the prepared baking sheet and roast for 35 minutes, or until crispy, flipping halfway through.

4. Meanwhile, in a large skillet, combine the ground "beef" with the black beans, onion, red bell pepper, garlic, cumin, chili powder, and the water. Sauté over medium heat for 5 minutes, or until the onion starts to turn translucent.

5. Assemble on a serving platter with the fries on the bottom, topped with the ground beef mixture and your desired toppings.

Save the Scraps: Onion peels for Onion Peel Powder (page 336), Scrappy Broth (page 102), or Bouilliant Bouillon Powder (page 336).

POTATOES

GARLIC POWDER

VEGAN GROUND BEEF

BLACK BEANS

YELLOW ONION

RED BELL PEPPER

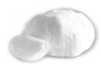

GARLIC

CHILI POWDER

CUMIN

OPTIONAL TOPPINGS:
TOMATO, JALAPEÑO, CILANTRO, LIME, SUNFLOWER CREAM SAUCE

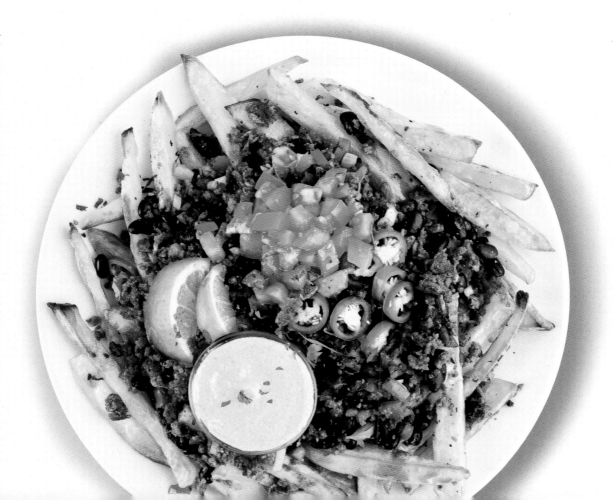

We-Got-the-Beet Chips

Drumroll, please . . . We gotta add beet leaves to the "never discard" list. Just like kale chips, beet leaves can be transformed into the crispy snack of your dreams with a bit of spice and an oven roast. Have them on their own, or serve as a crispy topping to my Whatever Sheet-Pan Soup (page 84).

MAKES 2 to 4 servings ✦ **START TO FINISH:** 30 minutes

5 cups beet leaves or kale

1 teaspoon paprika

¼ cup nutritional yeast

2 teaspoons Apple Scrap Vinegar (page 350) or store-bought apple cider vinegar or extra-virgin olive oil

½ teaspoon garlic powder

1 teaspoon salt

1. Preheat the oven to 300°F, and line two baking sheets with reusable baking mats or parchment paper.

2. Chop the beet leaves into bite-size pieces and place in a bowl, along with the rest of the ingredients.

3. Toss with your hands until coated, then evenly spread out on the prepared pans. Bake for 25 to 30 minutes, or until crispy.

Storage: Once cooled, store in an airtight container at room temperature for 2 to 3 days.

BEET LEAVES

PAPRIKA

NUTRITIONAL YEAST

APPLE CIDER VINEGAR

GARLIC POWDER

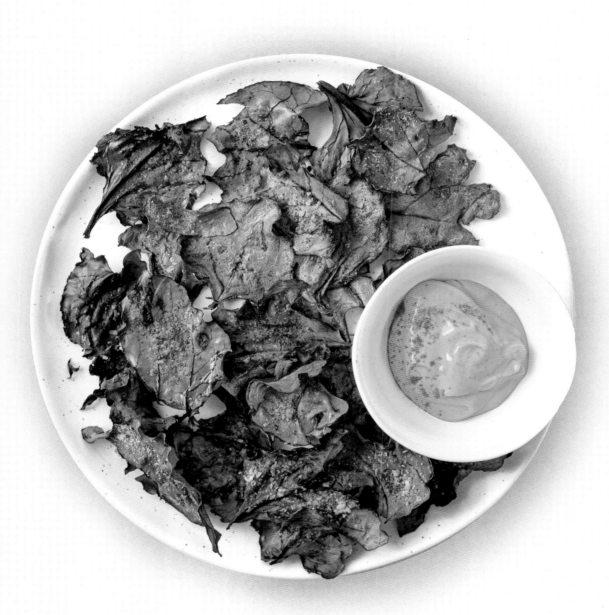

Crispy Crunches

Turn your kitchen scraps into a snack of champions with these potato peel chips—or what I love to call "crispy crunches." Whenever you find yourself peeling potatoes, save those skins and load 'em up with your favorite spices. So, go ahead, I dare you: eat just one!

MAKES 4 servings ✦ **START TO FINISH:** 35 minutes

2 cups potato skins, from 6 to 8 peeled potatoes (sweet potato skins work too)

3 tablespoons nutritional yeast

1 tablespoon vegetable broth or extra-virgin olive oil

1 teaspoon dried parsley

½ teaspoon salt

FOR SERVING

Flaky sea salt

Fresh chives

Creamy Vegan Tzatziki (page 276) or ketchup

1. Preheat the oven to 400°F, and line a baking sheet with a reusable baking mat or parchment paper.

2. In a bowl, combine the potato skins with nutritional yeast, broth, parsley, and salt. Mix until the skins are coated with the liquid and seasonings. Arrange in a single layer on the prepared baking sheet.

3. Bake for 25 minutes, or until crispy, tossing halfway through. Garnish with sea salt and chives. Serve with vegan tzatziki or ketchup.

Storage: Once cooled, store in an airtight container at room temperature for 1 to 2 weeks.

POTATOES

NUTRITIONAL YEAST

VEGETABLE BROTH OR OLIVE OIL

DRIED PARSLEY

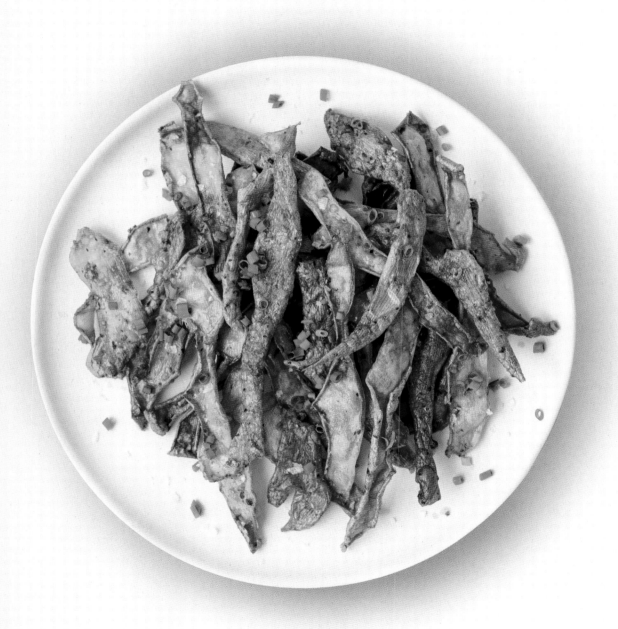

Dill Pickle Chips

As evidenced by my Pickled Tennessee Tenders (page 226) and Dilly Orzo Soup (page 100), I'm plum-crazy for pickle juice in the *Scrappy* kitchen. This incredibly versatile ingredient injects big flavor into even the most humble of dishes, including your new favorite snack: homemade Dill Pickle Chips. Tangy, crunchy, and ever so delicious!

MAKES 2 servings ✦ **START TO FINISH:** 1 hour 40 minutes

3 russet potatoes

2 cups pickle juice, or 2 cups Apple Scrap Vinegar (page 350) or store-bought apple cider vinegar mixed with a handful of fresh dill plus 1 teaspoon salt

1 tablespoon dried dill

Olive oil spray (optional)

¼ cup Roasted Red Pepper Sauce (page 276; optional)

1. Using a mandoline or a sharp knife, slice the potatoes thinly, around ¹⁄₁₆ inch thick. Pat dry to remove some of the moisture.

2. In a bowl, combine the sliced potatoes and the pickle juice, making sure the slices are fully submerged. Allow to marinate for an hour.

3. Preheat the oven to 400°F, and line a baking sheet with a reusable baking mat or parchment paper.

4. Drain and pat the potatoes dry. Place the dried dill on a dry plate and toss the potato slices in the dill. Distribute the slices evenly on the prepared baking sheet. Spray with olive oil, if desired, for a crispy result. Bake for 30 minutes, flipping halfway through.

5. Enjoy immediately with a dip of choice, such as my Roasted Red Pepper Sauce.

   Storage: Once cooled, store in an airtight container at room temperature for 1 to 2 weeks.

POTATOES

PICKLE JUICE

DRIED DILL

ROASTED RED PEPPER SAUCE

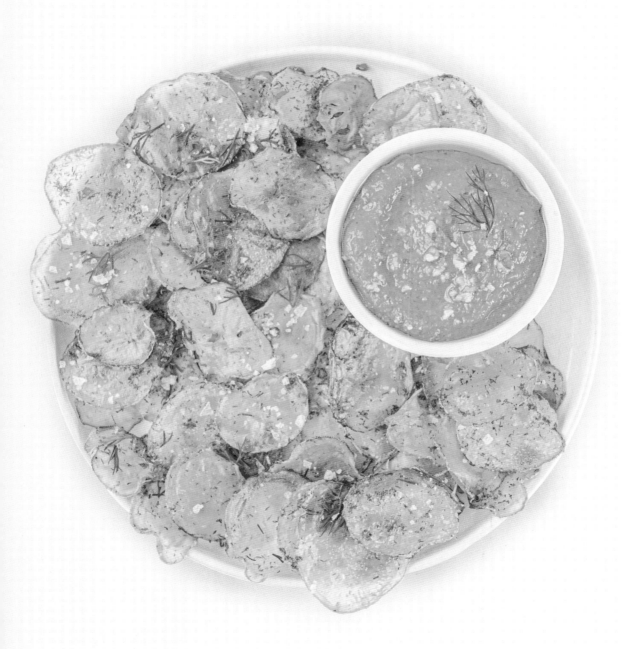

The Knead for Flatbread

You will be shocked and amazed at how easy it is to make your own pillowy soft, quick-and-delicious flatbread. The best part? This simple recipe can be used as a pizza dough, a naan replacement, or as a wrap for any of your favorite sandwich ingredients. Looking for more bread recipes? Check out the Small Sourdough Loaf (page 320) and Sourdough Discard Crackers (page 322).

MAKES 4 servings ✦ **START TO FINISH:** 20 minutes

2 cups self-rising flour or gluten-free self-rising flour, plus more for dusting

1 cup unsweetened Cultured Vegan Yogurt (page 48) or store-bought coconut or soy yogurt

OPTIONAL

Fresh parsley, garlic, flaky salt, and a touch of olive oil, for a naan-style flatbread

1. Preheat the oven to 400°F, and line two baking sheets with reusable baking mats or parchment paper.

2. In a bowl, combine the flour and vegan yogurt with a spoon. It will be clumpy. Transfer to a floured surface and knead until a dough is formed, about 5 minutes.

3. Slice the dough into four equal pieces. Roll out each piece of dough into a circular flatbread 7 to 8 inches in diameter and around ¼ inch thick.

4. Transfer to the prepared baking sheets and bake for 15 to 17 minutes, or until the flatbread is slightly browned on the outside and cooked through.

5. Use for dipping with Perfect Peanut Butter Curry (page 190), as the base for Life-Altering Mediterranean Wraps (page 110), or instead of sandwich bread in any of my sandwich recipes.

Storage: Once cooled, store in an airtight container at room temperature for 2 days, or freeze for up to 1 month.

SELF-RISING FLOUR

YOGURT

**OPTIONAL: FRESH PARSLEY
OR CILANTRO**

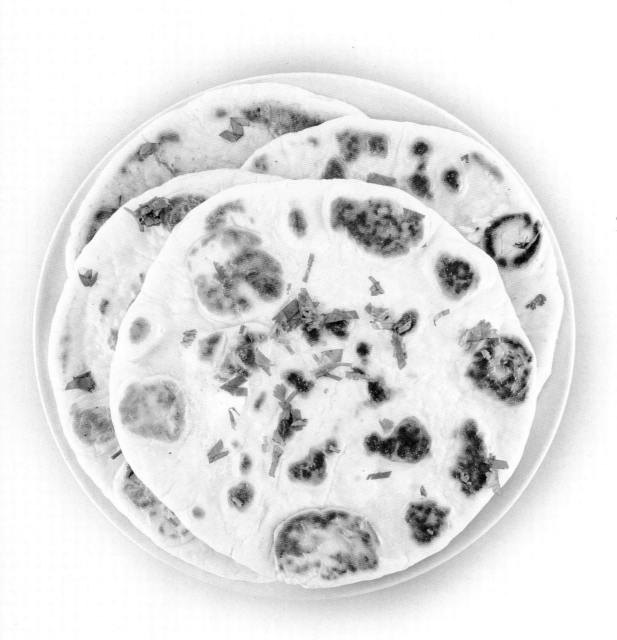

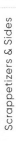

It's a (Flax) Wrap

You're craving a delicious wrap. But you *really* don't want to head to the grocery store (or grab a plastic package of tortillas). Problem solved with these wondrous two-ingredient flax wraps! They're high in fiber, easy to make, and so tasty (especially with my Sproutichoke Wrap, page 112). Use them in place of bread in any of the sandwich recipes here or to dip into any of the sauces.

MAKES 4 wraps ✦ **START TO FINISH:** 30 minutes

1 cup water

1½ cups ground flaxseed

1 teaspoon paprika

½ teaspoon salt

OPTIONAL FOR SAVORY

1 tablespoon nutritional yeast

1 teaspoon garlic powder

OPTIONAL FOR SWEET

1 teaspoon ground cinnamon

1 tablespoon light brown sugar

1. Bring the water to a boil in a medium-size saucepan. Turn off the heat, then add the ground flaxseed and your choice of the savory or sweet flavorings.

2. Stir with a wooden spoon until you begin to form a ball of dough in the middle of the saucepan. This will take about 90 seconds.

3. Transfer the dough ball to a cutting board and slice into four equal pieces.

4. Take two sheets of parchment paper. Place a dough piece on one piece of parchment and flatten it down with your hands. Place the other sheet of parchment on top and use a rolling pin (or empty wine bottle) to roll out the dough, creating a round tortilla shape, only about as thick as cardboard, ⅛ inch. Repeat with the remaining three pieces of dough.

5. In a large nonstick skillet over medium heat, cook a flax round on each side for about 2 minutes, until dry. Repeat with the other rounds. Allow to cool and use for your favorite wrap recipes, or for a sweet crepe-like snack.

Storage: Once cooled, store in an airtight container in the fridge for 4 days, or freeze for up to 1 month.

GROUND FLAXSEED

NUTRITIONAL YEAST

GARLIC POWDER

PAPRIKA

SALT

── **SWEET** ──

GROUND FLAXSEED

CINNAMON

BROWN SUGAR

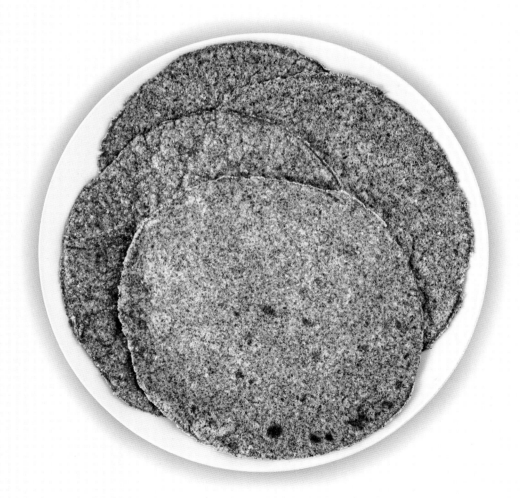

Save the Seeds

Don't toss those squash and pumpkin seeds; transform them into a savory or sweet snack with this mouthwatering zero-waste recipe. Have them on their own, or serve over pasta for a crunchy topping in the Whole Darn Squash Pasta (page 146).

MAKES 2 to 4 servings ✦ **START TO FINISH:** 25 minutes

½ to 1 cup seeds from any squash or gourd

1 to 2 tablespoons extra-virgin olive oil

SWEET BLEND

1 tablespoon ground cinnamon

2 tablespoons brown sugar

1 teaspoon Homemade Vanilla Extract or store-bought pure vanilla extract

½ teaspoon salt

SAVORY BLEND

1 teaspoon garlic powder

1 tablespoon paprika

2 tablespoons nutritional yeast

½ teaspoon salt

SPICY BLEND

1 teaspoon cayenne pepper

1 tablespoon garlic powder

1 teaspoon Onion Peel Powder (page 336) or onion powder

½ teaspoon freshly ground black pepper

½ teaspoon salt

1. Preheat the oven to 400°F, and line a baking sheet with a reusable baking mat or parchment paper.

2. Remove the guts and seeds from your squash or gourd. Separate the seeds from the guts. (I find this easiest by submerging in a bowl of water; dunk the seeds and work them with your hands to loosen from the stringy bits.)

3. Rinse the seeds and then dry in a clean cloth. Not all residue needs to be removed. Just do your best. Transfer to a bowl and toss in the olive the oil and your desired blend, either sweet, savory, or spicy. Transfer to your prepared baking sheet.

4. Roast for 10 to 20 minutes, or until crispy. Enjoy!

Storage: Store in an airtight container at room temperature for up to 2 weeks, or freeze for up to 3 months.

Scrappetizers & Sides

SWEET BLEND

CINNAMON

BROWN SUGAR

VANILLA EXTRACT

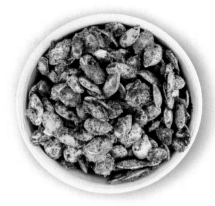

SAVORY BLEND

GARLIC POWDER

PAPRIKA

NUTRITIONAL YEAST

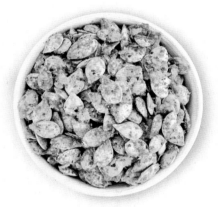

SPICY BLEND

CAYENNE PEPPER

GARLIC POWDER

ONION PEEL POWDER

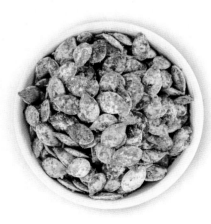

Cornmeal Biscuits

No kneading, rising, or fancy ingredients. These cornmeal drop biscuits are as easy as they are delicious! Throw everything in a bowl and then plop on a baking sheet, like playing Bingo. Or try them on top of my Chickpea Potpie (page 212). They rise to cornmeal perfection—soft, buttery, and so satisfying.

MAKES 8 or 9 biscuits ✦ **START TO FINISH:** 20 minutes

1 cup cornmeal

1 cup all-purpose or gluten-free flour

3 tablespoons nutritional yeast

2 teaspoons dried parsley

¼ teaspoon garlic powder

2½ teaspoons baking powder

½ teaspoon salt

2 teaspoons Apple Scrap Vinegar (page 350) or store-bought apple cider vinegar

1 cup + 1 tablespoon canned full-fat coconut milk or full-fat oat milk

1. Preheat the oven to 350°F, and line a baking sheet with a reusable baking mat or parchment paper.

2. In a bowl, combine the cornmeal, flour, yeast, parsley, garlic powder, baking powder, and salt. Then pour in the Apple Scrap Vinegar and coconut milk. Gently stir until a dough is formed.

3. Using a cookie scoop or a tablespoon, form about 2 tablespoons of dough into rounds on the prepared baking sheet, spacing them at least 1 inch apart.

4. Bake for 13 minutes, or until lightly browned. Remove from the oven and allow to cool before enjoying.

Storage: Store in a sealed container at room temperature for up to 3 days, or refrigerate for up to 4 days.

Save the Scraps: Coconut milk for Firecracker Tofu with Coconut Rice (page 184).

CORNMEAL

FLOUR

NUTRITIONAL YEAST

DRIED PARSLEY

GARLIC POWDER

BAKING POWDER

APPLE CIDER VINEGAR

COCONUT MILK

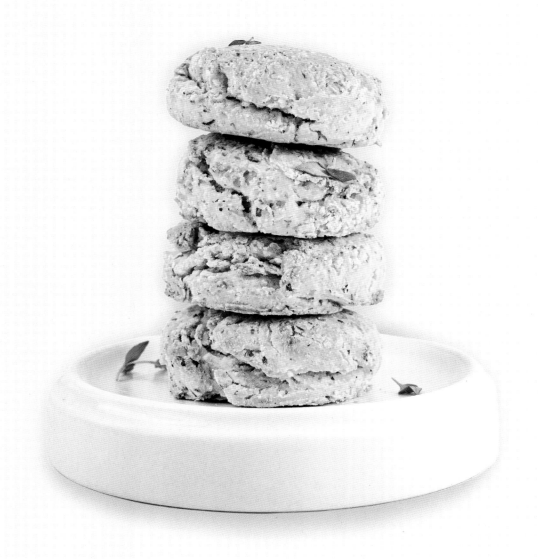

Sweet & Spicy Carrot Showstopper

Say good-bye to bland limp carrots and say hello to a sweet-and-spicy side dish sensation. Chili and hoisin-glazed heirloom carrots are served over a tangy whipped feta, dipped and drizzled with a Carrot Top Chimichurri to make for a "complete" eating experience you won't be able to get enough of.

MAKES 4 servings ✦ **START TO FINISH:** 40 minutes

7 to 10 medium-size heirloom or regular carrots, with tops if available

½ teaspoon ground cinnamon

½ teaspoon ground cumin

½ teaspoon salt

2 tablespoons garlic chili sauce

1 tablespoon pure maple syrup

1 tablespoon hoisin sauce

1 (14-ounce) can brown lentils, drained and rinsed, or canned bean of choice

1½ cups Whipped Feta Dip with Roasted Tomatoes (page 286), prepared without the tomatoes, or 1½ cups Sunflower Cream Sauce (page 272)

½ cup Carrot Top Chimichurri (page 272)

1. Preheat the oven to 400°F, and line a baking sheet with a reusable baking mat or parchment paper.

2. Cut the green tops off the carrots and reserve them for the Carrot Top Chimichurri, then place the carrots on the prepared baking pan. Sprinkle with the cinnamon, cumin, and salt until coated. Roast for 30 minutes, or until softened.

3. While the carrots roast, in a medium-size bowl or jar, combine the garlic chili sauce, maple syrup, and hoisin sauce. Add the lentils.

4. Remove the baking sheet from the oven, pour the lentil mixture over the cooked carrots, and toss until coated. Return the pan to the oven and roast for 5 more minutes.

5. Spoon the Whipped Feta Dip onto a serving plate and top with the carrots. Top with the Carrot Top Chimichurri. Serve.

Storage: Store in an airtight container in the fridge for up to 3 days.

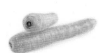

CARROT

CINNAMON

CUMIN

GARLIC CHILI SAUCE

MAPLE SYRUP

HOISIN SAUCE

BROWN LENTILS

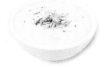

SUNFLOWER CREAM SAUCE
OR WHIPPED FETA DIP

CARROT TOP CHIMICHURRI

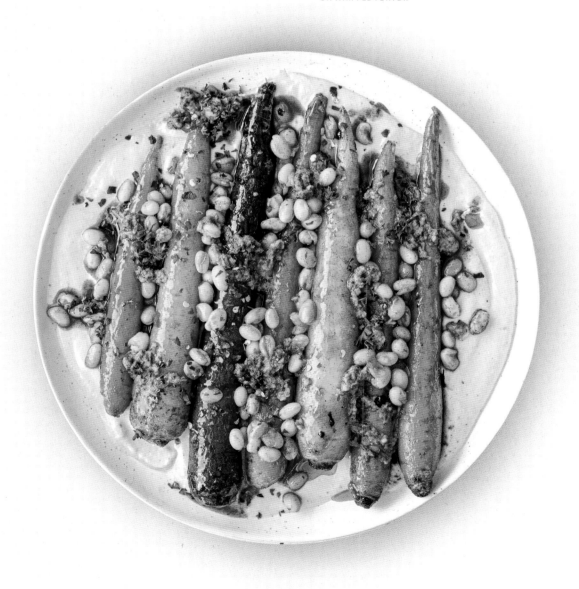

Greek Lemon Smashed Potatoes

Don't worry—no spuds were harmed in the making of this recipe. Instead, they're lovingly transformed into garlicky, lemony, crispy bites of heaven! The secret to the fluffiest, melt-in-your-mouth smashed potatoes is boiling them before baking.

MAKES 4 servings ✦ **START TO FINISH:** 40 minutes

1½ pounds mini yellow potatoes

Juice of 1 lemon

2 tablespoons extra-virgin olive oil

1 teaspoon garlic powder

2 teaspoons salt

1 teaspoon freshly ground black pepper

FOR SERVING

Fresh herbs

Creamy Vegan Tzatziki (page 276; optional)

1. Place the potatoes in a large pot. Add water to cover, and add half the lemon juice to the pot. Bring to a boil and cook until fork-tender, about 20 minutes.

2. While the potatoes are boiling, make the garlic lemon marinade by combining the olive oil, remaining lemon juice, garlic powder, salt, and pepper in a bowl.

3. Drain the potatoes and allow them to cool for 5 minutes. Transfer them to a baking sheet. Using a potato masher or the bottom of a cup, gently smash the potatoes until each is flattened.

4. Using a barbecue brush, brush the garlic lemon marinade over the potatoes. Bake at 425°F for 20 to 25 minutes, or until the potatoes are golden and crispy. Garnish with fresh herbs. Eat immediately with vegan tzatziki as a dip, if desired.

Note: To achieve a crispy smashed potato, oil is necessary for this recipe. For an oil-free version, you can replace the oil with vegetable broth; however, the potato will be softer.

Save the Scraps: Lemon peels for Citrus Peel Powder (page 332).

**MINI YELLOW
POTATOES**

LEMON

OLIVE OIL

GARLIC POWDER

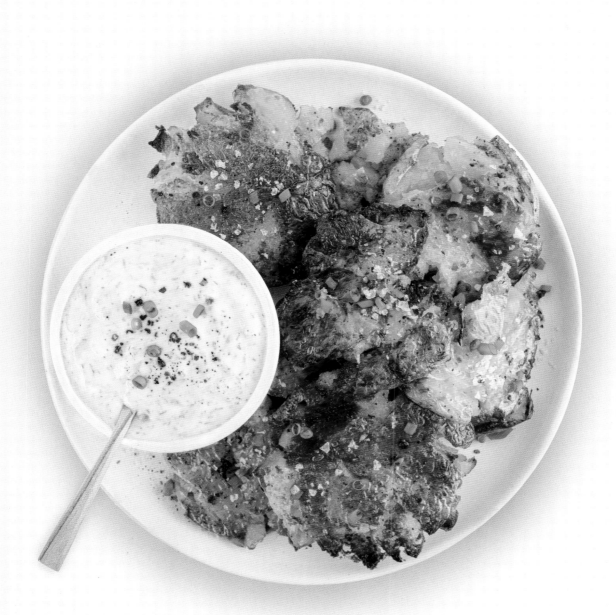

Scrappacia

A scarpaccia is a delicious rustic zucchini tart, originally hailing from Italy. For my *Scrappacia* version, nothing goes to waste, as we utilize the drained zucchini juice for the creamy batter. Best served warm as an appetizer or side dish, and especially delicious dipped into my Creamy Vegan Tzatziki (page 276).

MAKES 12 servings ✦ **START TO FINISH:** 3 hours (with resting time)

3 medium zucchinis, around 1½ pounds

1 small red onion

1 teaspoon salt

1 cup all-purpose flour, or gluten-free all-purpose flour

¼ cup cornmeal

½ teaspoon dried rosemary

2 tablespoons nutritional yeast (optional)

½ cup water, or up to ¾ cup

1. Using a mandoline, if possible, slice the zucchini and red onion very thinly into ⅛-inch rounds. If you do not have a mandoline, use a sharp knife and slice as thinly as possible. Transfer to a large bowl, sprinkle with the salt, and toss to coat. Place something heavy, such as a small cast-iron pan or plate with cans on top, on the zucchini-onion mixture to promote drainage.

2. Once 2 hours have passed, preheat the oven to 400°F and line a baking sheet (I use a 13 x 18–inch baking sheet) with parchment paper or spray with oil.

3. Transfer the zucchini and onions to a cheese cloth or thin kitchen cloth, and drain as much liquid as possible into the bowl where the mixture set. Put the drained zucchini and onions aside. The juice will be used as the liquid base for the scarpaccia.

4. Add the flour, cornmeal, dried rosemary, and nutritional yeast (if using) to the bowl with the zucchini juice. Mix to form a thick batter, similar to a pancake-batter consistency. Add ½ to ¾ cup of additional water as needed to thin.

5. Fold in the drained onions and zucchini and gently mix until evenly dispersed. Pour the batter onto the prepared baking sheet, and, using a spatula, spread the mix evenly, around ½ inch thick. For a crispy scarpaccia, spray the top with olive oil.

6. Bake for 35 to 40 minutes, until browned. Remove from the oven and allow to cool before transferring from the baking sheet and slicing into 12 squares.

Up the Veggies: Add 1 cup of chopped fresh herbs, green onions, or chopped zucchini blossoms to the batter when mixing.

Storage: Store in a sealed container in the fridge for up to 4 days.

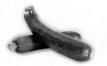
ZUCCHINI

RED ONION

ALL-PURPOSE
FLOUR

CORNMEAL

DRIED ROSEMARY

NUTRITIONAL
YEAST

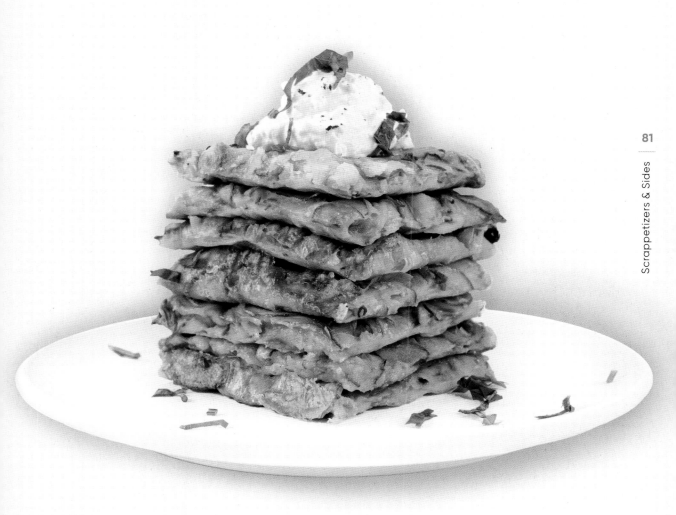

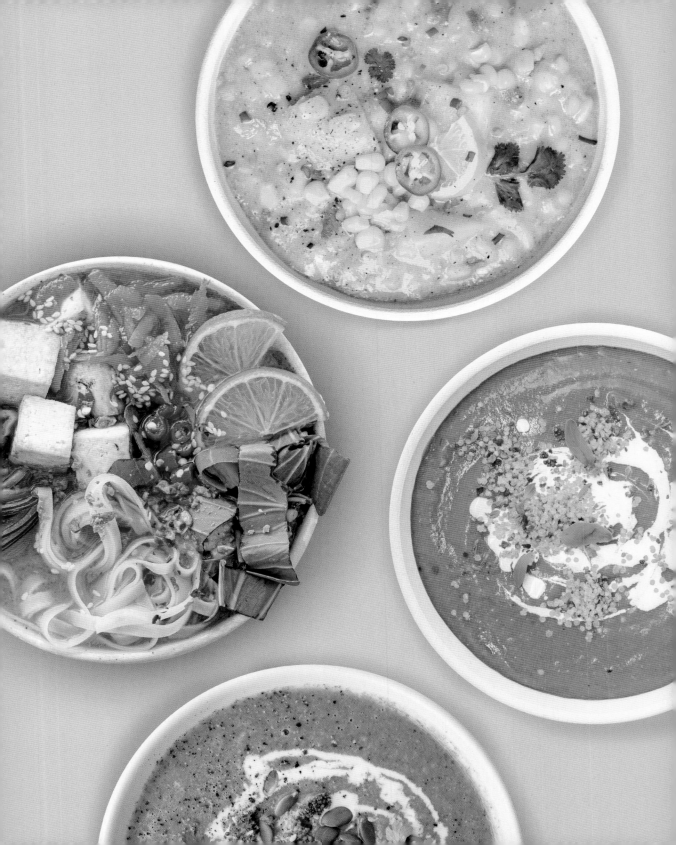

CHAPTER 3

Souperb Soups

Minimize waste and maximize flavor
with these simple, delicious, and
nourishing plant-based soup recipes.

Whatever Sheet-Pan Soup

Gather around for the soup that makes cooking easier, cleaner, and—dare I say—fun. Introducing my lazy chef's secret weapon to a scrumptious, low-waste, and nutritious meal. You take any—whatever—of your favorite vegetables, throw them on a sheet pan, and roast them until soft. Blend them into a velvety soup that's rich and flavorful, and top off with my crispy We-Got-the-Beet Chips for the perfect weeknight meal.

MAKES 4 to 6 servings ✦ **START TO FINISH:** 45 minutes

3 cups chopped butternut squash or pumpkin, seeded and skinned, or sweet potato, peeled

2 cups chopped cauliflower or potato

1 carrot, chopped

2 celery ribs, chopped

1 yellow onion, peeled and chopped

1 garlic head, skins on, top sliced off

1 teaspoon paprika

½ teaspoon ground cumin

½ teaspoon red pepper flakes

1 teaspoon salt

1 cup vegetable broth

1 cup coconut milk or Sunflower Cream Sauce (page 272)

Juice of ½ lemon

Handful of We-Got-the-Beet Chips (page 62; optional)

1. Preheat the oven to 400°F, and line a baking sheet with a reusable baking mat or parchment paper.

2. Arrange all the fresh vegetables and the garlic head in a single layer on the prepared baking sheet and sprinkle with the paprika, cumin, red pepper flakes, and salt. Roast for 30 minutes, or until the vegetables are fork-tender.

3. When safe to handle, transfer all the cooked vegetables, except the garlic head, to a high-speed blender along with the vegetable broth and most of the coconut milk (reserve 3 tablespoons for swirling on top). Squeeze the roasted cloves of garlic into the blender, omitting and composting the skins. Blend until a soup is formed, adding water or more broth to thin, if desired.

4. Serve with crusty sourdough bread, a squeeze of lemon, and, if desired, We-Got-the-Beet Chips on top.

Storage: Store in the fridge for 3 to 4 days, or in the freezer for up to 3 months.

Save the Scraps: Squash or pumpkin seeds for Save the Seeds (page 72). Carrot tops for the Carrot Top Chimichurri (page 272). Onion peels for Onion Peel Powder (page 336), Scrappy Broth (page 102), or Bouilliant Bouillon Powder (page 336). Leftover coconut milk for Coo-Coo for Coconut Caramel (page 260) or Firecracker Tofu with Coconut Rice (page 184).

BUTTERNUT SQUASH

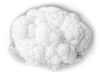

CAULIFLOWER

CARROT

CELERY

YELLOW ONION

GARLIC

PAPRIKA

CUMIN

RED PEPPER FLAKES

VEGETABLE BROTH

COCONUT MILK

OPTIONAL: BEETROOT CHIPS

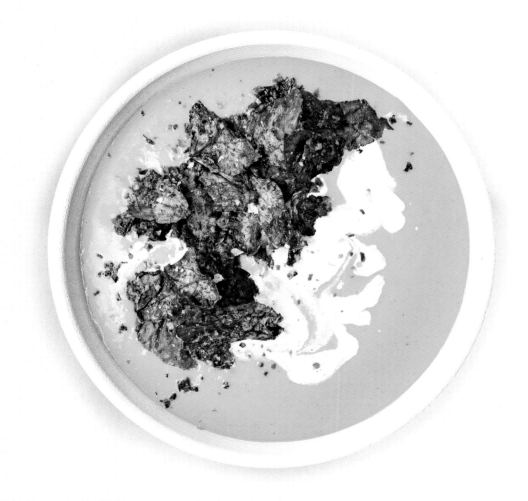

Green Goddess Soup

Never let a broccoli stem go to waste again. Not only are the stems extremely nutritious (gram for gram, they contain more vitamin C, calcium, and iron than the florets), they're also absolutely delicious when prepared right—and this glowing soup is a perfect example. The stems are combined with antioxidant-rich ginger, zucchini, and spinach for a velvety broth that will make you feel like a goddess!

MAKES 6 servings ✦ **START TO FINISH:** 20 minutes

1 medium yellow onion, chopped

3 garlic cloves, minced

1 (1-inch) piece fresh ginger, minced

1½ teaspoons green curry paste (optional)

3 to 4 tablespoons water, or 1 to 2
  tablespoons extra-virgin olive oil

1 broccoli head, broken into florets

2 broccoli stems, chopped

1 medium-size zucchini, chopped

4 cups vegetable broth

½ cup unsweetened coconut milk, soy milk, or
  any other plant-based milk

3 cups spinach or kale

¾ teaspoon salt

Handful of fresh cilantro, parsley, or chives

Juice of 1 lime

For topping: more coconut milk, pumpkin
  seeds, freshly ground black pepper, broccoli
  florets, or fresh herbs

1. In a large pot over medium heat, combine the onion, garlic, ginger, and green curry paste (if using), along with 1 to 2 tablespoons of the water. Sauté until the onion is translucent, about 3 minutes.

2. Add the broccoli florets, broccoli stems, and zucchini to the pot with the remaining 2 tablespoons of water. Cover the pot and allow to steam for 3 to 5 minutes, or until the florets are bright green.

3. Add the vegetable broth, coconut milk, spinach, and salt to the pot. Bring to a boil, then simmer until the greens are wilted, about 2 minutes.

4. When safe to handle, transfer the contents of the pot to a high-speed blender, along with a handful of fresh herbs of choice, and the lime juice. Alternatively, use an immersion blender directly in the pot. Blend until completely smooth.

5. Serve immediately, garnished with a swirl of coconut milk, pumpkin seeds, freshly ground black pepper, broccoli florets, or fresh herbs, as desired. This soup also pairs well with rice.

Storage: Store in the fridge for 3 to 4 days, or in the freezer for up to 3 months.

Save the Scraps: Onion peels for Onion Peel Powder (page 336), Scrappy Broth (page 102), or Bouilliant Bouillon Powder (page 336). Leftover coconut milk for Coo-Coo for Coconut Caramel (page 260) or Firecracker Tofu with Coconut Rice (page 184).

YELLOW ONION

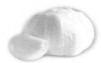
GARLIC

GINGER ROOT

GREEN CURRY PASTE

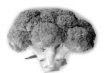
BROCCOLI

ZUCCHINI

VEGETABLE BROTH

SOY MILK

SPINACH

CILANTRO

LIME

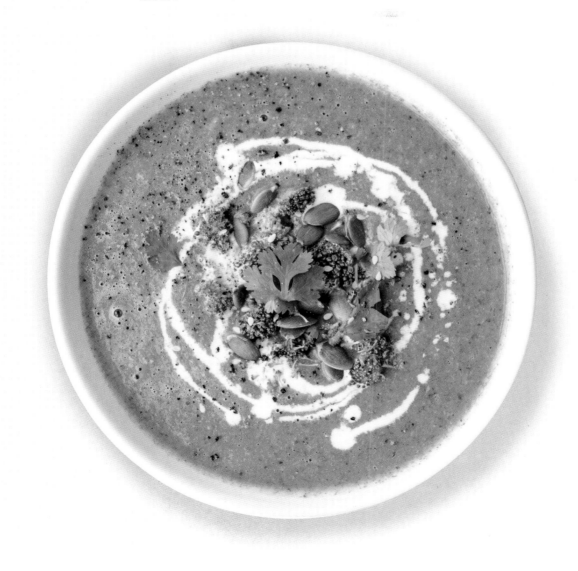

Raid-the-Fridge Noodle Soup

Get ready to slurp up some serious flavor with this creamy noodle soup recipe. I make this soup almost every week, utilizing the bits and bobs of vegetables left over from the week before. With an umami-rich soy milk broth, tender noodles, and bright toppings, this is the perfect balance of comfort and nourishment.

MAKES 4 servings ✦ **START TO FINISH:** 30 minutes

TOFU

1 (14-ounce) block extra-firm tofu, sliced into cubes, or Soy-Free Tofu (page 236)

½ teaspoon salt

¼ teaspoon freshly ground black pepper

BROTH AND NOODLES

1 to 2 tablespoons water or extra-virgin olive oil

2 garlic cloves, minced

1 (1-inch) piece fresh ginger, minced

1 yellow onion, diced finely

1½ teaspoons sweet chili sauce

2 tablespoons miso paste

1 teaspoon curry powder

1 tablespoon soy sauce

4 cups vegetable broth

2 cups unsweetened soy milk, coconut, almond, or cashew milk (do not use oat milk)

1 (8-ounce) package vermicelli, ramen noodles, or whole wheat spaghetti

FOR SERVING

1 cup fresh vegetables of choice (I used: 1 carrot, julienned; 1½ cups baby bok choy, chopped roughly; 2 green onions, diced)

1 lime, sliced into wedges

½ cup chopped fresh cilantro (optional)

Sesame seeds, for topping

1 teaspoon red pepper flakes

1. Make the tofu: Preheat the oven to 400°F, and line a baking sheet with a reusable baking mat or parchment paper. Slice the tofu into cubes, and sprinkle with salt and black pepper. Bake for 25 minutes, or until slightly crispy.

2. Meanwhile, make the broth: Heat the water in a large pot over medium heat. Add the garlic, ginger, and onion, and sauté until fragrant, about 2 minutes.

3. Add the chili sauce, miso paste, curry powder, and soy sauce. Stir until the onion, garlic, and ginger are covered in the sauce.

4. Pour in the vegetable broth and soy milk. Bring to a boil and then simmer, uncovered, for 8 minutes.

5. Meanwhile, prepare the noodles in a separate pot according to the package directions.

6. To serve, separate the noodles into four bowls. Pour the broth over them, then add the fresh vegetables, baked tofu, lime wedges, cilantro (if using), sesame seeds, and red pepper flakes to taste.

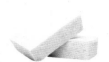

TOFU

PEPPER

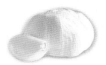

GARLIC

GINGER ROOT

YELLOW ONION

SWEET CHILI SAUCE

MISO PASTE

CURRY POWDER

SOY SAUCE

VEGETABLE BROTH

COCONUT MILK

VERMICELLI

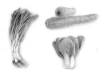

VEGGIES OF CHOICE

FOR SERVING

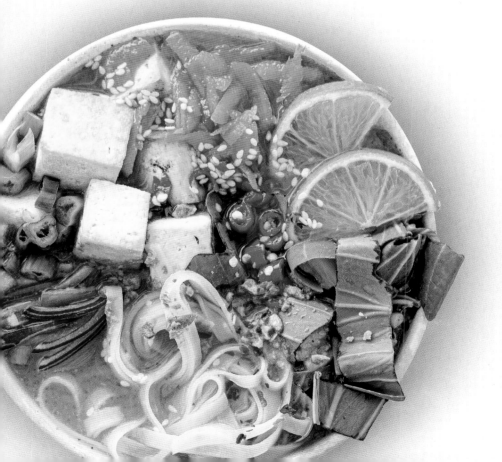

Storage: Store the broth in the fridge for 3 to 4 days, or in the freezer for up to 3 months.

Save the Scraps: Onion peels for Onion Peel Powder (page 336), Scrappy Broth (page 102), or Bouilliant Bouillon Powder (page 336).

Roasted Tomato Soup with Crispy Quinoa

When it comes to tomatoes, they all tend to get ripe at the same time. If you find yourself with an overabundance of the cherubic orbs, this soul-warming soup is the perfect solution. Once you see how easy it is to make a perfect bowl of tomato soup from scratch, you'll never go back. Topped with crispy quinoa, this scrumptious dish is equal parts simple and sophisticated.

MAKES 4 to 6 servings ✦ **START TO FINISH:** 40 minutes

CRISPY QUINOA

¾ cup uncooked quinoa

1 tablespoon vegetable broth or water

1 tablespoon nutritional yeast

¼ teaspoon ground turmeric

¼ teaspoon garlic powder

¼ teaspoon salt

SOUP

12 vine-ripened tomatoes, or 1 (28-ounce) can diced tomatoes (see note)

1 small yellow onion, chopped roughly

1 small Yukon Gold potato, peeled and chopped roughly

1 cup cherry tomatoes

2 thyme sprigs

1 garlic head, top sliced off

1½ teaspoons salt

½ teaspoon freshly ground black pepper

2 cups vegetable broth

1 tablespoon nutritional yeast

¼ cup fresh basil

Coconut milk, for drizzling (optional)

1. Preheat the oven to 400°F, and line two baking sheets with reusable baking mats or parchment paper.

2. Meanwhile, make the quinoa: Cook the quinoa according to the package directions.

3. For the soup, arrange the vine-ripened tomatoes, onion, potato, cherry tomatoes, thyme sprigs, garlic, salt, and pepper on one of the prepared baking sheets. Bake on the lower rack for 40 minutes, or until the tomatoes are roasted and the garlic is soft.

4. Meanwhile, once the quinoa is cooked, stir in the tablespoon of vegetable broth, nutritional yeast, turmeric, garlic powder, and salt. Transfer to the second baking sheet, and bake for 20 minutes, until slightly crispy.

5. Back to the soup: Transfer the roasted vegetable mixture to a high-speed blender along with the vegetable broth, nutritional yeast, and basil (reserving some for topping), and blend until smooth. Taste, and adjust the salt as needed.

6. Serve in bowls with the crispy quinoa, like croutons on top. If desired, drizzle with coconut milk for extra creaminess.

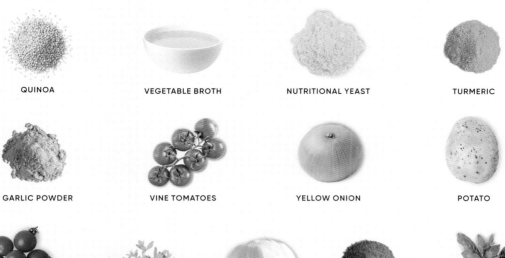

QUINOA

VEGETABLE BROTH

NUTRITIONAL YEAST

TURMERIC

GARLIC POWDER

VINE TOMATOES

YELLOW ONION

POTATO

CHERRY TOMATOES

THYME

GARLIC

BLACK PEPPER

BASIL

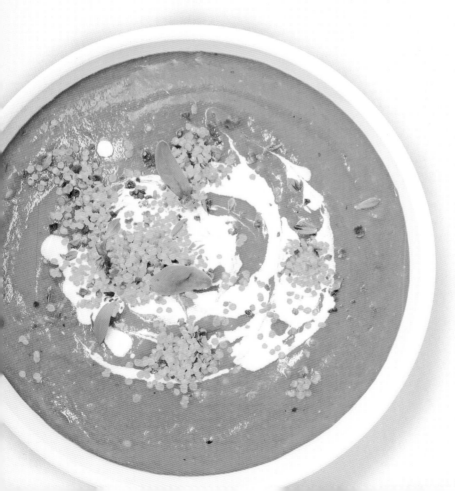

Note: If you don't have access to vine-ripened tomatoes, you can roast all the other ingredients, then add them to a blender with one (28-ounce) can of diced tomatoes.

Storage: Store the soup in the fridge for 3 to 4 days, or in a sealed container in the freezer for up to 2 months.

Save the Scraps: Onion peels for Onion Peel Powder (page 336), Scrappy Broth (page 102), or Bouilliant Bouillon Powder (page 336). Potato Peels for Crispy Crunches (page 64).

Leeky Tuscan Minestrone

The greens on leeks are often discarded, but with a little tender loving care, they can be equally as scrumptious as the white stems. This wildly delicious Tuscan minestrone allows both parts of the leek to shine, with the greens browned in the oven for an unexpected crispy topping. Seasonal vegetables provide the perfect base to this thick, creamy soup that is meal-prep- and freezer-friendly.

MAKES 6 servings ✦ **START TO FINISH:** 45 minutes

1 leek, white parts minced, green parts sliced thinly

Salt and freshly ground black pepper

1 carrot, diced

1½ cups diced zucchini, potato, cauliflower, celery, or bell pepper

3 garlic cloves, minced

6 cups + 1 to 2 tablespoons vegetable broth

2 tablespoons tomato paste

1 tablespoon dried parsley

1 tablespoon nutritional yeast

1 (14.5-ounce) can crushed tomatoes

1 (15-ounce) can white beans, chickpeas, or navy beans, drained and rinsed, or 1½ cups homemade

1 cup Sunflower Cream Sauce (page 272) or canned full-fat coconut milk

¾ cup uncooked small whole wheat or brown rice pasta shells

2 cups chopped kale, spinach, beet leaves, or chard

1. Preheat the oven to 375°F, and line a baking sheet with a reusable baking mat or parchment paper. Place the green parts of the sliced leeks on the baking sheet along with some salt and pepper. Bake until crispy, for 7 to 10 minutes.

2. Meanwhile, in a large pot over medium heat, combine the minced white leeks, carrot, diced vegetables, and garlic along with a tablespoon or two of the vegetable broth. Sauté until softened, about 3 minutes.

3. Add the tomato paste, parsley, and nutritional yeast. Stir until the vegetables are covered, another 2 minutes.

4. Add the crushed tomatoes, white beans, and remaining 6 cups of vegetable broth. Stir, then bring to a boil. Simmer, uncovered, for 5 minutes.

5. Pour in the Sunflower Cream Sauce and stir. Add the pasta shells and cook for 10 minutes, until they reach your desired tenderness. Add the chopped kale.

6. Serve with the crispy green leeks on top for crunch.

Storage: If preparing for meal prep, cook and store the pasta separately so it doesn't soak up the broth in the fridge. If this is done, you can store the soup in a sealed container in the fridge for 3 to 4 days, or in the freezer for up to 2 months.

LEEK

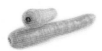
CARROT

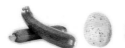
VEGGIES OF CHOICE: ZUCCHINI, POTATO, CAULIFLOWER, CELERY, BELL PEPPER

GARLIC

VEGETABLE BROTH

TOMATO PASTE

PARSLEY

NUTRITIONAL YEAST

CRUSHED TOMATOES

WHITE BEANS

SUNFLOWER CREAM SAUCE

WHOLE WHEAT SHELLS

KALE

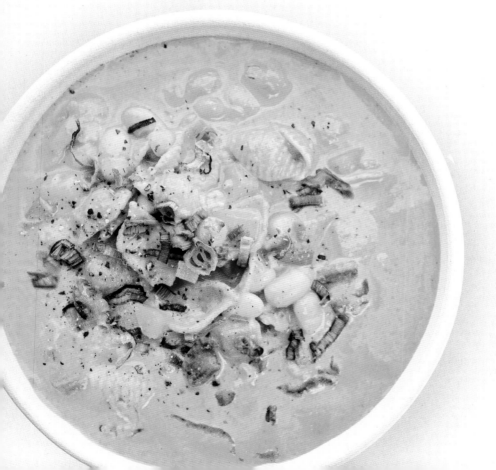

Gluten & Nut–Free Substitutions: Use brown rice pasta shells in place of whole wheat.

Save the Scraps: Carrot tops for the Carrot Top Chimichurri (page 272).

Cobby Chick'n Broth

Are you looking for a simple and sustainable way to add depth and flavor to your soups and stews? Stop discarding your corncobs, and make this amazing broth instead. The combination of the sweetness from the cobs, herbaceousness from the fresh thyme and parsley, and earthiness of the turmeric create a rich broth that tastes eerily similar to a traditional chicken broth. Use it in any recipe in this book that calls for broth.

MAKES 8 to 12 cups ✦ **START TO FINISH:** 3 hours

4 corncobs, kernels removed with knife and reserved (see Save the Scraps, below)

4 thyme sprigs

2 bay leaves

3 garlic cloves

Handful of fresh parsley, chopped

2 teaspoons celery salt

½ teaspoon ground turmeric

1 teaspoon garlic powder

8 to 12 cups filtered water

1. In a large pot, combine all the ingredients. Bring to a boil, then simmer for 1 to 3 hours. Remove the bay leaves and leftover corncobs for compost.

Storage: Store the cobby broth in an airtight container in the fridge for up to 5 days, or in the freezer for up to 3 months.

Save the Scraps: Corn kernels for the Smoky Corncob Chowder (page 96) or Street Corn Pasta Salad (page 132).

CORNCOB

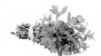

THYME

BAY LEAVES

GARLIC

PARSLEY

CELERY SALT

TURMERIC

GARLIC POWDER

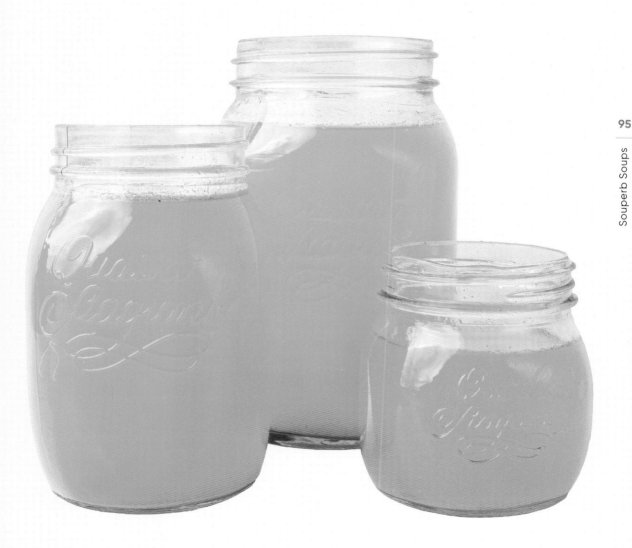

Smoky Corncob Chowder

Tired of the same old boring soups? Want something bold, something daring, something . . . corny? Look no further, because this smoky corncob chowder is about to take your taste buds on a wild ride. Juicy kernels of corn combined with creamy Yukon Gold potatoes, jalapeños, and pickle juice make for a soup that is equal parts comforting and adventurous.

MAKES 4 to 6 servings ✦ **START TO FINISH:** 40 minutes

1 yellow onion, diced

2 garlic cloves, minced

1 jalapeño pepper, seeded and diced (if desired)

1 red bell pepper, seeded and diced

1 to 2 tablespoons water or extra-virgin olive oil

4 cups corn kernels, frozen and thawed, or fresh

3 Yukon Gold potatoes, cubed

3 tablespoons pickle juice or Apple Scrap Vinegar (page 350) or store-bought apple cider vinegar

1 teaspoon smoked or regular paprika

¼ teaspoon freshly ground black pepper

½ teaspoon salt, plus more as needed

4 cups Cobby Chick'n Broth (page 94) or vegetable broth

1 cup unsweetened plant-based milk (soy, almond, or cashew [I don't recommend oat or coconut milk here])

2 tablespoons chopped fresh chives, for garnish

1. In a large pot over medium heat, combine the onion, garlic, jalapeño, and bell pepper with the water. Sauté until softened, about 5 minutes.

2. Add the corn, potatoes, pickle juice, smoked paprika, black pepper, and salt. Stir until the corn and potatoes are covered in the spices and have cooked slightly, about 5 minutes. Add the chick'n broth and plant-based milk. Bring to a boil, then simmer, uncovered, for about 20 minutes, until the potatoes are cooked.

3. Using an immersion blender, blend up to half of the soup until smooth, to create a creamy texture with chunks of corn and vegetables. Alternatively, when cool enough to handle, transfer one-quarter of the soup to a regular blender, blend until smooth, then transfer back to the soup pot, blending more, as desired. Garnish with chives.

Storage: Store in an airtight container in the fridge for 3 to 4 days, or in the freezer for up to 2 months.

Save the Scraps: Onion peels for Onion Peel Powder (page 336), Scrappy Broth (page 102), or Bouilliant Bouillon Powder (page 336). Corncobs for Cobby Chick'n Broth (page 94).

YELLOW ONION

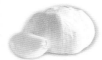

GARLIC

JALAPEÑO

RED BELL PEPPER

CORN KERNELS

POTATO

PICKLE JUICE

SMOKED PAPRIKA

BLACK PEPPER

VEGETABLE BROTH

PLANT-BASED MILK

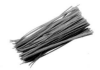

CHIVES

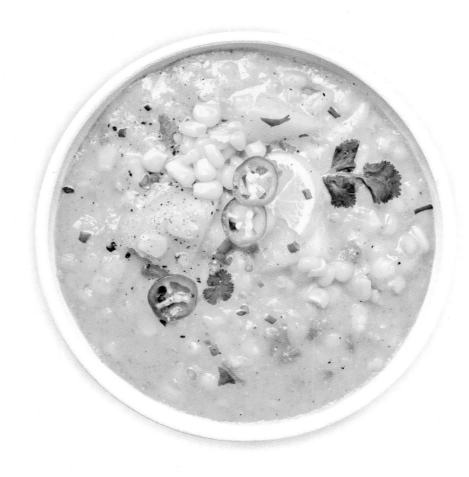

Caramelized French Onion Soup

This, my friends, is a flavor explosion, using eight yellow onions in one fell swoop. Although caramelizing onions is a labor—of love, for me—it's well worth the effort for a soup that's true comfort in a bowl. Top it off with a vegan cashew mozzarella and you'll be transported straight to France without ever leaving your kitchen.

MAKES 4 to 6 servings ✦ **START TO FINISH:** 90 minutes

8 large yellow onions, about 5 pounds

4 thyme sprigs

2 teaspoons salt

2 teaspoons light or dark brown sugar

2 to 4 tablespoons vegetable broth or extra-virgin olive oil, for caramelizing onions

2 tablespoons balsamic vinegar

1 tablespoon all-purpose or gluten-free flour

4 garlic cloves, minced

¼ teaspoon freshly ground black pepper

7 cups vegetable broth

8 slices stale baguette, sliced

VEGAN "MOZZARELLA"

1½ cups sunflower seeds or cashews, soaked in water overnight or boiled for 15 minutes

¾ cup unsweetened Cultured Vegan Yogurt (page 48) or store-bought coconut yogurt

2 teaspoons Apple Scrap Vinegar (page 350) or store-bought apple cider vinegar

1½ teaspoons cornstarch

¾ teaspoon sea salt

2 tablespoons unsweetened plant-based milk, any kind

1. In a large Dutch oven or pot, combine the onions, thyme, 1 teaspoon of the salt, and the brown sugar, along with the 2 to 4 tablespoons of vegetable broth.

2. Cook, uncovered, stirring occasionally, until the onions are caramelized and falling apart, for 45 to 50 minutes.

3. Add the balsamic vinegar, flour, garlic, and pepper. Stir until fragrant and incorporated, about 3 minutes.

4. Add the 7 cups of vegetable broth to the pot and bring to a boil. Then simmer, covered, for 25 minutes. Taste, and add the additional teaspoon of salt if needed.

5. Meanwhile, make the vegan "mozzarella" by combining all its ingredients in a blender and blending until smooth. Add more milk as needed to thin.

6. Preheat the broiler.

7. Ladle the soup into individual oven-safe bowls. Add the baguette slices on top of the soup, followed by 3 tablespoons of the vegan mozzarella and a sprig of thyme. Place the bowls in the oven for 2 to 3 minutes under the broiler, until the cheez is bubbly and browned. Enjoy immediately.

YELLOW ONION

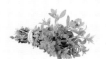

THYME

BROWN SUGAR

VEGETABLE BROTH

BALSAMIC VINEGAR

FLOUR

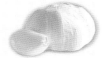

GARLIC

BLACK PEPPER

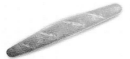

BAGUETTE

"CHEEZ" INGREDIENTS: SUNFLOWER SEEDS, YOGURT, CIDER VINEGAR, CORNSTARCH, PLANT-BASED MILK

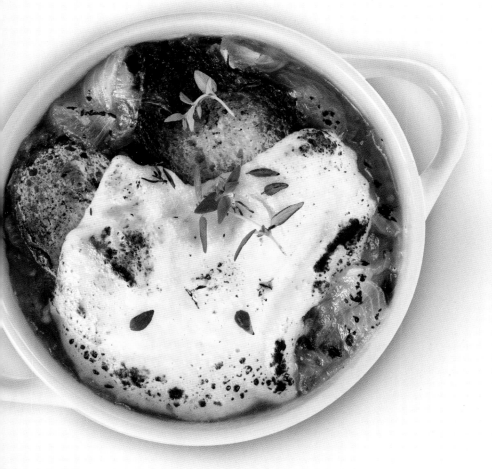

Storage: Store the soup in an airtight container in the fridge separate from the vegan mozzarella and baguette for 3 to 4 days, or in the freezer for up to 2 months. Store the vegan mozzarella in the fridge for up to 4 days.

Save the Scraps: Onion peels for Onion Peel Powder (page 336), Scrappy Broth (page 102), or Bouilliant Bouillon Powder (page 336).

Dilly Orzo Soup

Here's yet another delight to add to your "do not discard" list: pickle juice. Get ready to pucker up! This tangy and savory soup combines flavors of garlic, dill pickles, and turmeric for a gleaming bowl that will have you glowing from the inside out. Fiber filled and so delicious, this one will be on your weeknight rotation.

MAKES 4 servings ✦ **START TO FINISH:** 30 minutes

1 medium-size yellow onion, diced

1 large carrot, grated

1 to 2 tablespoons water or extra-virgin olive oil

1 teaspoon dried parsley

4 garlic cloves, minced

6 cups vegetable broth

1 cup pickle juice

1 (15-ounce) can navy beans, chickpeas, or white beans, drained and rinsed, or 1½ cups homemade

3 dill pickles, grated

¼ cup fresh dill, chopped

½ cup dried orzo, or 1 cup cooked rice

¼ cup tahini or Sunflower Cream Sauce (page 272)

1 teaspoon ground turmeric

¼ teaspoon freshly ground black pepper

½ teaspoon salt, or as needed

Small Sourdough Loaf (page 320), for serving

1. In a large pot over medium heat, combine the onion and carrot along with the water. Sauté until softened, about 3 minutes. Add the parsley and garlic, and stir for another 2 minutes, until fragrant.

2. Add the vegetable broth, pickle juice, navy beans, and grated pickles to the pot. Bring to a boil, then simmer, covered, for 15 minutes.

3. Add the dill and orzo to the pot and cook, uncovered, for 10 minutes, until the orzo is cooked through, stirring occasionally to prevent the pasta from sticking. If using cooked rice, add at this point and cook for 5 minutes, stirring occasionally to combine.

4. Stir in the tahini along with the turmeric, pepper, and salt as needed. Serve with homemade sourdough bread.

Storage: Store in an airtight container in the fridge for 3 to 4 days, or in the freezer for up to 2 months.

Save the Scraps: Onion peels for Onion Peel Powder (page 336), Scrappy Broth (page 102), or Bouilliant Bouillon Powder (page 336). Carrot tops for the Carrot Top Chimichurri (page 272).

YELLOW ONION

CARROT

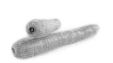

DRIED PARSLEY

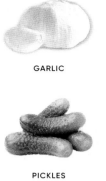

GARLIC

VEGETABLE BROTH

PICKLE JUICE

WHITE BEANS

PICKLES

DILL

ORZO

TAHINI

TURMERIC

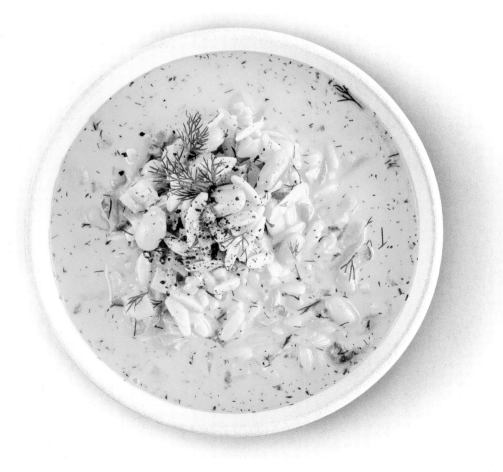

Scrappy Broth

Who knew that the key to delicious broth was hiding in your compost bin? Made, yes, from scraps—such as onion skins, carrot peels, and celery leaves—this is a full-bodied broth you can freeze and use for soups, stews, and pasta. Use it in any recipe in this book that calls for vegetable broth. To avoid sludgy or bitter broth, steer clear of members of the brassica family, such as broccoli, cauliflower, and cabbage, as well as mushy vegetables, such as cucumber or eggplant.

MAKES 8 to 12 cups ✦ **START TO FINISH:** 3 to 6 hours

1 gallon-size freezer bag vegetable scraps (onions, carrots, garlic, and potatoes work well)

1 teaspoon garlic powder

½ teaspoon ground turmeric

½ teaspoon freshly ground black pepper

½ teaspoon salt

1. In a large stockpot, combine the scraps. Add about 10 cups of water, enough so the vegetables are covered and begin to float. Add the garlic powder, turmeric, pepper, and salt.

2. Bring to a boil, then simmer. Cover and cook for 3 to 6 hours, or until the broth has a strong vegetable flavor and aroma. Alternatively, in a large slow cooker, you can cook this broth on HIGH for 4 to 5 hours. Once cooked, strain out the scraps, compost them, and keep the broth.

   Storage: Store in a sealed container in the fridge for 3 to 4 days, or in the freezer for up to 3 months.

VEGETABLE SCRAPS

GARLIC POWDER

TURMERIC

BLACK PEPPER

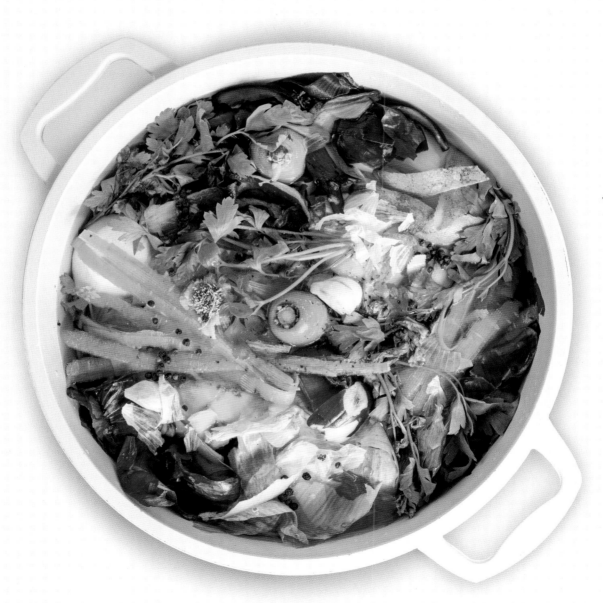

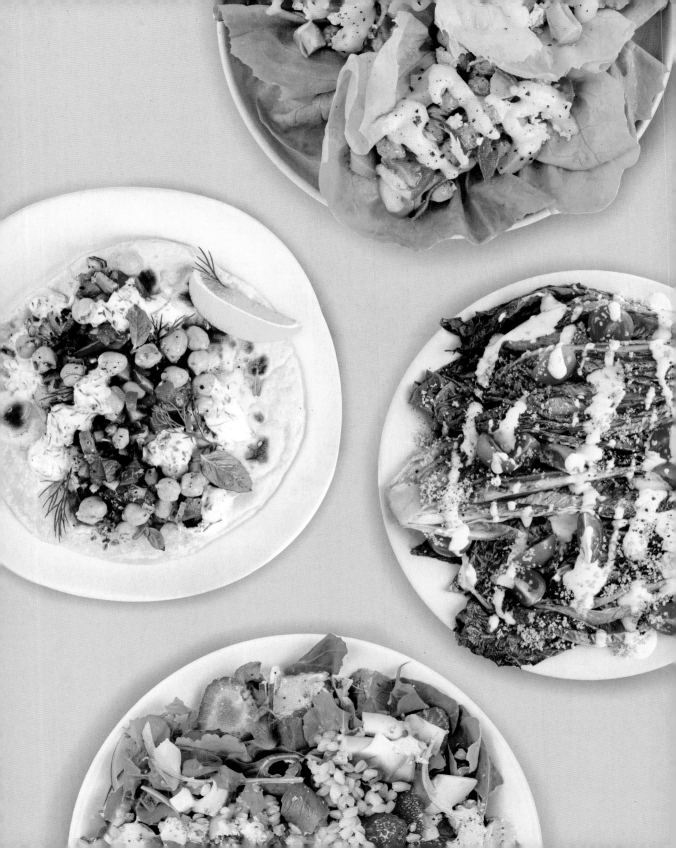

CHAPTER 4

Sustainable Sammies, Wraps & Salads

Low-waste luncheons (or anytime!)
that will make all your coworkers
green with envy.

Celery Leaf "Tabbouleh"

When I'm at the grocery store, I seek out the bundles of celery that have the most leaves intact. Not only are the leaves edible and delicious, but they have an amazingly fresh, almost lemony, flavor. They can be thrown into just about any soup or stew, but my favorite way to have celery leaves is in this tabbouleh-inspired salad.

MAKES 4 to 6 servings ✦ **START TO FINISH:** 25 minutes

1 cup water

¼ cup uncooked bulgur wheat

¼ cup uncooked quinoa

1 cup celery leaves, diced finely, or replace with an additional 1 cup chopped parsley

3 Roma tomatoes, diced

1 cup diced cucumber

2 bunches curly parsley, chopped

¼ cup fresh mint, chopped finely

2 green onions, chopped

Juice of 1 lemon, about ¼ cup

½ teaspoon sea salt

¼ teaspoon freshly ground black pepper

1. In a medium-size saucepan, bring the water to a boil. Stir in the bulgur wheat and quinoa. Return to a boil, then simmer, covered, for 10 minutes. Remove from the heat and allow to stand, covered, for 5 minutes. Fluff with a fork and allow to cool before serving.

2. In a bowl, combine the celery leaves, tomatoes, cucumber, parsley, mint, and green onions, along with the cooked bulgur and quinoa mixture. Season with the lemon juice, salt, and pepper. Serve with pita chips or another desired side dish.

Storage: Store in an airtight container in the fridge for 3 to 4 days.

Gluten-Free Substitution: In place of the bulgur wheat, use an additional ¼ cup of uncooked quinoa.

Save the Scraps: Lemon peels for Candied Citrus Peels (page 254) or Citrus Peel Powder (page 332).

BULGUR WHEAT

QUINOA

CELERY LEAVES

ROMA TOMATOES

CUCUMBER

PARSLEY

MINT

GREEN ONIONS

LEMON

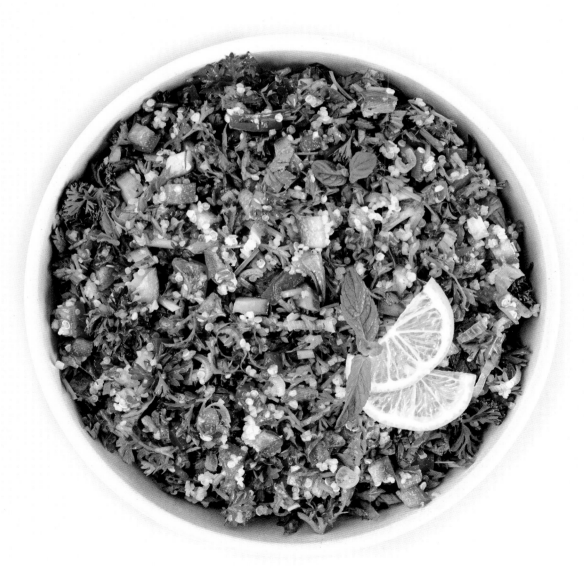

Sustainable Sammies, Wraps & Salads

Broccoli Stem Summer Rolls

Let's get ready to roll, baby. No need to compost those broccoli stems. They are the crisp and crunch in this amazing summer roll recipe—dipped in my delectable Mango Peanut Sauce.

MAKES 4 servings ✦ START TO FINISH: 30 minutes

12 edible rice paper sheets

2 broccoli stems, peeled and sliced into thin matchsticks

1 cup cooked vermicelli noodles (about 2 ounces dried)

1 carrot, peeled and sliced into thin matchsticks

1 red bell pepper, seeded and sliced into thin matchsticks

1 radish, sliced thinly

½ cup fresh mint, basil, or cilantro, chopped roughly

1 cup roughly chopped purple cabbage

FOR SERVING

½ cup Mango Peanut Sauce (page 274; optional)

2 tablespoons sesame seeds (optional)

1. You need to prepare summer rolls one at a time. Pour warm water into a shallow dish and add a sheet of rice paper for just 10 seconds, to soften slightly. Carefully transfer to a cutting board.

2. Add a small portion of the broccoli stems, cooked noodles, carrot, bell pepper, radish, herb of choice, and purple cabbage to the rice paper sheet. Gently fold over once, tuck in the edges, then continue to roll until the seam is sealed.

3. Place, seam side down, on a serving platter. Repeat until all the fillings are used up.

4. Serve with mango peanut sauce and/or a sprinkle of sesame seeds, as desired.

Storage: Store in a sealed container in the fridge for up to 3 days.

Save the Scraps: Radish tops for Scrappy Pesto (page 274). Onion peels for Onion Peel Powder (page 336), Scrappy Broth (page 102), or Bouilliant Bouillon Powder (page 336). Carrot tops for the Carrot Top Chimichurri (page 272).

RICE PAPER SHEETS

BROCCOLI STEMS

VERMICELLI NOODLES

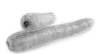

CARROT

RED BELL PEPPER

RADISH

MINT

PURPLE CABBAGE

MANGO PEANUT
SAUCE

SESAME SEEDS

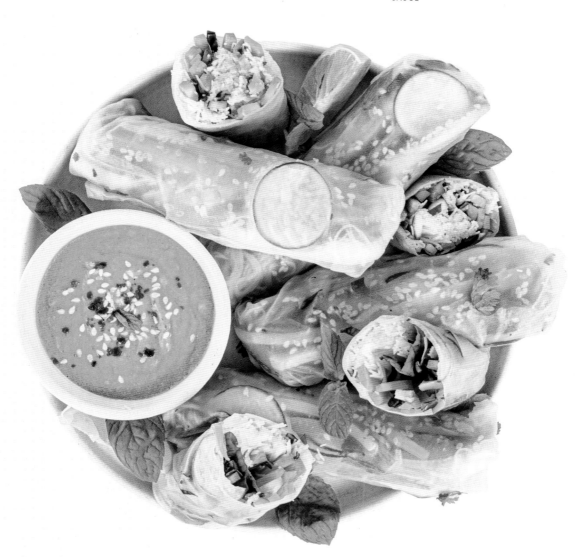

Life-Altering Mediterranean Wraps

Don't let anyone tell you that a wrap can't change your life. These unbelievable Mediterranean-inspired chickpea wraps are the perfect 15-minute lunch that you'll want to put on repeat. Experience a flavor explosion with Creamy Vegan Tzatziki, chickpeas, and a killer combination of fresh tomatoes, cucumber, red onion, and olives—all slathered on a flatbread.

MAKES 4 servings ✦ **START TO FINISH:** 15 minutes

SALAD

2 (15-ounce) cans chickpeas, drained and rinsed, or 3 cups homemade

4 Roma tomatoes, diced finely

1½ cups finely diced cucumber (about 1 large cucumber)

1 large red onion, diced finely

½ cup black olives, pitted and finely diced

Juice of 1 lemon

½ teaspoon sea salt

1 tablespoon oregano

½ cup Tofu Feta (page 288) or store-bought vegan feta

Freshly ground black pepper

FOR SERVING

½ cup Creamy Vegan Tzatziki (page 276) or store-bought vegan tzatziki

4 The Knead for Flatbread (page 68), It's a (Flax) Wrap wraps (page 70), or store-bought pitas

1. Make the salad: In a bowl, combine the chickpeas, tomatoes, cucumber, red onion, black olives, lemon juice, salt, oregano, vegan feta, and pepper to taste.

2. Add a heaping scoop of the tzatziki to each flatbread, followed by a cup of the chickpea salad mixture. Enjoy immediately.

Storage: Store the salad ingredients in an airtight container in the fridge for 2 to 3 days.

Gluten-Free Substitute: Use a store-bought gluten-free flatbread or It's a (Flax) Wrap wraps (page 70).

Save the Scraps: Lemon peels for Candied Citrus Peels (page 254) or Citrus Peel Powder (page 332). Aquafaba (chickpea water) for Mousse on the Loose (page 264) or Mini Aquafaba Pavlovas (page 266).

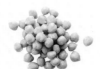

CHICKPEAS

ROMA TOMATOES

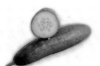

CUCUMBER

RED ONION

BLACK OLIVES

LEMON

OREGANO

VEGAN FETA

TZATZIKI

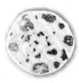

PITAS OR WRAPS

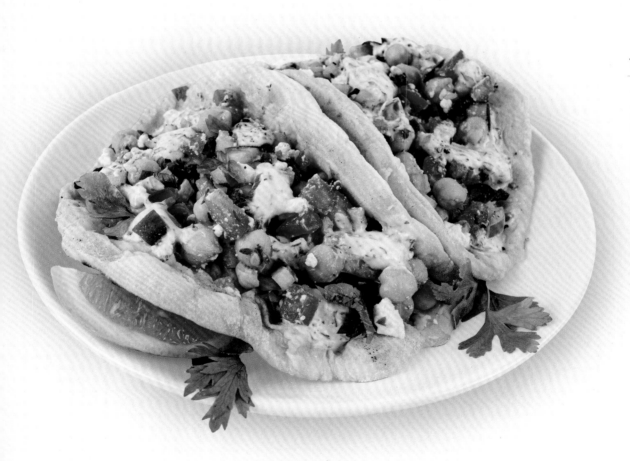

Sustainable Sammies, Wraps & Salads

Sproutichoke Wrap

Get ready to sprout into flavor town with this unusual (and delicious) wrap, featuring all the green vegetables you can find in your fridge, nestled in a bed of cooked quinoa. With greens, pickled artichokes, and my creamy Green Goddess Dressing, it's the perfect combination of crunchy, tangy, and healthy.

MAKES 2 wraps ✦ **START TO FINISH:** 15 minutes

¼ cup uncooked quinoa

1 cup spinach

1 cup finely chopped iceberg lettuce, or whatever lettuce you have on hand

½ cup Lentil Sprouts (page 338) or broccoli sprouts

¼ cucumber, chopped

½ cup frozen edamame, thawed

½ cup diced marinated artichokes

2 green onions, chopped

1 tablespoon crushed walnuts, peanuts, or pumpkin seeds

¼ cup Green Goddess Dressing (page 280) or vegan dressing of choice

2 It's a (Flax) Wrap wraps (page 70) or whole-grain wraps

1. Cook the quinoa according to the package directions and set aside to cool until room temperature.

2. In a bowl, combine everything, except the wraps, and toss until well combined.

3. Divide the salad mixture between each wrap. Fold the two side ends in, then wrap tightly.

Storage: Store the salad mixture separately from the wraps in the fridge for up to 3 days. When ready to eat, fold in a vegan wrap of choice.

QUINOA

SPINACH

ICEBERG LETTUCE

LENTIL SPROUTS

CUCUMBER

EDAMAME

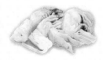

MARINATED ARTICHOKES

GREEN ONIONS

WALNUTS

GREEN GODDESS
DRESSING

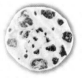

PITAS OR WRAPS

Sustainable Sammies, Wraps & Salads

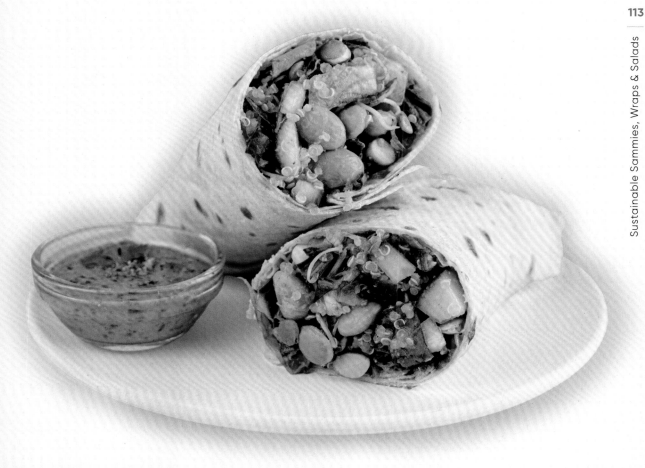

A-Better-Burger Wrap

Don't be surprised if you find yourself making excuses to eat this loaded cheeseburger wrap every day. After all—it's got Vegan Ground Beef and melty Sunflower Cream Sauce all wrapped in a tortilla. What's not to make excuses for?!

MAKES 4 servings ✦ **START TO FINISH:** 20 minutes

2 tablespoons water or extra-virgin olive oil

1 yellow onion, diced

2 garlic cloves, minced

2 cups Vegan Ground Beef (page 222) or your favorite vegan ground beef substitute

2 tablespoons ketchup

1 teaspoon prepared mustard

FOR ASSEMBLY

4 whole wheat tortillas or It's a (Flax) Wrap wraps (page 70)

1 Roma tomato, diced

¼ head iceberg lettuce, shredded

¼ cup Quick 'n' Easy Homemade Pickles (page 344) or store-bought pickles, diced

½ cup Sunflower Cream Sauce (page 272)

1. In a large skillet over medium heat, boil the water. Put in the onion and garlic, and sauté until softened, about 3 minutes. Add the cooked Vegan Ground Beef crumble along with the ketchup and mustard. Mix well and sauté for 3 to 5 minutes, or until the mixture is combined.

2. Assemble the wraps with the vegan ground beef mixture, tomato, lettuce, pickles, and Sunflower Cream Sauce. Grill, as desired, for a crispy wrap.

Storage: Store ingredients separately in an airtight container in the fridge for up to 5 days, or assembled without lettuce in the freezer for up to 1 month. Reheat in a microwave in 1-minute intervals, or grill in a skillet on the stove top.

Gluten-Free Substitution: This wrap is also excellent served on a bed of iceberg lettuce as a salad. Alternatively, use my It's a (Flax) Wrap wraps (page 70) or a store-bought gluten-free wrap.

Save the Scraps: Onion peels for Onion Peel Powder (page 336), Scrappy Broth (page 102), or Bouilliant Bouillon Powder (page 336).

YELLOW ONION

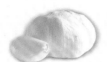

GARLIC

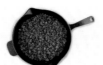

VEGAN HOMEMADE
GROUND BEEF

KETCHUP

MUSTARD

WHOLE WHEAT
TORTILLAS

ROMA TOMATOES

ICEBERG LETTUCE

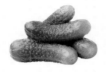

PICKLES

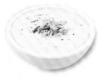

SUNFLOWER CHEESE
SAUCE

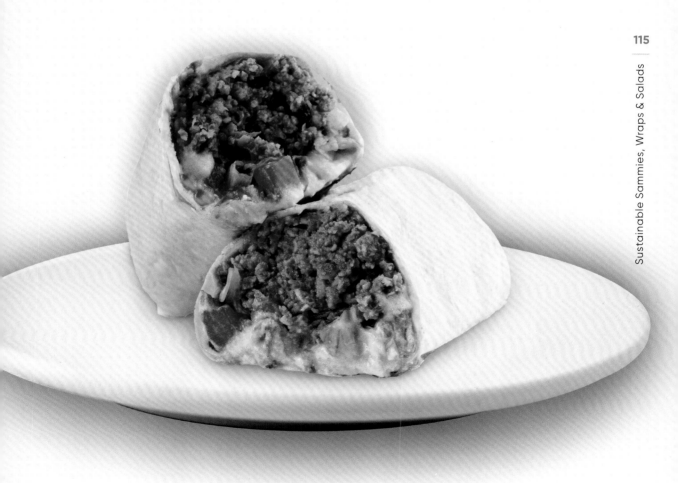

Stacked Veggie Sandwich

A sandwich so stacked that it may tip like the Leaning Tower of Pisa itself! This Wich is a symphony of flavors, using up just about every vegetable you have on hand, heaped between two delicious slices of sourdough and a tangy zero-waste pesto that will make your taste buds do the cha-cha. Go ahead, take a big bite, and let the good times roll—or better yet, let the good veggies STACK.

MAKES 4 servings ◆ **START TO FINISH:** 1 hour

MARINADE

½ cup vegetable broth

1 tablespoon red wine vinegar

2 teaspoons dried basil

1 teaspoon paprika

1 teaspoon garlic powder

1 teaspoon dried oregano

½ teaspoon salt

VEGGIES

1 small eggplant, sliced into ½-inch-thick rounds

2 red bell peppers, cut into wedges

1 medium-size zucchini, cut into ½-inch round slices

FOR SANDWICHES

½ cup Scrappy Pesto (page 274) or store-bought pesto

8 crusty slices of Small Sourdough Loaf (page 320), vegan baguette, or vegan gluten-free bread

½ cup Scratch Tomato Sauce (page 164) or store-bought marinara

½ cup Spicy Pickled Red Onions (page 342)

1 cup arugula

1. Preheat the oven to 400°F, and line two baking sheets with reusable baking mats or parchment paper.

2. Make the marinade: In a large bowl, combine the vegetable broth, red wine vinegar, basil, paprika, garlic powder, oregano, and salt.

3. Marinate the veggies: Add the eggplant, bell pepper, and zucchini slices to the bowl of marinade and toss to coat. Allow to soak for 20 minutes if you have time.

4. Transfer the vegetable slices to the prepared baking sheet, brush with any remaining marinade from the bowl, and roast for 30 minutes, until softened.

5. Once the vegetables are roasted, assemble the sandwiches. Spread the pesto on four slices of the bread, and spread the other four slices with the marinara. Add the grilled vegetables, pickled onions, and arugula to the pesto-coated slices, top with the marinara-coated slices, and enjoy.

Storage: Store the roasted vegetables in an airtight container in the fridge for 2 to 3 days. Assemble when ready to eat.

Sustainable Sammies, Wraps & Salads

VEGETABLE BROTH

RED WINE VINEGAR

DRIED BASIL

PAPRIKA

GARLIC POWDER

DRIED OREGANO

EGGPLANT

RED BELL PEPPER

ZUCCHINI

SCRAPPY PESTO

TOMATO SAUCE

PICKLED ONIONS

ARUGULA

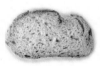

SOURDOUGH BREAD

Sustainable Sammies, Wraps & Salads

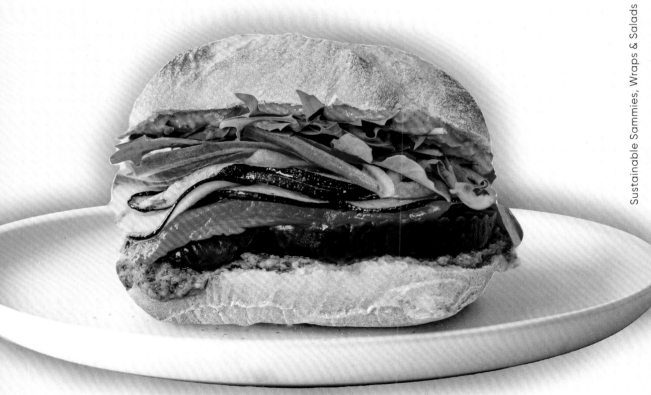

White Bean "Tuna" Sandwich

This is a sandwich that's good not only for you but also for the oceans. This beauty packs a protein punch, with bean fiber and flavor that will make you feel that you can take on the world . . . or at least the day ahead. So take a bite, close your eyes, and imagine yourself on a beach, sipping a cold one and enjoying life's simple pleasures. Or just relish this "tuna" treat at your desk. Either way, you can't go wrong.

MAKES 4 to 6 servings ✦ **START TO FINISH:** 15 minutes

1 (15-ounce) can white beans or chickpeas, drained and rinsed, or 2 cups homemade

½ small red onion, diced

1 pickle, diced

1 tablespoon vegan Dijon mustard

1 tablespoon unsweetened Cultured Vegan Yogurt (page 48) or store-bought soy or coconut yogurt

1 tablespoon tahini

1 teaspoon fresh dill

2 large nori sheets, crumbled

½ cup marinated artichokes

1 teaspoon pickle juice or artichoke marinade

½ teaspoon salt

FOR SERVING

8 slices Small Sourdough Loaf (page 320), vegan gluten-free bread, or 8 lettuce cups

¼ cup Scrappy Pesto (page 274)

¼ cup vegan Dijon mustard

1. In a food processor or blender, combine all the "tuna" ingredients. Pulse until incorporated but still chunky.

2. Serve on a sandwich with pesto and Dijon mustard, as desired.

Storage: Store the white bean "tuna" in an airtight container in the fridge for 3 to 4 days.

Save the Scraps: Aquafaba (chickpea water) for Mousse on the Loose (page 264) or Mini Aquafaba Pavlovas (page 266). Onion for Strawberry Farro Salad (page 136). Onion peels for Onion Peel Powder (page 336), Scrappy Broth (page 102), or Bouilliant Bouillon Powder (page 336).

WHITE BEANS

RED ONION

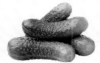

PICKLES

DIJON MUSTARD

YOGURT

TAHINI

DILL

NORI SHEETS

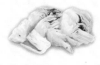

MARINATED ARTICHOKES

PICKLE JUICE

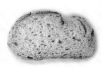

SOURDOUGH BREAD

SCRAPPY PESTO

119

Sustainable Sammies, Wraps & Salads

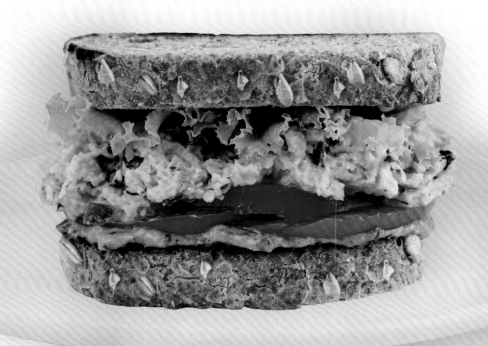

Buffalo Chickpea Lettuce Cups

These spicy and crisp Buffalo cups are the perfect way to use up leftover lettuce and add some plant-based protein to your diet. It's a delicious and satisfying meal that comes together in less than 25 minutes, with minimal cleanup and maximum flavor.

MAKES 4 servings ✦ **START TO FINISH:** 25 minutes

1 (15-ounce) can chickpeas, drained and rinsed, or 1½ cups homemade

¼ cup hot sauce of choice

1½ tablespoons unsweetened Cultured Vegan Yogurt (page 48) or store-bought soy or coconut yogurt

1 teaspoon pure maple syrup

8 lettuce leaves (butter, iceberg, or romaine), for serving

¼ cup cherry tomatoes, quartered

1 avocado, peeled, pitted, and diced

¼ cup Tofu Feta (page 288) or store-bought vegan feta

½ red onion, sliced thinly

1 cup Creamy Hummus Caesar (page 278) or vegan dressing of your choice

1. Preheat the oven to 400°F, and line a baking sheet with a reusable baking mat or parchment paper. Put the chickpeas on the sheet and roast for 20 minutes, or until slightly crispy.

2. Meanwhile, make the Buffalo sauce: In a medium-size bowl, stir the hot sauce with the vegan yogurt and maple syrup until smooth. Once the chickpeas are out of the oven, toss them with the sauce.

3. Serve the chickpeas in lettuce cups, along with the cherry tomatoes, avocado, vegan feta, and red onion, drizzled with the hummus Caesar or your dressing of choice.

Storage: Store the Buffalo chickpeas in an airtight container in the fridge for 2 to 3 days.

Save the Scraps: Aquafaba (chickpea water) for Mousse on the Loose (page 264) or Mini Aquafaba Pavlovas (page 266). Onion peels for Onion Peel Powder (page 336), Scrappy Broth (page 102), or Bouilliant Bouillon Powder (page 336).

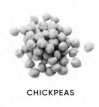

CHICKPEAS

HOT SAUCE

YOGURT

MAPLE SYRUP

BUTTER LETTUCE

CHERRY TOMATOES

AVOCADO

TOFU FETA

RED ONION

CREAMY HUMMUS
CAESAR

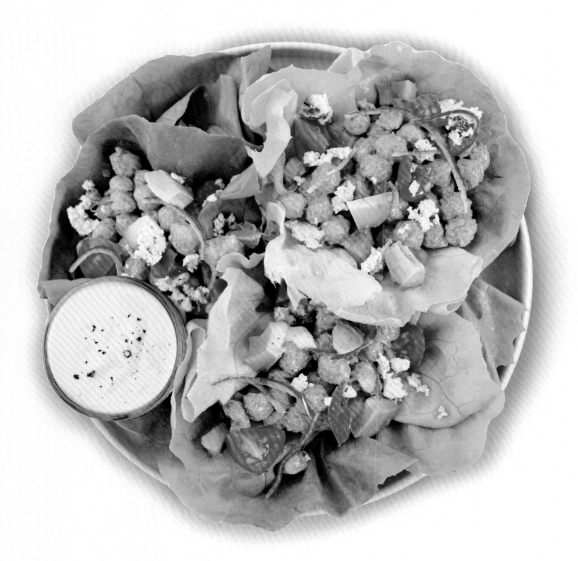

Sustainable Sammies, Wraps & Salads

Citrus Cabbage Slaw

This slaw is crunchy, crisp, and refreshing—and the perfect pairing to any plant-filled meal (try it on my Veggie Masala Burgers, page 232). Better yet, it uses up an entire head of cabbage, along with carrot, green onions, and a full broccoli stem. Get ready for a slaw-some adventure!

MAKES 4 servings ✦ **START TO FINISH:** 10 minutes

1 small red cabbage, sliced thinly (about 8 cups)

1 red onion, sliced thinly

1 large carrot, grated

6 green onions, sliced thinly

1 broccoli stem, grated

CITRUS DRESSING

3 tablespoons Apple Scrap Vinegar (page 350) or store-bought apple cider vinegar

1½ tablespoons pure maple syrup

1 tablespoon soy sauce

1 teaspoon grated fresh ginger

1 garlic clove, minced

Juice of 1 orange

1 teaspoon orange zest

1 teaspoon sesame oil (optional but recommended)

1 teaspoon salt

1. In a bowl, combine the cabbage, red onion, carrot, green onions, and grated broccoli stem.

2. Make the dressing: In a jar or other container, whisk together all the dressing ingredients until combined. Pour the dressing over the salad, toss until coated, and enjoy.

Storage: Store, fully prepared, in the fridge for up to 5 days.

Save the Scraps: Carrot tops for the Carrot Top Chimichurri (page 272). Onion peels for Onion Peel Powder (page 336), Scrappy Broth (page 102), or Bouilliant Bouillon Powder (page 336). Orange peel for Citrus Peel Powder (page 332) or Candied Citrus Peels (page 254).

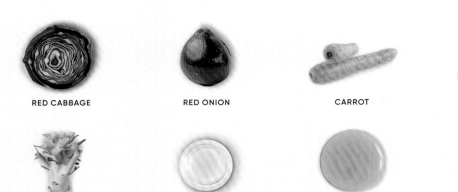

RED CABBAGE   RED ONION   CARROT   GREEN ONIONS

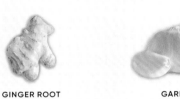

BROCCOLI STEMS   APPLE CIDER VINEGAR   MAPLE SYRUP   SOY SAUCE

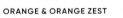

GINGER ROOT   GARLIC   ORANGE & ORANGE ZEST   SESAME OIL

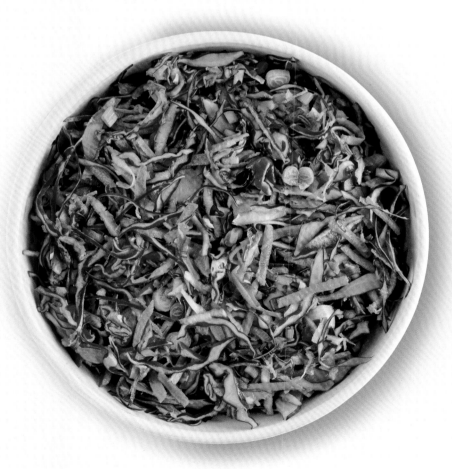

Grilled Romaine Salad

What do you do when you have a package of romaine wasting away in the back of the fridge? Transform it into this delicious salad. With a little char, and lots of flavor, this simple salad will make you forget everything you ever knew about lettuce. Well . . . almost everything!

MAKES 4 servings ✦ **START TO FINISH:** 15 minutes

2 heads romaine lettuce

1 tablespoon vegan Dijon mustard

2 tablespoons balsamic vinegar

½ teaspoon salt

½ teaspoon garlic powder

¾ cup Creamy Hummus Caesar (page 278)

FOR SERVING

¼ cup Vegan Nutty "Parm" (page 290) or store-bought vegan bread crumbs

1 cup cherry tomatoes, halved

Balsamic Glaze (page 290) or balsamic reduction (optional)

1. Slice the romaine heads in half lengthwise. Use a clean cloth to dry the romaine, and clean off any debris or dirt.

2. In a bowl, combine the Dijon mustard, balsamic vinegar, salt, and garlic powder. Using a brush, liberally coat the romaine with the marinade.

3. Turn your gas grill to high, or heat a cast-iron skillet over high heat. Grill the romaine lettuce on the grill or in the skillet until lightly charred on all sides, turning every minute or two until done.

4. Plate and drizzle the hummus Caesar over the lettuce, followed by a hefty helping of vegan "Parm," the halved cherry tomatoes, and balsamic glaze. Serve immediately.

ROMAINE LETTUCE

DIJON MUSTARD

BALSAMIC VINEGAR

GARLIC POWDER

VEGAN CAESAR DRESSING

VEGAN PARM

CHERRY TOMATOES

BALSAMIC GLAZE

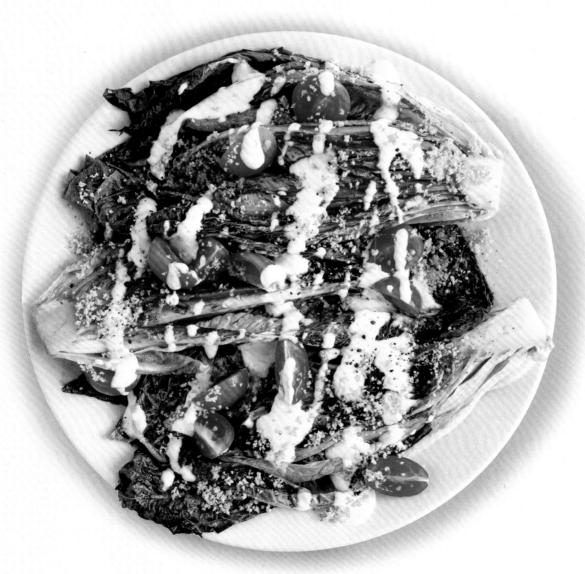

That's-a-Panzanella

Got bread that's seen better days? Good. Let's transform it into a salad delicacy. Originating in Tuscany, traditional panzanella utilizes stale bread in a simple salad with olive oil, vinegar, and salt. This panzanella salad has a creamy twist, with a red wine vinegar and tahini dressing that makes even stale bread taste gourmet.

MAKES 4 to 6 servings ✦ START TO FINISH: 30 minutes

3 cups hard, stale vegan sourdough bread or baguette, gluten-free if needed, torn into 1-inch cubes

3 garlic cloves, minced

3 cups cherry tomatoes

1 teaspoon salt

¼ cup water

1 small red onion, sliced

2 large handfuls of fresh basil, torn

½ cup Tofu Feta (page 288) or store-bought vegan feta (optional)

DRESSING

2 tablespoons red wine vinegar

1 tablespoon tahini

1 tablespoon vegan Dijon mustard

½ teaspoon salt

½ cup reserved tomato juices

1. Preheat the oven to 350°F, and line a baking sheet with a reusable baking mat or parchment paper.

2. Rub a garlic clove across the chunks of stale bread and assemble in a single layer on the prepared baking sheet. Bake on the center rack until crunchy, about 20 minutes, checking intermittently to avoid burning.

3. In a medium-size saucepan over medium heat, combine the cherry tomatoes, salt, garlic, and water. Allow to sweat over low to medium heat for 15 minutes, stirring halfway through. Using a spatula, help the tomatoes burst and release their juices. Remove the burst tomatoes from the saucepan and place in a salad bowl, reserving ½ cup of the remaining juices in the saucepan.

4. Make the dressing: Add the red wine vinegar, tahini, Dijon mustard, and salt to the tomato juices in the pan, and stir until a dressing is formed, adding water a tablespoon at a time as needed, to thin.

5. Assemble the salad: Add the bread, red onion, basil, and vegan feta (if using) to the bowl of tomatoes and toss. Pour the dressing on the salad 10 minutes before serving and enjoy.

Storage: Store the salad base and dressing separately in the fridge for up to 2 days.

Save the Scraps: Onion peels for Onion Peel Powder (page 336), Scrappy Broth (page 102), or Bouilliant Bouillon Powder (page 336).

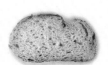

SOURDOUGH BREAD

CHERRY TOMATOES

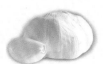

GARLIC

RED ONION

BASIL

TOFU FETA

RED WINE VINEGAR

TAHINI

DIJON MUSTARD

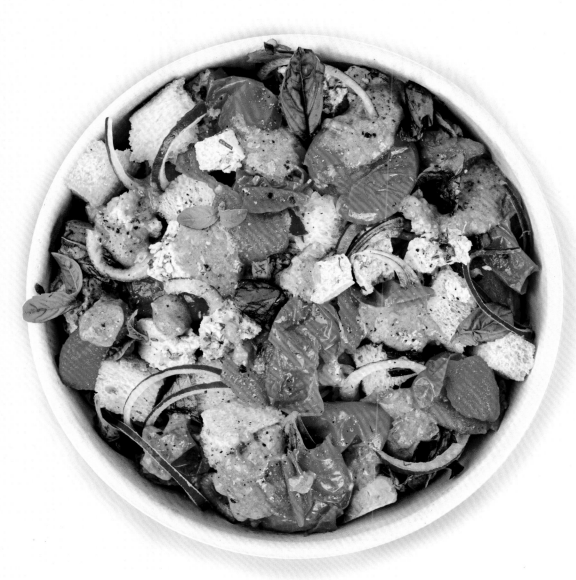

The Saucy Kale

This ain't your average salad. It's saucy, sassy, and a wee bit spicy. Plus, it's ready in just 10 minutes: you can whip it up with any base of greens and beans you have on hand. With the dressing on the side, it also makes the perfect meal-prep lunch!

MAKES 4 to 6 servings ✦ **START TO FINISH:** 10 minutes

5 cups curly kale, chopped finely (about 1 bunch), or finely chopped greens of choice

Juice of 1 lemon

½ cup chopped Sun-Dried Tomatoes (page 328)

1 red onion, chopped finely

1 avocado, peeled, pitted, and diced

1 (15-ounce) can white beans, chickpeas, or navy beans, drained and rinsed, or homemade

3 tablespoons hemp hearts

½ cup Everything Tahini Dressing, spicy option (page 278)

3 tablespoons crushed peanuts (optional)

1. In a bowl, combine the kale and lemon juice and massage until tender, about 3 minutes. Add the Sun-Dried Tomatoes, red onion, avocado, white beans, and hemp hearts.

2. Pour the dressing over the salad, toss, and top with the crushed peanuts (if using), for crunch.

Storage: Store the salad base and dressing separately in the fridge for up to 3 days.

Save the Scraps: Lemon peels for Candied Citrus Peels (page 254) or Citrus Peel Powder (page 332). Onion peels for Onion Peel Powder (page 336), Scrappy Broth (page 102), or Bouilliant Bouillon Powder (page 336).

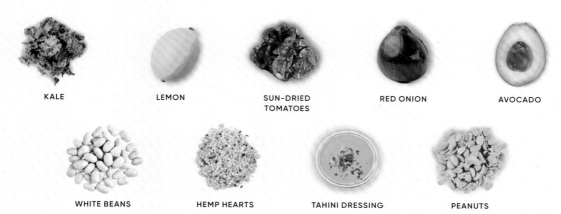

KALE   LEMON   SUN-DRIED TOMATOES   RED ONION   AVOCADO

WHITE BEANS   HEMP HEARTS   TAHINI DRESSING   PEANUTS

Sustainable Sammies, Wraps & Salads

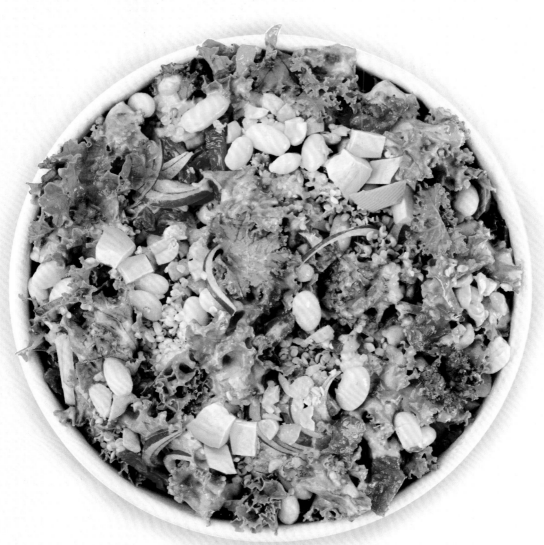

Brussels Sprouts Caesar Salad

Did you know brussels sprouts are just mini cabbages?! Love 'em or hate 'em, this vegan Caesar salad will make you forget everything you thought you knew about the diminutive cousin. Many people, unfortunately, waste half the sprout when they slice off the end, but for this scrumptious salad, you throw the entire thing in the food processor and whirl away. Serve warmed with crispy garlic croutons and a to-die-for homemade vegan Caesar dressing.

MAKES 4 servings ✦ **START TO FINISH:** 30 minutes

1 garlic clove

2 cups torn (1-inch cubes) hard or fresh Small Sourdough Loaf (page 320), vegan baguette, or vegan gluten-free bread

¼ cup sunflower seeds

2 pounds brussels sprouts (about 4 cups)

1 cup chopped dinosaur (a.k.a. lacinato) kale, curly kale, or spinach

½ teaspoon salt

2 tablespoons water or extra-virgin olive oil

¾ cup Creamy Hummus Caesar (page 278) or store-bought vegan Caesar dressing

1. Preheat the oven to 350°F, and line a baking sheet with a reusable baking mat or parchment paper. Rub a garlic clove across the bread pieces and assemble in a single layer on the prepared baking sheet along with the sunflower seeds. Bake on the center rack until crunchy, about 20 minutes.

2. Put the brussels sprouts, stems intact, in a food processor or blender, and pulse until shredded.

3. In a large skillet, combine the shredded brussels sprouts, kale, salt, and water, and fry over low to medium heat for 10 to 15 minutes, or until the mixture is crisp and tender.

4. Transfer the fried brussels sprouts mixture to a large bowl and toss with the dressing. Pour the baked croutons and sunflower seeds on top. Serve immediately.

Storage: Allow to cool, then store the salad base in the fridge, separate from the dressing, for up to 3 days.

GARLIC

**SOURDOUGH
BREAD**

**SUNFLOWER
SEEDS**

**BRUSSELS
SPROUTS**

KALE

**CREAMY
HUMMUS CAESAR**

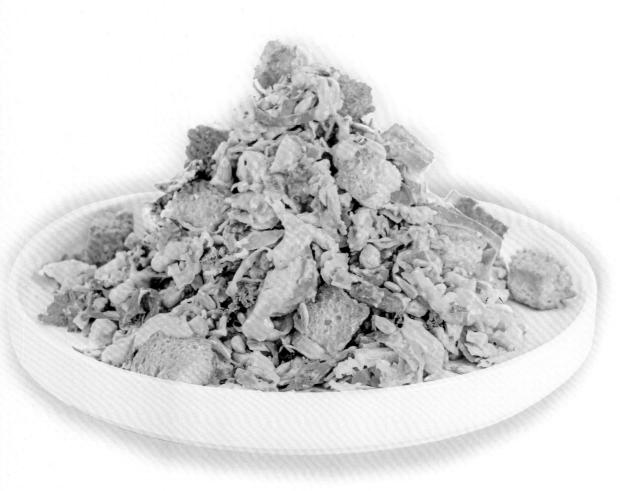

Sustainable Sammies, Wraps & Salads

Street Corn Pasta Salad

This salad is the love child of street corn and macaroni. Inspired by Mexican street corn, traditionally known as *elote*, this incredible pasta salad is a delicious medley of spicy, creamy, and cheesy flavors that will have you doing the salsa on your plate. Perfect for a plant-based barbecue or a meal-prep workweek lunch.

MAKES 6 servings ✦ **START TO FINISH:** 30 minutes

1 (16-ounce) package whole wheat or brown rice macaroni

1 tablespoon water or extra-virgin olive oil

3 cups frozen corn, thawed

1 teaspoon garlic powder

1 teaspoon chili powder

½ teaspoon Tajín (optional)

1 red onion, chopped

2 jalapeño peppers, seeded and diced

2 Roma tomatoes, diced

1 cup chopped fresh cilantro

½ cup crumbled Tofu Feta (page 288) or store-bought vegan feta (optional)

1¼ cups Sunflower Cream Sauce (page 272; nearly double the recipe, or double it if you like things saucy) or store-bought vegan mayonnaise

1. Cook the macaroni according to the package directions. Drain the pasta and let it cool.

2. In a large skillet, combine the water with the corn, garlic powder, chili powder, and Tajín (if using). Roast over medium to high heat for 5 minutes, or until the corn is slightly charred.

3. Transfer the cooked macaroni to a bowl, along with the charred corn, red onion, jalapeño, tomatoes, cilantro, and tofu feta. Pour the Sunflower Cream Sauce over all and mix. Store in the fridge for up to 4 days or enjoy immediately.

Storage: Store, fully prepared, in the fridge for up to 4 days.

Save the Scraps: Onion peels for Onion Peel Powder (page 336), Scrappy Broth (page 102), or Bouilliant Bouillon Powder (page 336).

MACARONI

CORN KERNELS

GARLIC POWDER

CHILI POWDER

RED ONION

JALAPEÑO

ROMA TOMATOES

CILANTRO

TOFU FETA

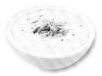

SUNFLOWER CREAM SAUCE

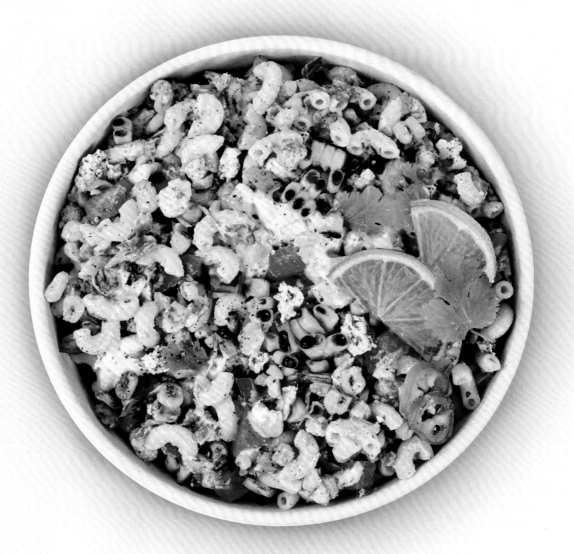

Sustainable Sammies, Wraps & Salads

Pantry Bean Salad

Eating plant-based, healthy, and low-waste food doesn't have to be expensive, time-consuming, or complicated, and this simple salad is living proof. It takes just 10 minutes to throw everything in a bowl and dig in. Just about any canned bean will do, but my favorite is cannellini white beans!

MAKES 1 to 2 servings ✦ **START TO FINISH:** 10 minutes

1 (15-ounce) can cannellini white beans, chickpeas, black beans, kidney beans, or navy beans, drained and rinsed, or 1½ cups homemade

½ cup chopped marinated artichokes

¼ cup chopped Sun-Dried Tomatoes (page 328)

1 Perfect Preserved Lemon (page 326), diced (optional)

¼ cup roasted red pepper from a jar, diced

½ red onion, sliced thinly (optional)

Handful of fresh parsley, cilantro, dill, or other fresh herb, chopped

½ cup Luscious Lemon Dressing (page 282) or store-bought vegan vinaigrette

1. In a bowl, combine all the salad ingredients, and pour the dressing over the top. It's that simple!

Storage: Store, fully prepared, in the fridge for up to 4 days.

Save the Scraps: Lemon peels for Candied Citrus Peels (page 254) or Citrus Peel Powder (page 332). Onion peels for Onion Peel Powder (page 336), Scrappy Broth (page 102), or Bouilliant Bouillon Powder (page 336).

WHITE BEANS

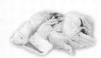

MARINATED ARTICHOKES

SUN-DRIED TOMATOES

PERFECT PRESERVED LEMONS

ROASTED RED PEPPERS

RED ONION

PARSLEY

LUSCIOUS LEMON DRESSING

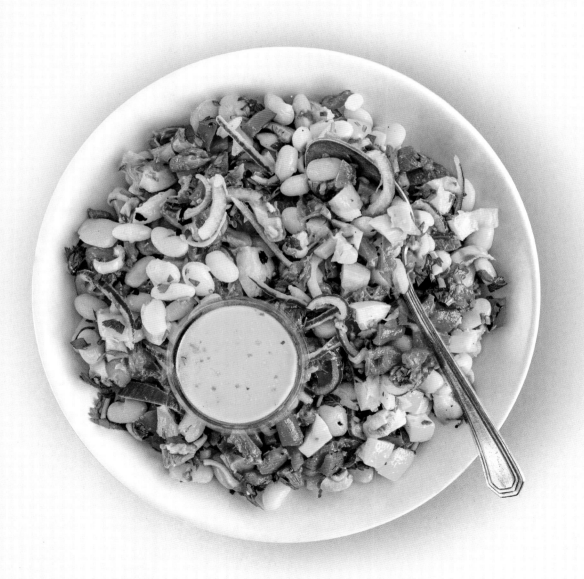

Sustainable Sammies, Wraps & Salads

Strawberry Farro Salad

Did you know strawberry tops are edible? Whether you're throwing them into a smoothie or making a salad, you can leave the tops intact—or use them to make Strawberry Top Vinegar (page 348) and Strawberry Top Vinaigrette. Either way, this salad is forever a nourishing summer delight, with fresh strawberries, nutty farro, and crisp arugula, finished off with my poppy seed–studded Strawberry Top Vinaigrette.

MAKES 4 servings ✦ **START TO FINISH:** 15 minutes

SALAD

1 cup uncooked farro or quinoa

4 cups arugula

2 cups fresh strawberries, hulled and sliced in half

¼ red onion, sliced thinly

1 avocado, peeled, pitted, and chopped

¼ cup crushed walnuts or hemp hearts

DRESSING

¼ cup Strawberry Top Vinaigrette (page 280) or store-bought vegan poppy seed dressing

1. Make the salad: Cook the farro or quinoa according to the package directions.

2. Assemble the salad with the leafy greens on the bottom, followed by the farro or quinoa, strawberries, red onion, avocado, and crushed walnuts.

3. Pour the dressing over the top and serve immediately.

Storage: Store the salad base and dressing separately in the fridge for up to 3 days.

Save the Scraps: Strawberry tops for Strawberry Top Vinaigrette (page 280). Onion peels for Onion Peel Powder (page 336), Scrappy Broth (page 102), or Bouilliant Bouillon Powder (page 336).

FARRO

ARUGULA

STRAWBERRIES

RED ONION

AVOCADO

WALNUTS

**STRAWBERRY TOP
VINAIGRETTE**

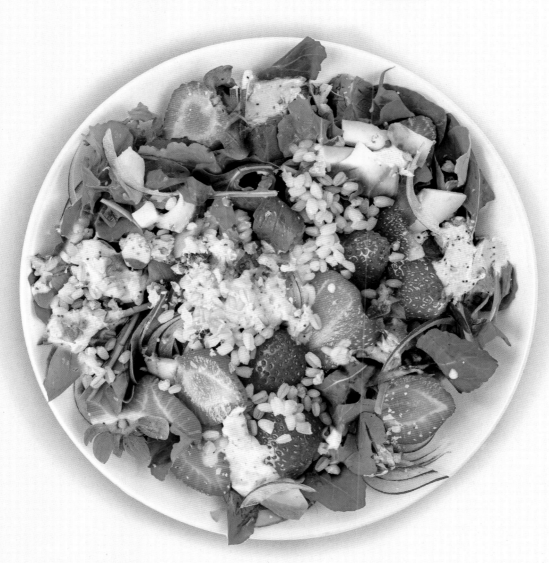

Sustainable Sammies, Wraps & Salads

Beaming Lentil Lemon Salad

Why do I say this salad beams? Because it is like sunshine in a bowl. Hearty lentils, juicy cherry tomatoes, crunchy cucumber, and creamy vegan feta come together with a zesty preserved lemon dressing for a refreshing protein- and fiber-rich meal. This is something you can prep on Monday and enjoy all week, as it keeps beautifully in the fridge.

MAKES 4 servings ✦ **START TO FINISH:** 15 minutes

1 cup halved cherry tomatoes

1 red bell pepper, seeded and diced

1 cup pitted and diced kalamata olives

1 medium-size red onion, diced

½ cup chopped fresh parsley

½ cup crumbled Tofu Feta (page 288) or store-bought vegan feta (optional)

8 ounces dried orzo, cooked and cooled (omit if gluten-free)

1 (15-ounce) can brown lentils, drained and rinsed, or 1½ cups homemade

¼ cup Luscious Lemon Dressing, page (282) or store-bought vegan vinaigrette

1. In a bowl, combine all the salad ingredients in a bowl, drizzled with the dressing. Toss and serve.

Storage: Store, fully prepared, in the fridge for up to 4 days.

Save the Scraps: Onion peels for Onion Peel Powder (page 336), Scrappy Broth (page 102), or Bouilliant Bouillon Powder (page 336).

CHERRY TOMATOES

RED BELL PEPPER

OLIVES

RED ONION

PARSLEY

TOFU FETA

ORZO

BROWN LENTILS

LUSCIOUS LEMON DRESSING

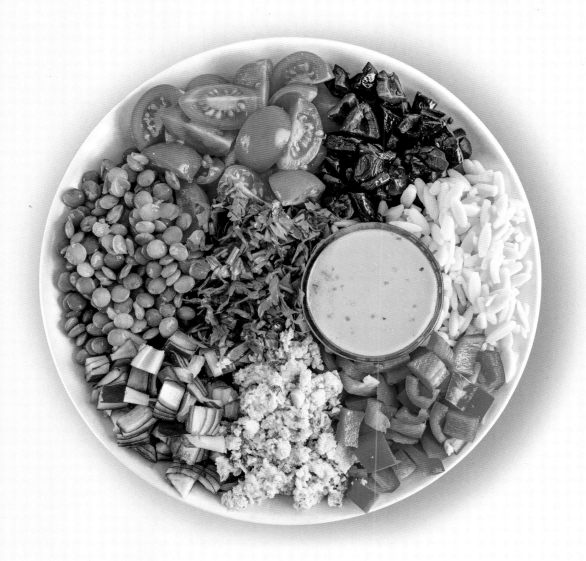

139

Sustainable Sammies, Wraps & Salads

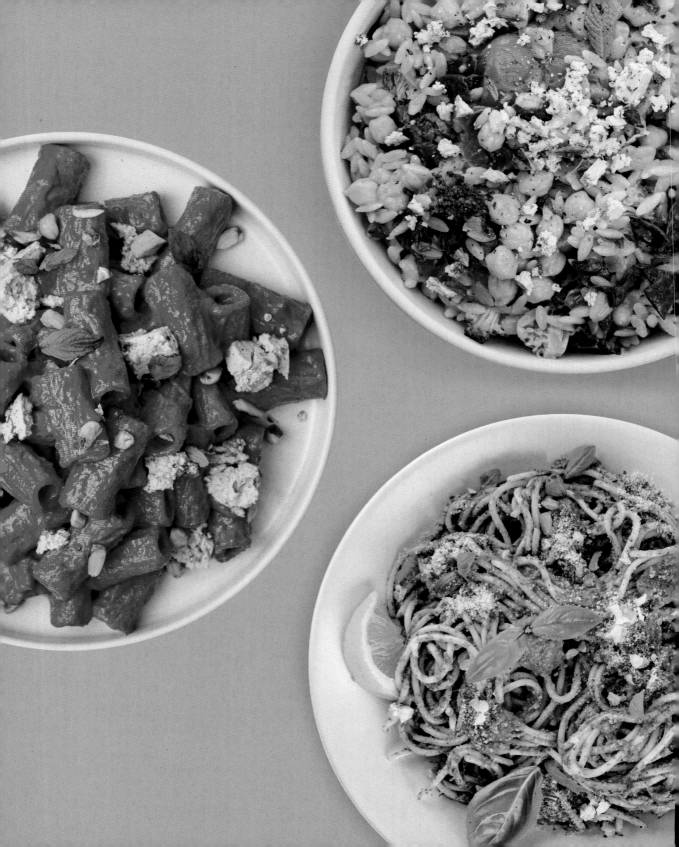

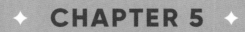

CHAPTER 5

No-Waste Noodles

Grab your colander and prepare to cook up some pasta magic, *Scrappy* style.

Tuscan Sweet Potato Gnocchi

If you have two sweet potatoes and some flour in your pantry, you can whip up a bowl of this deliciously creamy gnocchi. Don't let the lengthy instruction list make you run for the Tuscan hills. Once you get the hang of making gnocchi, you'll want to put this simple yet gourmet-tasting dish on repeat. Oh, yeah—and don't toss those sweet potato skins; they make an amazing snack, Crispy Crunches (page 64).

MAKES 2 servings ✦ **START TO FINISH:** 60 minutes

2 medium-size sweet potatoes

½ teaspoon salt

1¾ cups + 2 tablespoons spelt flour, or all-purpose or gluten-free flour

2 cups chopped kale

¾ cup Sunflower Cream Sauce (page 272)

½ cup chopped Sun-Dried Tomatoes (page 328)

1. Preheat the oven to 400°F, and line a baking sheet with a reusable baking mat or parchment paper.

2. Stab the sweet potatoes all over with a fork, then place on the prepared baking sheet and bake until tender, about 50 minutes. Once the sweet potatoes are crispy on the outside and soft on the inside, set aside to cool. Alternatively, microwave the sweet potatoes for 5 minutes each until soft.

3. When the potatoes are safe to handle, peel and transfer their insides to a bowl. (Reserve the skins for Crispy Crunches, page 64.) Add the salt, then mash until completely smooth.

4. Meanwhile, pour 1¾ cups of the flour onto a clean work surface and make a well in the center. Pour the sweet potato mash into the center.

5. Massage the mash into the flour until it is fully combined. The dough should be dry, not sticky; adjust the quantity of flour accordingly.

6. Once combined, slice the dough into six equal-size pieces. Roll out each piece until it forms a ½-inch-thick rod. Then slice the gnocchi into ½-inch lengths. Using the back of a fork, press grooves into the gnocchi. Once the gnocchi are formed, sprinkle them with the remaining flour to prevent them from sticking.

7. Meanwhile, bring a pot of salted water to a boil. Drop in the gnocchi and cook for about 3 minutes, until they rise to the top. Drain, reserving 1 cup of the pasta water.

8. Heat a large nonstick skillet over medium heat. Add the kale and gnocchi, plus 1 to 2 tablespoons of the reserved pasta water. Sauté until the kale has softened and the gnocchi have a slight golden color. Pour in the Sunflower Cream Sauce, along with ¾ cup of the reserved pasta water and the Sun-Dried Tomatoes, and toss until the sauce is warm and the gnocchi are covered. Taste and adjust the salt, as desired.

SWEET POTATOES

SPELT FLOUR

KALE

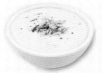

SUNFLOWER CREAM SAUCE

SUN-DRIED TOMATOES

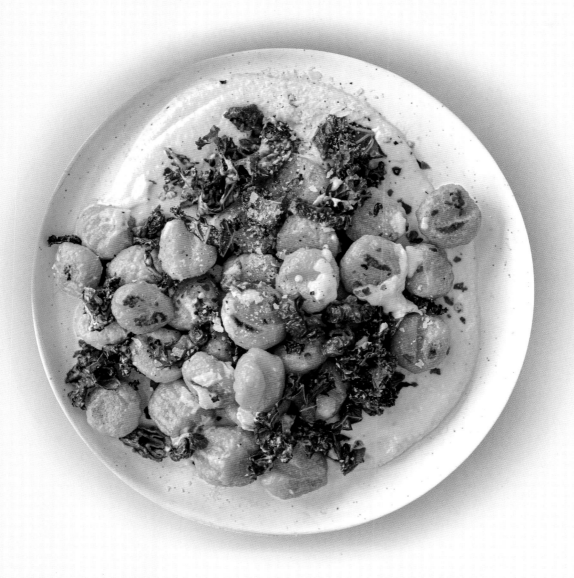

Storage: Store, fully prepared, in the fridge for up to 3 days.

Save the Scraps: Sweet potato peels for Crispy Crunches (page 64).

Hot-Pink Pasta

Despite its vibrant pink hue, this pasta recipe requires zero food coloring. Instead, it uses the magic of beets to create a rich, colorful, and delicious pasta dish that's ready in under 25 minutes. If you're a bit timid because of the earthiness of beets, this sauce is the perfect entry point, creating a balance of sweet, salty, garlicky, and tangy with the slightest touch of beet flavor. And don't throw out those beet leaves! Reserve them for one of my favorite snacks, We-Got-the-Beet Chips (page 62).

MAKES 4 servings ✦ **START TO FINISH:** 25 minutes

2 small beets, roasted, peeled, and chopped, or 2½ tablespoons Beet Powder (page 334)

1 pound dried rigatoni pasta or gluten-free pasta of choice

¾ cup sunflower seeds or cashews, soaked in water overnight or boiled for 10 minutes

¼ cup canned full-fat coconut milk or water, or soy milk if desired

2 garlic cloves, peeled

½ teaspoon sea salt

½ cup vegetable broth or water

Juice of 1 lemon

½ cup crumbled Tofu Feta (page 288) or store-bought vegan feta (optional)

FOR SERVING

⅓ cup pistachios, crushed

Fresh mint or basil

1. You can buy canned beets that are roasted and peeled. If roasting from scratch, preheat the oven to 400°F and wrap the beet in foil. Roast for 1½ hours, or until the beets are soft and tender. Remove from the oven, allow to cool, then peel off the skin and slice the beets into chunks.

2. Boil the pasta according to the package directions and drain, reserving ⅓ cup of the pasta water.

3. Meanwhile, in a blender, start by putting in just one of the beets, then the sunflower seeds, coconut milk, garlic, salt, and vegetable broth. Blend, then add the second beet gradually, to achieve your desired color, and the lemon juice.

4. Transfer the pink sauce, cooked pasta, and reserved pasta water to a large skillet over medium-low heat, and stir until coated. Serve immediately with vegan feta, garnished with crushed pistachios and mint.

Storage: Store, fully prepared, in the fridge for up to 3 days.

Save the Scraps: Lemon peels for Candied Citrus Peels (page 254) or Citrus Peel Powder (page 332). Beet skins for Beet Powder (page 334). Beet leaves for We-Got-the-Beet Chips (page 62). Leftover coconut milk for Coo-Coo for Coconut Caramel (page 260) or Firecracker Tofu with Coconut Rice (page 184).

BEET

RIGATONI

SUNFLOWER SEEDS

COCONUT MILK

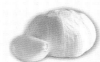

GARLIC

VEGETABLE BROTH

LEMON

TOFU FETA

PISTACHIOS

MINT

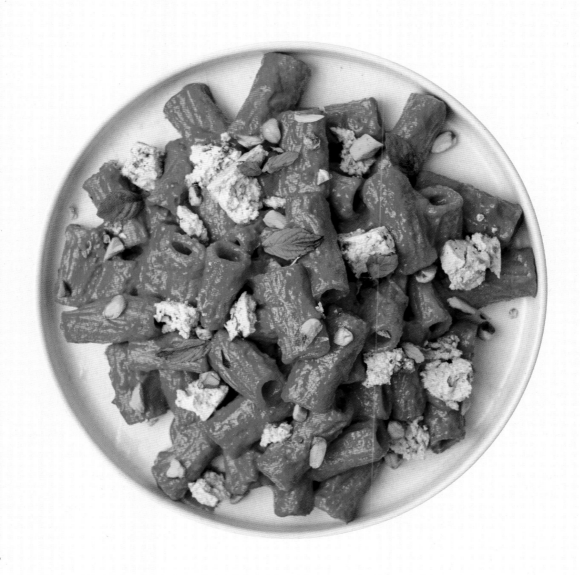

The Whole Darn Squash Pasta

I'm a big believer that there's a lot of unnecessary peeling going on in the culinary world. Take this butternut squash pasta, for example. When you slow-roast squash until it's pillowy soft, there's no harm in throwing the whole thing, skin and all, into a blender for a smooth, creamy pasta sauce with extra fiber. Better yet, utilize the seeds for a crispy topping, reminiscent of toasted bread crumbs.

MAKES 4 to 6 servings ✦ **START TO FINISH:** 45 minutes

1 medium-size butternut squash (about 2 pounds), cut into 1-inch cubes, unpeeled, seeds removed and reserved

1 red bell pepper

3 garlic cloves, minced

1 teaspoon salt

1 teaspoon freshly ground black pepper

3 tablespoons nutritional yeast

1 teaspoon paprika

1 pound dried rigatoni or gluten-free pasta of choice

1 cup vegetable broth

TOASTED SEED CRUMB

½ cup butternut squash seeds

1 teaspoon paprika

½ teaspoon garlic powder

½ teaspoon onion powder

¼ cup crushed walnuts or raw sunflower seeds

½ cup fresh sage, chopped

FOR SERVING

Juice of 1 lemon

1. Preheat the oven to 400°F, and line two baking sheets with reusable baking mats or parchment paper.

2. Arrange the butternut squash, bell pepper, and garlic in a single layer on one of the prepared baking sheets. Season with salt, pepper, nutritional yeast, and paprika. Bake for 30 minutes, or until the squash is soft.

3. Make the toasted seed crumb: Rinse the squash seeds in warm water to remove most of the squash debris, then toss in a bowl with the paprika, garlic powder, and onion powder. Transfer to the second prepared baking sheet. Roast in the oven for 10 minutes. Remove from the oven, add the crushed walnuts and sage, and bake for an additional 5 minutes, or until crisp and golden brown.

4. Meanwhile, cook the pasta according to the package directions, reserving ½ cup of the pasta water.

5. In a high-speed blender, blend the cooked squash mixture and vegetable broth until smooth. Taste and adjust the seasonings as needed.

6. Pour the sauce over the pasta, along with the reserved pasta water and toasted seed crumb. Sprinkle all the lemon juice over the top and stir until all the noodles are coated.

BUTTERNUT SQUASH

RED BELL PEPPER

GARLIC

BLACK PEPPER

NUTRITIONAL YEAST

PAPRIKA

LEMON

RIGATONI

VEGETABLE BROTH

TOASTED SEED CRUMB: BUTTERNUT SQUASH SEEDS, WALNUTS, PAPRIKA, GARLIC POWDER, ONION POWDER, WALNUTS, SAGE

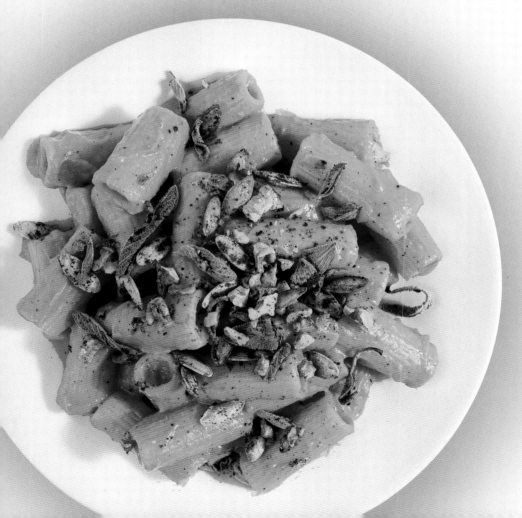

Storage: Store, fully prepared, in the fridge for up to 4 days, or freeze the sauce for up to 3 months.

Save the Scraps: Lemon peels for Candied Citrus Peels (page 254) or Citrus Peel Powder (page 332). Squash Seeds for Save the Seeds (page 72).

Skillet Lasagna

Say good-bye to hours of layering and oven time, and hello to the skillet lasagna! This simple, plant-packed recipe has quickly become a favorite in our household—so much so that I haven't made lasagna the regular way since first testing this out.

MAKES 6 servings ✦ **START TO FINISH:** 45 minutes

- 1 yellow onion, diced finely
- 1½ cups finely diced zucchini, carrot, eggplant, bell pepper, or cauliflower (or a combo of any) or ground with a food processor
- 1 to 2 tablespoons water, for sautéing
- 1 (14-ounce) block extra-firm tofu, crumbled; ½ cup crushed walnuts; or 1 cup finely chopped cremini mushrooms
- 3 garlic cloves, diced finely
- 1 (6-ounce) can tomato paste
- 3 tablespoons nutritional yeast
- 1 teaspoon garlic powder

- 1 tablespoon paprika
- 2 tablespoons soy sauce or gluten-free tamari
- 1 tablespoon Apple Scrap Vinegar (page 350) or store-bought apple cider vinegar
- 3 cups Scratch Tomato Sauce (page 164) or store-bought tomato sauce
- 6 to 8 oven-ready whole wheat or brown rice lasagna noodles
- ¾ cup Sunflower Cream Sauce (page 272)
- ½ cup Scrappy Pesto (page 274) or store-bought vegan pesto (optional)

1. In a large skillet over medium heat, combine the onion, veggies, and water. Sauté until slightly softened, about 3 minutes. Add the crumbled tofu to the skillet, along with the garlic, tomato paste, nutritional yeast, garlic powder, paprika, soy sauce, and apple scrap vinegar. Stir until everything is coated, and the tofu begins to brown, about 5 minutes.

2. Pour in the tomato sauce and stir. Bring to a boil, then simmer for 5 minutes. Break the lasagna noodles into large chunks, about 3 inches long, and add them to the skillet, making sure they are submerged in the sauce. If needed, add ½ cup to 1 cup of water or vegetable broth to the sauce to ensure the noodles are covered. Cover and simmer for 12 to 15 minutes, or until the lasagna noodles are half cooked. Stir to make sure everything is evenly distributed.

3. Using a spoon, dollop the Sunflower Cream Sauce and pesto (if using) on top of the mixture in the skillet, and then cover and cook for an additional 10 minutes. Serve.

Storage: Store, fully prepared, in the fridge for up to 4 days, or freeze for up to 2 months.

Save the Scraps: Carrot tops for the Carrot Top Chimichurri (page 272). Onion peels for Onion Peel Powder (page 336), Scrappy Broth (page 102), or Bouilliant Bouillon Powder (page 336).

YELLOW ONION

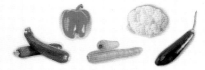

VEGETABLES OF CHOICE: ZUCCHINI, CARROT, EGGPLANT, RED BELL PEPPER, CAULIFLOWER

TOFU

GARLIC

TOMATO PASTE

NUTRITIONAL YEAST

GARLIC POWDER

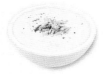

PAPRIKA

SOY SAUCE

APPLE CIDER VINEGAR

TOMATO SAUCE

LASAGNA NOODLES

SUNFLOWER CREAM SAUCE

SCRAPPY PESTO

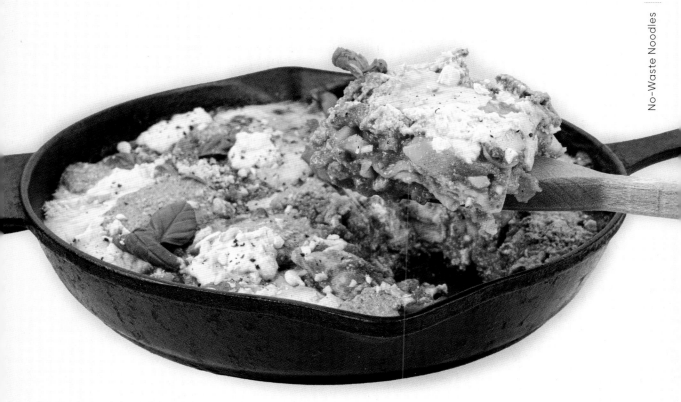

One-Pan Orzo Casserole

Dishes piling up in your sink like a clown car? No worries—this one-pan orzo casserole is the veggie-packed dish you need for those busy weeknights. Just dump everything into a casserole dish and plop it in the oven. Thirty-five minutes later, you have dinner on the table—and a single dish to wash. How's that for saving water?!

MAKES 4 to 6 servings ✦ **START TO FINISH:** 1 hour

1 red onion, chopped

2 cups diced zucchini, broccoli, bell pepper, eggplant, or cauliflower (or a combo of any)

1 (15-ounce) can chickpeas, white beans, or navy beans, drained and rinsed, or 1½ cups homemade

1½ cups cherry tomatoes

¼ cup Sun-Dried Tomatoes (page 328), chopped

2 garlic cloves, minced

1 teaspoon salt

2 tablespoons tomato paste

1¾ cups vegetable broth

¼ cup canned full-fat coconut milk

8 ounces dried orzo or gluten-free orzo

2 cups baby spinach, chopped

¼ cup crumbled Tofu Feta (page 288), or store-bought vegan feta (optional)

1. Preheat the oven to 400°F.

2. In a 9 x 13–inch casserole dish, combine the red onion, diced veggies, chickpeas, cherry tomatoes, Sun-Dried Tomatoes, garlic, salt, tomato paste, and ¼ cup of the vegetable broth. Bake for 25 minutes, or until the vegetables are soft.

3. Add the remaining 1½ cups of vegetable broth, coconut milk, and orzo to the dish, and stir. Cover with tinfoil or a lid and bake for 15 minutes, or until the orzo is cooked.

4. Remove from the oven and stir in the spinach. Enjoy immediately—with vegan feta, if desired.

Storage: Store, fully prepared, in the fridge for up to 3 days.

Save the Scraps: Aquafaba (chickpea water) for Mousse on the Loose (page 264) or Mini Aquafaba Pavlovas (page 266). Onion peels for Onion Peel Powder (page 336), Scrappy Broth (page 102), or Bouilliant Bouillon Powder (page 336). Broccoli stems for Broccoli Stem Summer Rolls (page 108) or Citrus Cabbage Slaw (page 122). Leftover coconut milk for Coo-Coo for Coconut Caramel (page 260) or Firecracker Tofu with Coconut Rice (page 184).

RED ONION

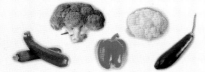

VEGGIES OF CHOICE: ZUCCHINI, BROCCOLI, RED BELL PEPPER, EGGPLANT, CAULIFLOWER

CHICKPEAS

CHERRY TOMATOES

SUN-DRIED TOMATOES

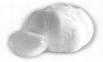

GARLIC

TOMATO PASTE

VEGETABLE BROTH

COCONUT MILK

ORZO

SPINACH

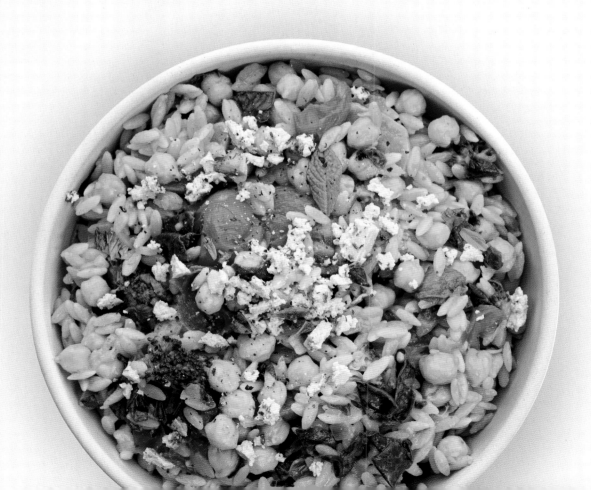

Vodka Penne with Broccolini

Pick up a fork—and maybe a shot glass. This vodka penne (alcohol optional) is the life of the party. You'll be smitten with this time-saving—and water-saving—hack, which involves cooking your broccolini in the same boiling water as the pasta to make this a quick, efficient, and off-the-beaten-path dish!

MAKES 4 servings ✦ **START TO FINISH:** 20 minutes

1 pound dried whole wheat or brown rice penne

1 bunch broccolini or broccoli florets, chopped

½ yellow onion, diced

4 garlic cloves, minced

1 to 2 tablespoons water or extra-virgin olive oil

½ cup tomato paste

1 tablespoon vodka or freshly squeezed lemon juice

1 cup unsweetened plant-based milk (soy, almond, cashew, or other)

¼ cup canned full-fat coconut milk

1 teaspoon red pepper flakes (optional)

½ teaspoon salt

½ teaspoon freshly ground black pepper

Handful of spinach or fresh basil

FOR SERVING

More red pepper flakes and Vegan Nutty "Parm" (page 290)

1. Cook the pasta according to the package directions. Two minutes before draining, add the broccolini to the pot to quickly blanch. Drain the pasta and broccoli, reserving ¼ cup of the pasta water for the sauce.

2. In a large skillet over medium heat, sauté the onion and garlic in water until translucent, about 3 minutes.

3. Add the tomato paste and stir, followed by the vodka, plant-based milk, and coconut milk. Mix until a sauce is formed, then add the red pepper flakes, salt, and black pepper.

4. Pour the reserved pasta water, broccolini, and cooked penne into the pan. Stir until the pasta is coated, adding a handful of spinach at the end. Serve with more red pepper flakes and Vegan Nutty "Parm," as desired.

Storage: Store in an airtight container in the fridge for up to 4 days.

Save the Scraps: Onion peels for Onion Peel Powder (page 336), Scrappy Broth (page 102), or Bouilliant Bouillon Powder (page 336). Broccoli stems for Broccoli Stem Summer Rolls (page 108) or Citrus Cabbage Slaw (page 122). Lemon peels for Candied Citrus Peels (page 254) or Citrus Peel Powder (page 332).

WHOLE WHEAT PENNE

BROCCOLINI

YELLOW ONION

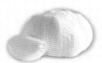

GARLIC

TOMATO PASTE

LEMON JUICE

PLANT-BASED MILK

COCONUT MILK

RED PEPPER FLAKES

PEPPER

SPINACH

VEGAN PARM

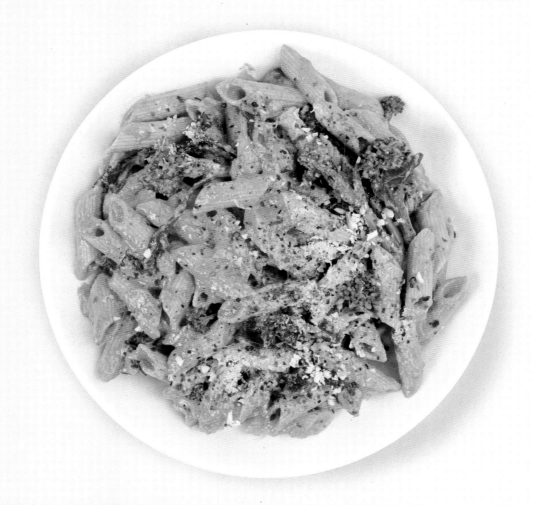

15-Minute Lemon Pepper Alfredo

A creamy, dairy-free pasta sauce made in 15 minutes flat? Yes, thanks to the superpowers of hummus (seriously, what *can't* chickpeas do?). Whether it's store-bought or homemade, when you dilute hummus with pasta water, it makes the creamiest base for a luscious dish fit for a vegan feast.

MAKES 4 to 6 servings ✦ **START TO FINISH:** 30 minutes

1 pound dried whole wheat fettuccine or brown rice pasta of choice

1 shallot, chopped finely

1 garlic clove, minced

1 to 2 tablespoons water, for sautéing

1 cup (Almost) the Whole Can Hummus (page 282) or store-bought hummus

Juice of large lemon, or ¼ cup freshly squeezed lemon juice

1 teaspoon lemon zest

8 to 10 slices Two-Way "Bacon" Street, oyster mushroom variation (page 50; optional)

½ cup fresh parsley

1 teaspoon freshly ground black pepper

1. Bring a large pot of salted water to a boil. Cook the pasta according to the package directions, reserving at least 1 cup of pasta water before draining.

2. In a large skillet over medium heat, combine the shallot and garlic, as well as the (fresh) water. Sauté until fragrant, about 2 minutes.

3. Add the hummus, lemon juice, lemon zest, and ½ cup of the pasta water to the pan. Stir until a creamy sauce is formed, adding the remaining pasta water 1 tablespoon at a time until the sauce reaches your desired consistency.

4. Transfer the cooked pasta to the pan, and toss until coated. Sprinkle with the "bacon" bits, if desired, plus parsley and black pepper. Serve immediately.

Storage: Store in a sealed container in the fridge for up to 4 days.

Save the Scraps: Lemon peels for Candied Citrus Peels (page 254) or Citrus Peel Powder (page 332).

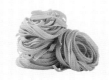

WHOLE WHEAT FETTUCCINE

SHALLOT

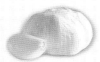

GARLIC

HUMMUS

LEMON

OYSTER MUSHROOM
BACON

PARSLEY

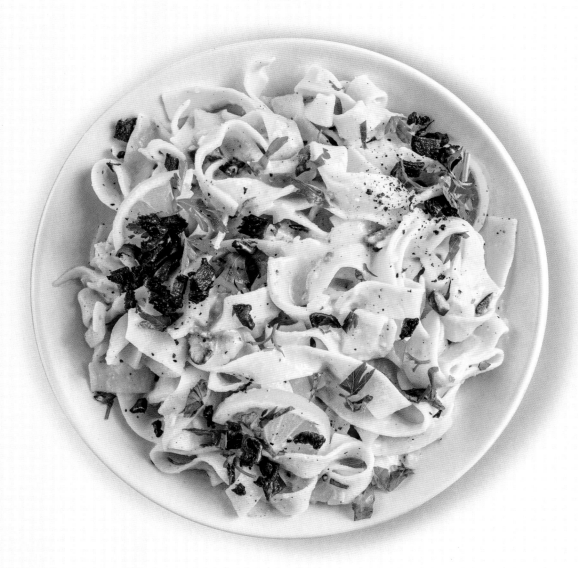

Rock-Your-Broc Mac & Cheez

Just one pot and 15 minutes . . . This rockin' broccoli mac and cheez will enliven your dinner table with a creamy sauce, tender macaroni, and a nutritious green twist. With two whole heads of broccoli (stems included) grated into the luscious sauce, it's nostalgic, comforting, and simply delicious. Mix it up by adding a grated carrot or cauliflower to the pot with the broccoli for a sneaky veggie-loaded mac.

MAKES 4 to 6 servings ✦ **START TO FINISH:** 15 minutes

1 pound dried whole-grain or brown rice macaroni

4 cups vegetable broth

3 garlic cloves, minced

2 broccoli heads with stems, grated

1 carrot, grated, or 1 cup grated cauliflower (optional, for more veggies)

1 cup canned full-fat coconut milk

½ teaspoon paprika

½ cup nutritional yeast

¼ teaspoon ground turmeric

Juice of 1 lemon

½ teaspoon salt

½ teaspoon freshly ground black pepper

Vegan bread crumbs, for serving (optional)

1. In a large pot over medium heat, combine the pasta, broth, garlic, broccoli, and carrot (if using). Stir. Bring to a boil, then cover and lower the heat to medium. Cook the pasta for 10 to 12 minutes, or until tender, stirring halfway through to ensure it's being evenly cooked.

2. Once the pasta is cooked, add the coconut milk, paprika, nutritional yeast, turmeric, lemon juice, salt, and pepper, and stir until creamy. Enjoy with vegan bread crumbs on top, if desired.

Storage: Store in a sealed container in the fridge for up to 4 days.

Save the Scraps: Lemon peels for Candied Citrus Peels (page 254) or Citrus Peel Powder (page 332). Leftover coconut milk for Coo-Coo for Coconut Caramel (page 260) or Firecracker Tofu with Coconut Rice (page 184).

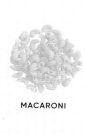

MACARONI

VEGETABLE BROTH

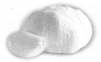

GARLIC

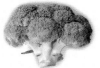

BROCCOLI

CARROT

COCONUT MILK

PAPRIKA

NUTRITIONAL YEAST

TURMERIC

LEMON

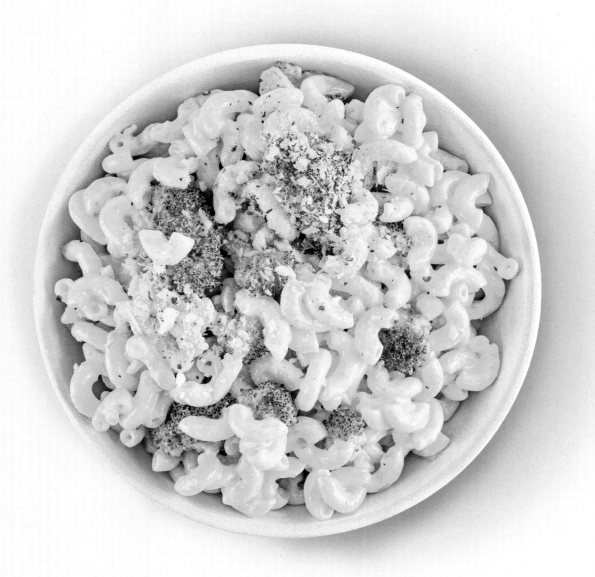

Instant Mac 'n' Cheez Powder

When I went plant-based, I'm almost ashamed to admit this, but one of the foods I missed the most was a nostalgic bowl of boxed mac 'n' cheese. You know the one with the fluorescent orange cheese powder? After several recipe tests, I was able to master a vegan version that can be stored in your pantry for a 20-minute dinner (or midnight bowl) of mac 'n' cheez. It's low-waste, simple to make, and ridiculously delicious.

MAKES enough for 4 batches mac 'n' cheez ✦ **FROM START TO FINISH:** 10 minutes

¾ cup nutritional yeast

¼ cup rolled oats

2 teaspoons garlic powder

2 teaspoons paprika

1½ teaspoons salt

1 teaspoon onion powder

¼ teaspoon freshly ground black pepper

1 teaspoon mustard powder

¼ teaspoon ground turmeric

½ teaspoon Citrus Peel Powder (page 332; optional)

1. In a high-speed blender or spice grinder, combine all the ingredients and blend until a smooth powder is formed.

   Storage: Store in an airtight container in the pantry for up to 1 month.

INSTANT MAC 'N' CHEEZ

MAKES 4 to 6 servings ✦ **FROM START TO FINISH:** 20 minutes

1 pound uncooked whole-grain or brown rice macaroni noodles

¼ cup Instant Mac 'n' Cheese Powder

½ cup unsweetened plant-based milk, plus more as needed

2 tablespoons vegan butter (optional, for a more indulgent mac)

1. Cook the macaroni according to the package directions. Drain the pasta, return it to the pot, and add the ¼ cup of Instant Mac 'n' Cheez Powder, plant-based milk, and vegan butter (if using). Stir until a smooth sauce is formed, adding more milk, as desired, to thin. Eat immediately.

   Storage: Store in an airtight container in the refrigerator for up to 3 days.

INSTANT MAC 'N' CHEEZ POWDER

NUTRITIONAL YEAST

ROLLED OATS

GARLIC POWDER

PAPRIKA

ONION POWDER

MUSTARD POWDER

TURMERIC

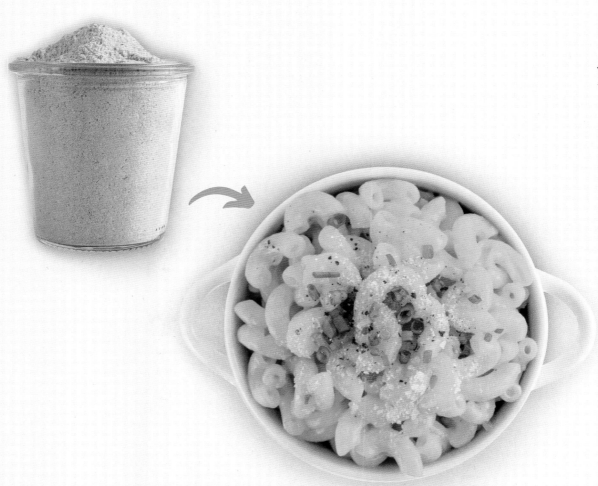

Green with Envy Spaghetti

It's time to put those wilting greens in your fridge to good use. Whether it's spinach, kale, or summer basil, you can whip up this delicious green 'ghetti in less than 20 minutes with just a few simple ingredients. Once you taste a bowl, you'll never let those wilted greens go to waste again!

MAKES 4 to 6 servings ✦ **START TO FINISH:** 20 minutes

1 pound dried whole-grain or brown rice spaghetti

1½ cups roughly chopped kale, chard, radish tops, or arugula

1½ cups spinach

2 garlic cloves

Juice of ½ lemon

½ teaspoon salt

½ teaspoon freshly ground black pepper

¼ cup walnuts or sunflower seeds, soaked in water overnight or boiled for 10 minutes

½ cup nutritional yeast

FOR SERVING

Vegan Nutty "Parm" (page 290)

Crushed walnuts

Red pepper flakes

Fresh basil

1. Bring a large pot of salted water to a boil.

2. Put in the pasta, then the kale and spinach. Allow the greens to blanch for 1 to 2 minutes, until bright green and vibrant. Using tongs, remove the greens and transfer them to a blender container as the pasta continues to cook.

3. In the blender container, add the garlic, lemon juice, salt, black pepper, walnuts, and nutritional yeast. Before draining the pasta, reserve 1½ cups of the salted pasta water. Add ¾ to 1 cup of the pasta water to the blender and blend until smooth. Add more pasta water as needed to reach your desired smooth consistency for the sauce.

4. Add the drained pasta back into its pot, along with the sauce. Toss until covered, and serve with Vegan Nutty "Parm," crushed walnuts, red pepper flakes, and fresh basil, as desired.

Storage: Store in a sealed container in the fridge for up to 4 days.

Save the Scraps: Lemon peels for Candied Citrus Peels (page 254) or Citrus Peel Powder (page 332).

WHOLE-GRAIN SPAGHETTI

KALE, CHARD, RADISH TOPS,
OR ARUGULA

SPINACH

GARLIC

LEMON

WALNUTS

NUTRITIONAL YEAST

FOR SERVING: VEGAN NUTTY "PARM," CRUSHED
WALNUTS, RED PEPPER FLAKES, BASIL

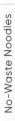

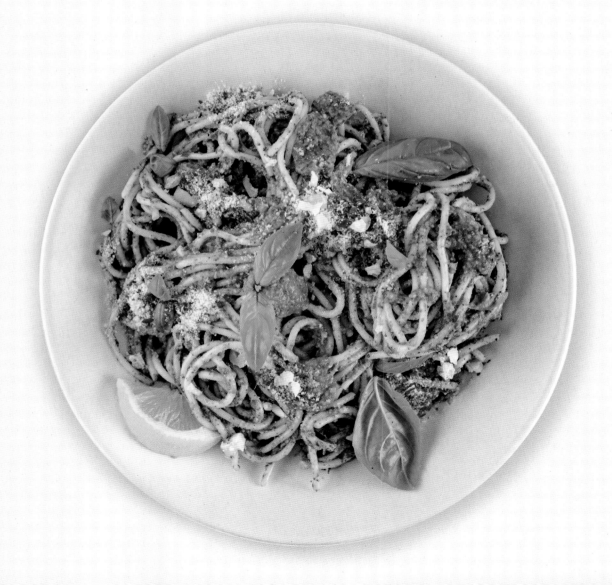

Sunday Sauce

For many folks, Sunday is for rest and relaxation, but in my kitchen, it's for whipping up a pot of sauce that will knock your socks off. Instead of slow-roasting ground beef for your Bolognese, opt for this meatless version with a lower carbon footprint. It's a vegan mince of veggies, walnuts, and lentils—big on plants and flavor. I promise, you won't miss the meat. Note: To make the chopping easier and efficient, add the veggies to a food processor and pulse until finely ground.

MAKES 6 to 8 servings ✦ **START TO FINISH:** 60 minutes

1 yellow onion, diced finely or ground in a food processor

1½ cups carrot, celery, bell pepper, cauliflower, or zucchini (or a combo of any), chopped finely or ground in a food processor

2 cups cremini, oyster, or portobello mushrooms, diced finely or ground in a food processor, or 1 (14-ounce) block extra firm tofu, crumb

1 to 2 tablespoons water

1½ teaspoons salt

½ teaspoon freshly ground black pepper

4 garlic cloves, minced

½ cup walnuts or sunflower seeds, crushed

2 teaspoons dried oregano

¼ cup tomato paste

3 tablespoons balsamic vinegar

1 tablespoon soy sauce or gluten-free tamari

2 tablespoons nutritional yeast

1 tablespoon light or dark brown sugar

1 (28-ounce) can crushed tomatoes, or 4 cups Scratch Tomato Sauce (page 164)

¼ cup dried brown lentils, or 1 cup canned lentils

1 pound dried pappardelle pasta, or gluten-free pasta of choice

FOR SERVING

Chopped fresh parsley

Vegan Nutty "Parm" (page 290)

1. In a large pot over medium heat, combine the diced onion, carrot, mushrooms, water, salt, and pepper. Cook, stirring occasionally, until the vegetables have softened, about 15 minutes.

2. Add the garlic, walnuts, oregano, tomato paste, balsamic vinegar, soy sauce, nutritional yeast, and brown sugar to the pot. Cook, stirring occasionally, until everything is combined, about 3 minutes.

3. Add the crushed tomatoes and brown lentils. Bring the ragù to a simmer, covered, stirring occasionally, for about 40 minutes, or until the lentils are soft and cooked. When safe to handle, use an immersion blender or countertop blender to puree half the sauce to your desired consistency. Taste and adjust the seasoning as needed.

4. Meanwhile, prepare the pasta according to the package directions.

5. Drain the pasta and top with the cooked ragù.

YELLOW ONION

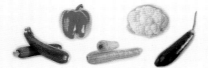

VEGETABLES OF CHOICE: ZUCCHINI, CARROT, EGGPLANT, RED BELL PEPPER, CAULIFLOWER

CREMINI MUSHROOMS

GARLIC

WALNUTS

OREGANO

TOMATO PASTE

BALSAMIC VINEGAR

SOY SAUCE

NUTRITIONAL YEAST

BROWN SUGAR

CRUSHED TOMATOES

BROWN LENTILS

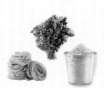

FOR SERVING: PAPPARDELLE PASTA, PARSLEY, VEGAN NUTTY "PARM"

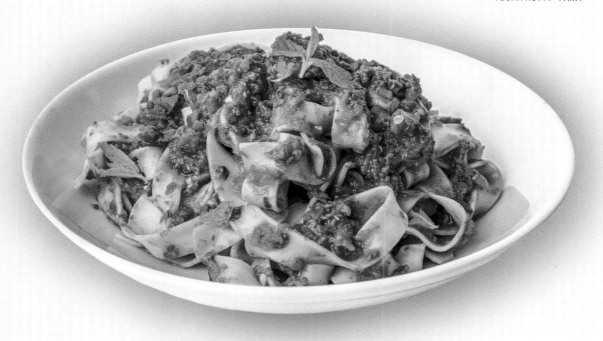

Storage: Store, fully prepared, in the fridge for up to 4 days, or freeze the sauce for up to 3 months.

Save the Scraps: Carrot tops for the Carrot Top Chimichurri (page 272). Onion peels for Onion Peel Powder (page 336), Scrappy Broth (page 102), or Bouilliant Bouillon Powder (page 336). Celery leaves in Celery Leaf "Tabbouleh" (page 106) or Scrappy Broth (page 102).

Scratch Tomato Sauce

It's time to get saucy in the *Scrappy* kitchen. Making homemade tomato sauce can seem intimidating, but once you try it, you may never buy the store stuff again. The only tedious part is removing the tomato skins, but that just gives you an excuse to make Tomato Peel Powder (page 332).

MAKES 4 servings ✦ **START TO FINISH:** 1 hour

3 pounds tomatoes

1 garlic head, top sliced off

1 teaspoon salt

½ teaspoon freshly ground black pepper

1 tablespoon light or dark brown sugar

1 teaspoon dried parsley

½ teaspoon red pepper flakes

1 tablespoon balsamic vinegar

Handful of fresh basil, chopped

1. Preheat the oven to 400°F, and line a baking sheet with a reusable baking mat or parchment paper.

2. Slice the tomatoes in half (remove the green stems) and place them, cut side down, on the prepared baking sheet, along with the head of garlic. Season with a pinch each of the salt and black pepper.

3. Roast in the oven for 40 minutes, or until the skins start to peel from the tomatoes.

4. Remove from the oven and allow to cool. Carefully remove the peels from the tomatoes, for a smooth sauce. Alternatively, you can leave the skins on, but they may stay slightly intact after blending. Place the tomato flesh in a large saucepan, along with the roasted garlic head, remaining salt and black pepper, brown sugar, parsley, red pepper flakes, balsamic vinegar, and basil. Using an immersion blender or a potato masher, blend or mash the ingredients until a sauce is formed.

Storage: Store in the fridge for up to 5 days, or use proper canning procedures to jar this sauce for later. It can also be frozen for up to 3 months.

Save the Scraps: Tomato peels for Tomato Peel Powder (page 332).

ROMA TOMATOES

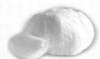

GARLIC

BROWN SUGAR

DRIED PARSLEY

RED PEPPER FLAKES

BALSAMIC VINEGAR

BASIL

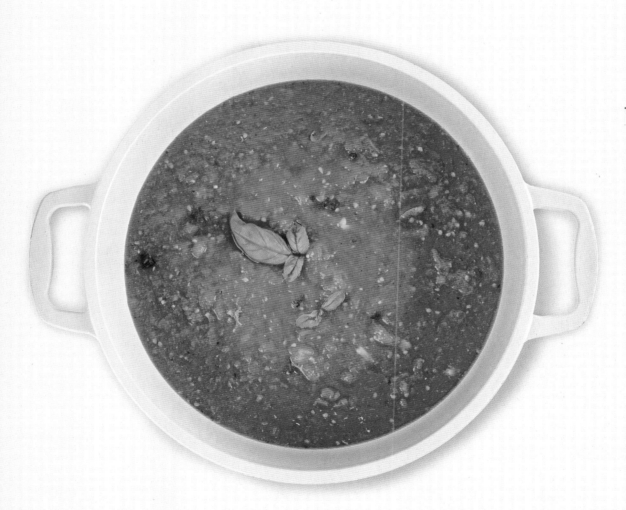

Lemon Peel Pesto

What happens when you replace the basil in my favorite vegan pesto recipe with lemon peels? Magic—that's what. This easy recipe utilizes the low-waste magic of pasta water (a.k.a. liquid gold) and two entire lemons to create the creamy plant-based sauce of your dreams. Quick enough for a weeknight meal and fancy enough for date night.

MAKES 4 servings ✦ **START TO FINISH:** 25 minutes

16 ounces fettuccine or gluten-free pasta of choice

2 whole lemons, preferably organic

1½ cups raw cashews, sunflower seeds, or pine nuts, soaked overnight or boiled for 10 minutes

3 cloves garlic

3 tablespoons nutritional yeast

1½ teaspoons salt

1 teaspoon pepper

FOR SERVING

Chopped parsley, Vegan Nutty "Parm" (page 290), and black pepper, if desired

1. Cook the pasta according to package directions. Drain, reserving 2 ½ cups of the pasta water. Set the pasta aside.

2. While the pasta cooks, peel the lemons, discarding as much of the white pith as you can, as it is bitter. I like to use a potato peeler for this.

3. In a blender or food processor, put in the cashews, lemon peels, juice of the lemons, garlic, nutritional yeast, 1¾ cups of the reserved pasta water, salt, and pepper. Blend until a smooth sauce is formed, adding more pasta water as needed to thin the sauce.

4. Put the pasta back into the pot it was cooked in, and pour the sauce over the top, as well as the remaining pasta water to thin if needed. Toss gently with tongs over medium heat until the sauce is evenly dispersed and the pasta is warm. Serve with chopped parsley, vegan parm, and black pepper, if desired.

Up the Veggies: Sauté 1 head of broccoli, 1 cup of cherry tomatoes, and ½ cup of green peas for 5 minutes over medium heat while the pasta is cooking and mix them into the pasta with the sauce at the end. This is also delicious with baked tofu.

Storage: Store in a sealed container for up to 4 days.

FETTUCCINE

CASHEWS

LEMONS

GARLIC

NUTRITIONAL YEAST

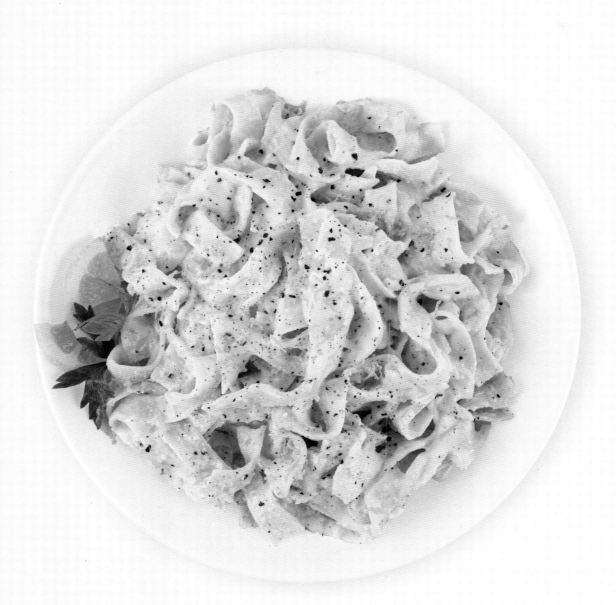

No-Waste Noodles

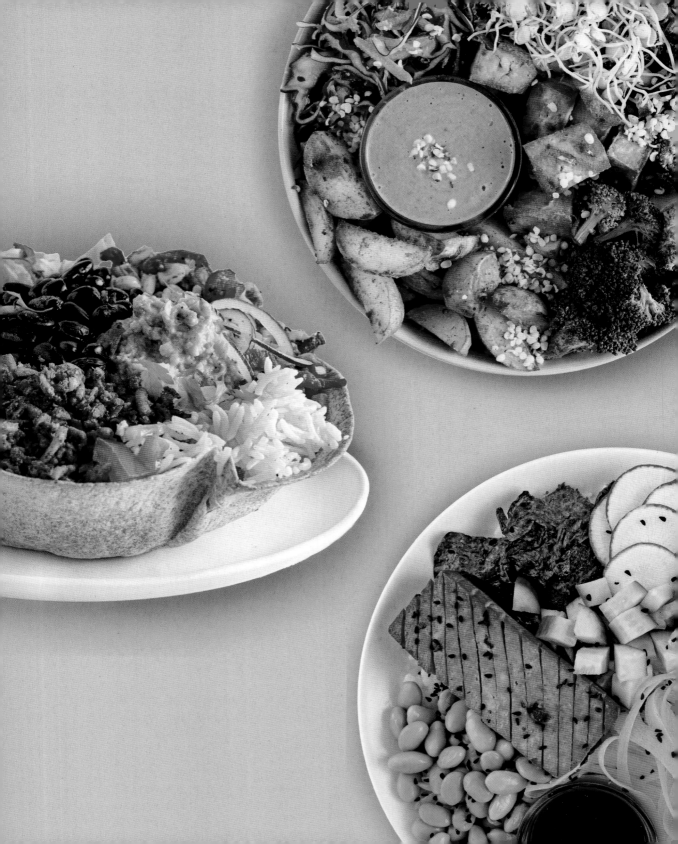

CHAPTER 6

The Main Bowl

I like big bowls and I cannot lie . . .
Serve these up for a perfect meal
prep lunch or hearty dinner.

Super Loaded Harvest Bowl

This harvest bowl is like a farmers' market on a plate. Packed with tenderized kale, roasted brussels sprouts, sweet potato, and crisp apple, it's got all the flavors of fall while also using up a bunch of seasonal ingredients in one hearty dish.

MAKES 4 servings ✦ **START TO FINISH:** 45 minutes

FOR SHEET PAN

2 cups quartered brussels sprouts, broccoli florets, or cauliflower florets

2 sweet potatoes, Yukon Gold potatoes, or 1 medium-size squash (any type), cut into small cubes

2 tablespoons soy sauce or gluten-free tamari

1 tablespoon paprika

1 teaspoon garlic powder

1 teaspoon dried thyme

FOR BOWL

½ cup uncooked wild rice blend or quinoa

1 bunch kale or chard

Juice of 1 lemon

1 red apple, cored and sliced

½ cup pomegranate seeds

¼ cup Save the Seeds, savory blend (page 72), or ¼ cup walnuts

¾ cup Everything Tahini Dressing (page 278) or store-bought vegan balsamic dressing

1. Roast the sheet-pan ingredients: Preheat the oven to 400°F, and line a baking sheet with a reusable baking mat or parchment paper. Add the brussels sprouts and sweet potatoes. Toss with the soy sauce, paprika, garlic powder, and thyme.

2. Bake for 15 minutes, then flip the vegetables and bake for another 15 minutes until the brussels sprouts are soft and the potatoes are cooked through.

3. Meanwhile, prepare the bowl ingredients: Cook the wild rice according to the package directions. Then place the kale in a large bowl with the lemon juice. Massage until the kale is tenderized. (If using chard, no need to tenderize.)

4. Assemble the salad: Place the sweet potatoes, brussels sprouts, cooked wild rice, apple, pomegranate seeds, and savory seeds on top of the kale. Drizzle with the dressing when ready to serve. If meal prepping, you can add lemon juice to the apple to prevent browning.

Storage: Store the salad base and dressing separately in the fridge for up to 3 days.

Save the Scraps: Lemon peels for Candied Citrus Peels (page 254) or Citrus Peel Powder (page 332). Pomegranate peel for Pomegranate Peel Powder (page 334). Extra quinoa for Leftover Quinoa Truffles (page 248). Apple scraps for Apple Scrap Vinegar (page 350) or Apple Scrap Honey (page 256). Squash seeds for Save the Seeds (page 72).

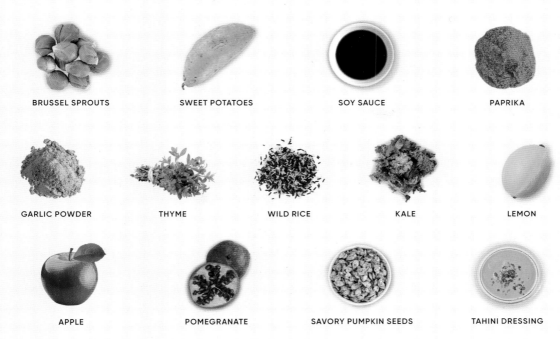

BRUSSEL SPROUTS

SWEET POTATOES

SOY SAUCE

PAPRIKA

GARLIC POWDER

THYME

WILD RICE

KALE

LEMON

APPLE

POMEGRANATE

SAVORY PUMPKIN SEEDS

TAHINI DRESSING

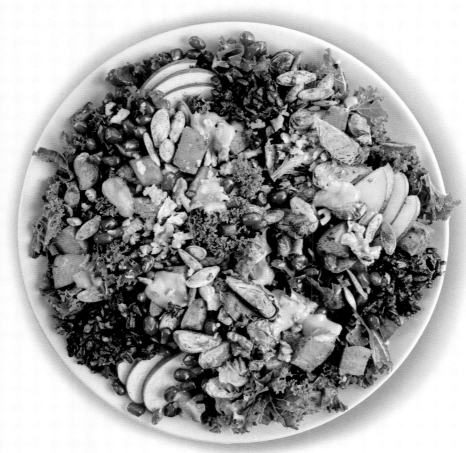

Microbiome Bowl

With a killer combo of fermented foods, fiber-rich plants, and a garlicky green dressing, this microbiome bowl is like a party for your gut! Eating probiotic- and fiber-rich foods regularly promotes a healthy digestive system, which enriches every other part of your body, including your mind. So give your gut a big hug by whipping up this biome bonanza, and it will thank you later (probably with a toot, but that's just love).

MAKES 4 servings ✦ **START TO FINISH:** 30 minutes

½ cup uncooked wild rice blend or quinoa

2 cups fingerling potatoes, halved or quartered

2 cups broccoli florets or brussels sprouts

1 (14-ounce) block extra-firm tofu, cubed

2 tablespoons soy sauce or gluten-free tamari

1 tablespoon paprika

1 teaspoon garlic powder

1 teaspoon dried thyme

SALAD

1 cup Lentil Sprouts (page 338) or broccoli sprouts

1 cup Citrus Cabbage Slaw (page 122), Turmeric Sauerkraut (page 340), or store-bought sauerkraut

¼ cup hemp hearts

Handful of fresh parsley or cilantro, for garnish

1 cup Green Goddess Dressing (page 280) or store-bought vegan vinaigrette

1. Cook the wild rice blend according to the package directions.

2. Preheat the oven to 400°F, and line a baking sheet with a reusable baking mat or parchment paper. Then place on the sheet the potatoes, broccoli, and tofu. Toss with the soy sauce, paprika, garlic powder, and thyme. Bake for 25 minutes, or until the broccoli is soft, the tofu is browned, and the potato is cooked through, tossing halfway through.

3. Assemble the salad: In a bowl, combine the Lentil Sprouts, wild rice, Citrus Cabbage Slaw, potatoes, broccoli florets, tofu, and hemp hearts. Garnish with parsley. Drizzle with the dressing when ready to serve.

Storage: Store the salad and dressing separately in the fridge for up to 3 days.

Save the Scraps: Lemon peels for Candied Citrus Peels (page 254) or Citrus Peel Powder (page 332). Broccoli stems for Broccoli Stem Summer Rolls (page 108) or Citrus Cabbage Slaw (page 122).

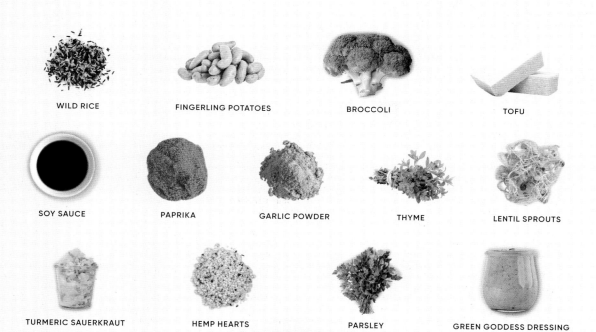

WILD RICE

FINGERLING POTATOES

BROCCOLI

TOFU

SOY SAUCE

PAPRIKA

GARLIC POWDER

THYME

LENTIL SPROUTS

TURMERIC SAUERKRAUT

HEMP HEARTS

PARSLEY

GREEN GODDESS DRESSING

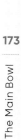

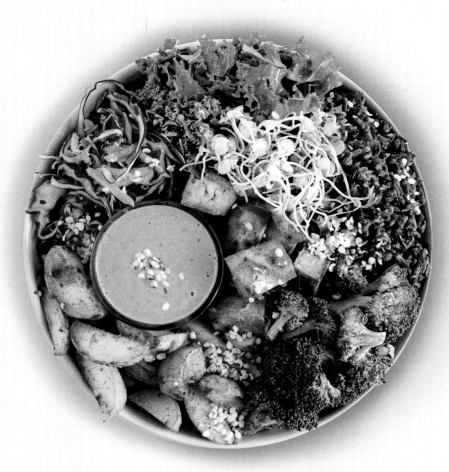

Pesto & Herb Vitality Bowl

If you're looking for a bowl of plant goodness loaded with protein, fiber, and layers of flavor, my Pesto & Herb Vitality Bowl has boldly entered the chat. Crispy chickpeas are nestled between whole-grain pasta, broccoli, kale, and green peas, all tossed in a creamy pesto sauce (made from whichever green you have on hand) for a bowl that will leave you energized and revitalized. Perfect for meal prep, date night, or a nourishing weeknight dinner.

MAKES 4 servings ✦ **START TO FINISH:** 40 minutes

CHICKPEAS
1 (15-ounce) can chickpeas, drained and rinsed, or 1½ cups homemade

1 teaspoon paprika

½ teaspoon onion powder

1 teaspoon garlic powder

½ teaspoon cayenne pepper

½ teaspoon dried oregano

1 teaspoon sea salt

PASTA AND VEGGIES
1 pound dried whole wheat penne

1 head broccoli, chopped into small florets

1½ cups chopped kale

1½ cups frozen green peas, thawed

2 tablespoons vegetable broth

½ teaspoon salt

1 tablespoon nutritional yeast

PESTO SAUCE
1 cup Scrappy Pesto (page 274) or store-bought vegan pesto

FOR SERVING
1 cup chopped fresh parsley

4 teaspoons hemp hearts

1. Preheat the oven to 400°F, and line a baking sheet with a reusable baking mat or parchment paper.

2. Make the chickpeas: In a bowl, combine the chickpeas, paprika, onion powder, garlic powder, cayenne, oregano, and salt until the chickpeas are coated. Transfer the coated chickpeas to the prepared baking sheet and roast in the oven for 30 minutes, or until crispy, stirring halfway through.

3. While the chickpeas roast, start the pasta and veggies: Cook the penne according to the package directions.

4. Meanwhile, in a large skillet over medium heat, combine the broccoli florets, kale, green peas, vegetable broth, salt, and nutritional yeast. Cover and steam for 3 to 5 minutes, or until cooked.

5. Now, assemble. Place the pasta in a bowl, with the greens and crispy chickpeas on top, followed by the Scrappy Pesto, as well as parsley and hemp hearts, as desired. Enjoy immediately or save for a meal-prep lunch.

Storage: Store in a sealed container in the fridge for up to 4 days.

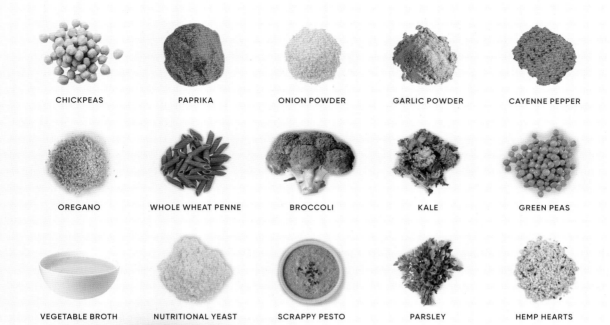

CHICKPEAS   PAPRIKA   ONION POWDER   GARLIC POWDER   CAYENNE PEPPER

OREGANO   WHOLE WHEAT PENNE   BROCCOLI   KALE   GREEN PEAS

VEGETABLE BROTH   NUTRITIONAL YEAST   SCRAPPY PESTO   PARSLEY   HEMP HEARTS

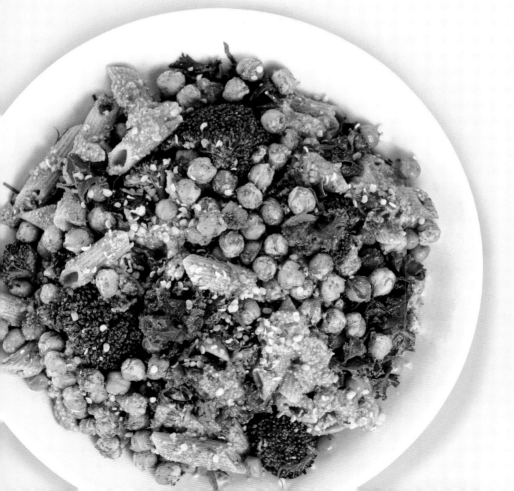

Save the Scraps:
Lemon peels for
Candied Citrus Peels
(page 254) or Citrus
Peel Powder (page
332). Broccoli stems for
Broccoli Stem Summer
Rolls (page 108) or
Citrus Cabbage Slaw
(page 122). Aquafaba
(chickpea water) for
Mousse on the Loose
(page 264) or Mini
Aquafaba Pavlovas
(page 266).

Sea-Saving "Salmon" Bowl

Seafood lovers—it's time to chuck down the fishing rod and grab a chunk of tofu. This delicious bowl is proof that you can enjoy the vibrant taste of salmon without harming a single fish. The secret ingredient here is nori, which gives a taste of the sea. Better for our oceans and also packs a flavor-punch with plant-powered protein.

MAKES 4 servings ✦ **START TO FINISH:** 60 minutes

"SALMON"

1 (14-ounce) block extra-firm tofu

1½ cups vegetable broth

1½ tablespoons Beet Powder (page 334), for color (optional)

2 tablespoons hoisin sauce

1 sheet nori—½ crushed, ½ reserved for serving, as desired

1 teaspoon rice vinegar

1 tablespoon extra-virgin olive oil (optional)

2 tablespoons soy sauce or gluten-free tamari

RICE

1½ cups uncooked sushi rice

1 cup frozen edamame, shelled

FOR SERVING (OPTIONAL)

Kimchi

Radish

Carrot

Cucumber

1. Make the "salmon": Slice your block of tofu in half. Flip on its side and slice in half again, so you have four equal slices. Using a sharp knife, carefully score the top of your slices diagonally to create a fishlike skin appearance.

2. In a bowl, prepare a marinade: Combine the vegetable broth, beet powder, hoisin sauce, crushed nori, rice vinegar, olive oil (if using), and soy sauce. Place the tofu in a sealable container or resealable bag along with the marinade. Soak for at least 30 minutes.

3. Cook your rice and edamame according to their package directions.

4. Preheat the oven to 400°F, and line a baking sheet with a reusable baking mat or parchment paper. Transfer the "salmon" slices to the prepared baking sheet, and bake for 20 minutes, or until slightly browned. For a char on the outside, you can broil the tofu in the oven for 2 to 3 minutes after baking.

5. When cooking is complete, divide the rice and edamame among four bowls, followed by the tofu "salmon" and your desired optional toppings.

Storage: Store the vegan "salmon" in a sealed container in the fridge for up to 4 days.

TOFU

VEGETABLE BROTH

BEET POWDER

HOISIN SAUCE

NORI SHEETS

RICE VINEGAR

SOY SAUCE

   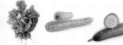

BOWL OPTIONALS: SUSHI RICE, EDAMAME, KIMCHI, RADISH, CARROT, CUCUMBER

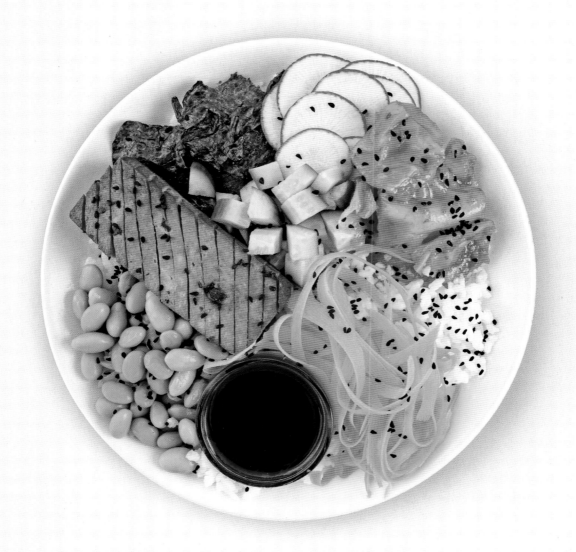

Loaded Tortilla Bowls

Get ready to take the art of the edible bowl to a whole new level with this loaded burrito–inspired masterpiece. If you have almost-stale tortillas sitting in your cupboard, we'll transform them into the perfect shell for all your taco-night favorites. As you dig in, you can break off the side of the bowl to use as tortilla crisps for the ultimate dipping experience.

MAKES 4 servings ✦ **START TO FINISH:** 40 minutes

TACO SEASONING

2 tablespoons chili powder

1 teaspoon paprika

1 teaspoon garlic powder

1 teaspoon onion powder

1 teaspoon dried oregano

TOFU TACO MEAT (FOR A SOY-FREE VERSION, CHECK OUT VEGAN GROUND BEEF, PAGE 222)

1 (14-ounce) block extra-firm tofu, drained

2 tablespoons tomato paste

1 tablespoon soy sauce

1 tablespoon hoisin sauce

ROASTED VEGETABLES

2 cups diced vegetables, such as bell pepper, corn, zucchini, and onion

TORTILLA BOWLS

4 whole wheat or gluten-free tortilla wraps (can be slightly hard or stale—but no mold)

FOR SERVING (OPTIONAL)

1 head iceberg lettuce, or greens of choice

2 cups cooked rice

Bunch of cilantro, chopped

1 (15-ounce) can black beans, pinto beans, or chickpeas, drained and rinsed, or 1½ cups homemade

Sunflower Cream Sauce, cheesy version (page 272), or salsa

1. Preheat the oven to 375°F, and line two baking sheets with reusable baking mats or parchment paper. In a small bowl, combine the taco seasoning ingredients.

2. Make the tofu taco meat: Using a cheese grater, grate the block of tofu into shreds. Alternatively, mash it with the back of a fork. Add half the taco seasoning mixture along with all the tomato paste, soy sauce, and hoisin sauce, and stir until coated. Transfer to one of the prepared baking sheets.

3. Roast the vegetables: On the other prepared baking sheet, arrange the diced vegetables in a single layer, sprinkled with the rest of the taco seasoning. Place both baking sheets in the oven and bake for 25 minutes, stirring halfway through.

4. Meanwhile, place a large tortilla at the bottom of an oven-safe bowl or small pot, allowing the edges of the tortilla to fold in on themselves to create a bowl shape. Place in the oven until crisped, for 12 to 15 minutes. Remove from the oven and allow to cool until able to safely remove from the bowl. Repeat with the other tortillas to create a total of four bowls.

5. Place the tofu taco meat, roasted vegetables, and your additional taco ingredients of choice in the bowls. Top with Sunflower Cream Sauce and serve.

TACO SEASONING: CHILI POWDER, PAPRIKA, GARLIC POWDER, ONION POWDER, OREGANO

TOFU TACO MEAT: TOFU, TOMATO PASTE, SOY SAUCE, HOISIN

ROASTED VEGETABLES: RED BELL PEPPER, CORN, ZUCCHINI, ONION

WHOLE WHEAT TORTILLA

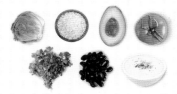

FOR SERVING: ICEBERG LETTUCE, JASMINE RICE, AVOCADO, TOMATO, CILANTRO, BLACK BEANS, SUNFLOWER CREAM SAUCE

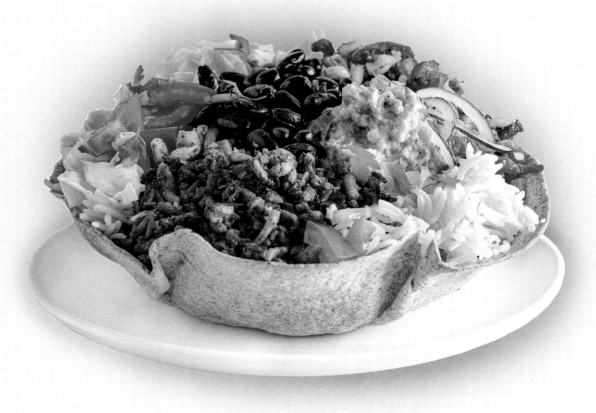

Storage: Store the tofu taco meat in the fridge for up to 4 days, or freeze for up to 2 months.

Save the Scraps: Onion peels for Onion Peel Powder (page 336), Scrappy Broth (page 102), or Bouilliant Bouillon Powder (page 336).

Nutty Noodle Bowl

Noodles have never tasted so nutty. Packed with crunchy peanuts, edamame for protein, and a tangy mango peanut sauce, this dish will have you doing cartwheels with every bite. (Have we lost our noodle?!) Serve it as the main event or as a savory side to such recipes as the Firecracker Tofu with Coconut Rice (page 184).

MAKES 4 servings ✦ **START TO FINISH:** 20 minutes

12 ounces whole wheat spaghetti or brown rice vermicelli noodles

1 cup shredded red cabbage

1 red bell pepper, seeded and thinly sliced into matchsticks

1 large carrot, julienned

1 cup edamame, thawed

6 green onions, diced

1 cup chopped fresh cilantro (optional)

¾ cup Mango Peanut Sauce (page 274)

FOR SERVING

¼ cup crushed peanuts

1 lime, sliced into wedges, for serving

1. Cook the spaghetti according to the package directions. Run under cold water and let cool to room temperature.

2. In a bowl, combine the noodles and vegetables and pour the sauce over the top. Toss until the noodles are coated in the sauce, then serve with the crushed peanuts and lime wedges.

Storage: Store, fully prepared, in the fridge for up to 4 days.

Save the Scraps: Carrot tops for the Carrot Top Chimichurri (page 272).

WHOLE WHEAT
SPAGHETTI

RED CABBAGE

RED BELL PEPPER

CARROT

EDAMAME

GREEN ONIONS

CILANTRO

MANGO PEANUT
SAUCE

PEANUTS

LIME

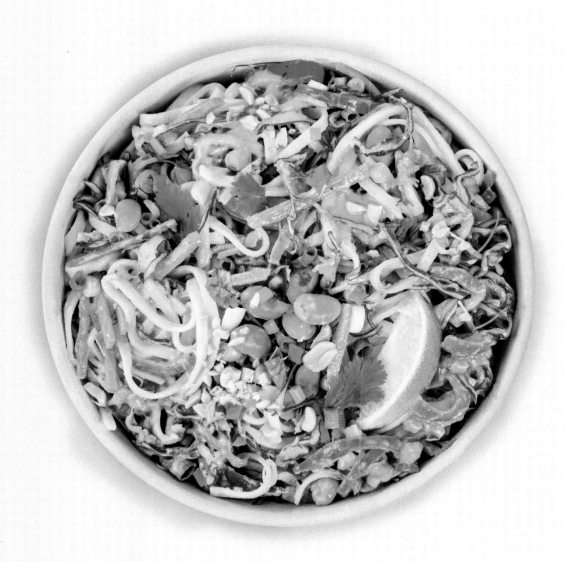

The Main Bowl

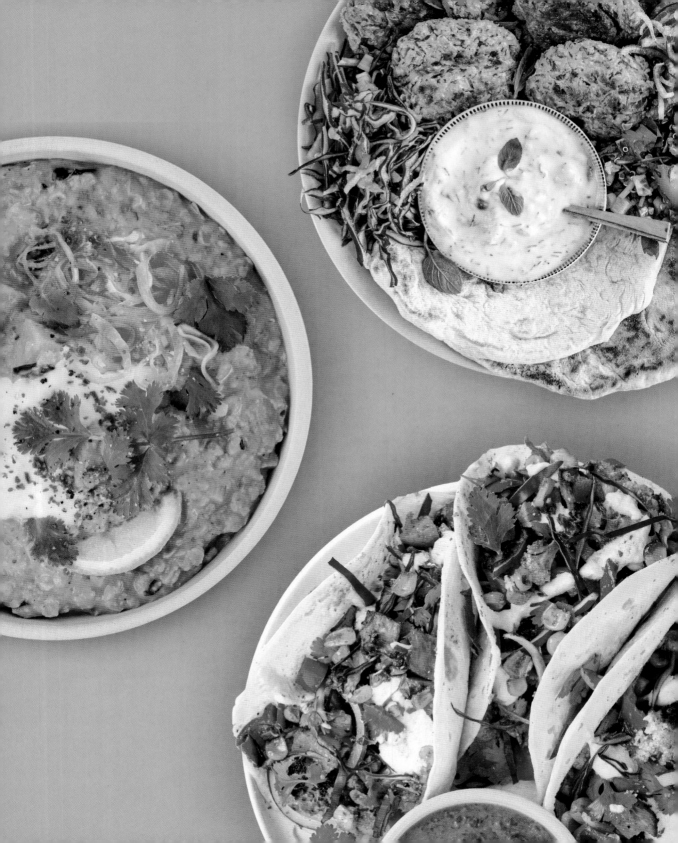

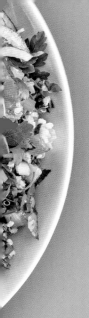

CHAPTER 7

Eco Entrées

Mouthwatering mains that make the most of everything in your kitchen.

Firecracker Tofu with Coconut Rice

Got leftover coconut milk? Let's whip up a batch of coconut rice for this firecracker tofu, which provides an explosive combination of spicy, sweet, and savory—for many dishes!

MAKES 4 servings ◆ **START TO FINISH:** 30 minutes

COCONUT RICE
1 cup uncooked jasmine rice

½ cup full-fat coconut milk

¾ cup water

Pinch of salt

TOFU
1 (14-ounce) block extra-firm tofu

2 tablespoons vegetable broth

4 tablespoons cornstarch, arrowroot powder, or flour

SAUCE
2 tablespoons all-purpose or gluten-free flour

½ cup water

2 tablespoons rice vinegar

¼ cup soy sauce or gluten-free tamari

3 tablespoons hoisin sauce

¼ cup sweet chili sauce or ketchup

1 (1-inch) piece fresh ginger, minced

½ teaspoon red pepper flakes

VEGGIES
2 garlic cloves, minced

¼ red onion, diced

1 red bell pepper, seeded and diced

4 baby bok choy, sliced vertically into quarters

FOR SERVING
Sesame seeds

Fresh cilantro

1. Make the coconut rice: Rinse the jasmine rice in a colander until the water runs clear. Transfer to a large pot, add the coconut milk, water, and salt, and bring to a boil. Simmer, covered, for 20 to 25 minutes.

2. Preheat the oven to 400°F, and line a baking sheet with a reusable baking mat or parchment paper.

3. Make the tofu: Set it on a cutting board, wrap it in a clean cloth, and then stack something heavy, such as books or a cast-iron pan, on top. Let press for 15 to 20 minutes.

4. After pressing the tofu, slice it into ten to twelve equal slices, about ½ inch thick. Toss with the vegetable broth and then with the cornstarch. Transfer to the prepared baking sheet and bake for 25 minutes, flipping halfway through.

5. Meanwhile, prepare the sauce: In a small bowl, whisk the flour with the water, then add the rice vinegar, soy sauce, hoisin sauce, sweet chili sauce, ginger, and red pepper flakes.

6. In a large skillet over medium heat, sauté the garlic, red onion, and bell pepper until softened, about 5 minutes. Pour in the sauce and simmer until thickened, about 3 minutes. Add the tofu and bok choy, and stir until the bok choy is vibrant and the tofu is coated with the sauce, about 2 minutes.

7. Serve over the coconut rice, garnished with sesame seeds and cilantro.

JASMINE RICE

COCONUT MILK

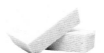

TOFU

VEGETABLE BROTH

CORNSTARCH

FLOUR

RICE VINEGAR

SOY SAUCE

HOISIN SAUCE

SWEET CHILI SAUCE

GINGER ROOT

RED PEPPER FLAKES

RED ONION

RED BELL PEPPER

BOK CHOY

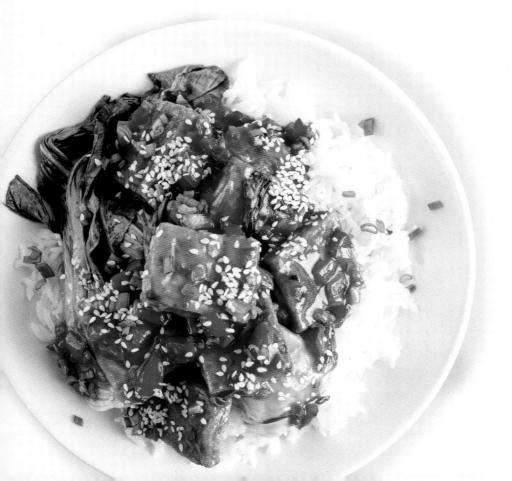

Storage: Store in a sealed container in the fridge for up to 4 days, or in the freezer for 3 months.

Save the Scraps: Onion peels for Onion Peel Powder (page 336), Scrappy Broth (page 102), or Bouilliant Bouillon Powder (page 336). Leftover coconut milk for Coo-Coo for Coconut Caramel (page 260).

Zucchini "Falafel" Fritters

Falafel is great, but here's a wonderful fritter twist on the splendid concoction. This recipe is a way to utilize that overabundance of zucchini at harvest time—and a terrific excuse for us to sneak in some nutritious, tasty, colorful greens. These fritters are also easy to make, with no food processor or blender needed! Best served with my Creamy Vegan Tzatziki, Citrus Cabbage Slaw, or Celery Leaf "Tabbouleh," for a vibrant bowl of *Scrappy* plant-based goodness.

MAKES 12 to 14 fritters ✦ **START TO FINISH:** 45 minutes

2 zucchini (about 1 pound total), grated (3½ to 4 cups)

½ teaspoon salt

1 cup chickpea flour

3 tablespoons nutritional yeast

1 teaspoon ground cumin

1 teaspoon ground coriander (optional)

3 garlic cloves, minced

Large handful of fresh parsley, chopped finely

Juice of 1 lemon

2 tablespoons tahini, plus more as needed

FOR SERVING (OPTIONAL)

Cooked rice

The Knead for Flatbread (page 68)

Creamy Vegan Tzatziki (page 276)

Citrus Cabbage Slaw (page 122)

Celery Leaf "Tabbouleh" (page 106)

1. Preheat the oven to 400°F, and line a baking sheet with a reusable baking mat or parchment paper.

2. Place the grated zucchini in a colander with a sprinkle of salt, and allow to drain for 15 minutes into your sink or into a bowl.

3. In a medium-size bowl, stir together the chickpea flour, nutritional yeast, cumin, coriander (if using), garlic, parsley, and salt until combined.

4. Using a piece of cheesecloth or a clean kitchen cloth, squeeze out as much liquid as possible from the grated zucchini. You can reserve this water for another recipe. Add the zucchini to the bowl, along with the lemon juice and tahini, and stir until a dough is formed. Add an additional tablespoon of tahini if the mixture is too dry to form.

5. Using your hands or a cookie scoop, divide the mixture into twelve to fourteen equal-size balls, each about 2 inches in diameter. Flatten into ovals about ½ inch thick.

6. Bake for 20 minutes, or until browned, flipping halfway through. Enjoy with rice, flatbread, vegan tzatziki, cabbage slaw, and tabbouleh, as desired.

Storage: Store in a sealed container in the fridge for up to 5 days, or in the freezer for 3 months.

Save the Scraps: Lemon peels for Candied Citrus Peels (page 254) or Citrus Peel Powder (page 332), reserved zucchini water for Tummy-Soothing Lemon, Ginger & Mint Ice Cubes (page 308).

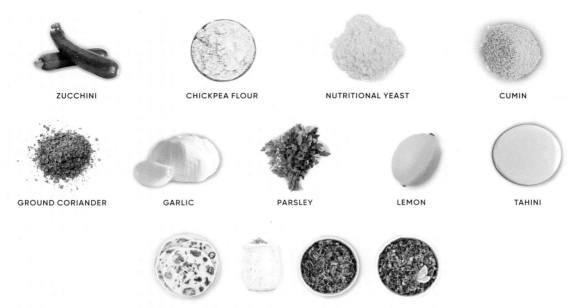

ZUCCHINI

CHICKPEA FLOUR

NUTRITIONAL YEAST

CUMIN

GROUND CORIANDER

GARLIC

PARSLEY

LEMON

TAHINI

FOR THE BOWL: FLATBREAD, TZATZIKI, CITRUS CABBAGE SLAW, CELERY LEAF TABBOULEH

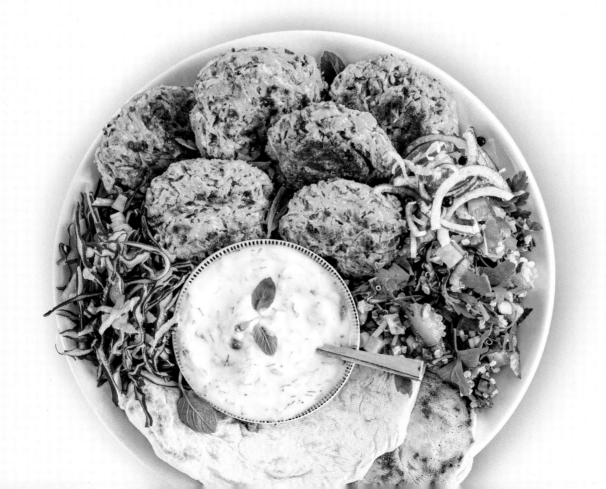

Any Vegetable Curry

It's time to raid your fridge (again) and turn leftover veggies into a cool meal. Inspired by the rich flavors of Indian butter chicken, this dish is wonderful served with basmati rice and vegan naan or the Knead for Flatbread (page 68).

MAKES 4 to 6 servings ✦ **START TO FINISH:** 40 minutes

1 cup uncooked basmati rice

TOFU

1 (14-ounce) block extra-firm tofu

1 tablespoon vegetable broth or extra-virgin olive oil

1 tablespoon cornstarch

Pinch of salt and black pepper

CURRY

1 yellow onion, diced

3 garlic cloves, minced

1 (1-inch) piece fresh ginger, minced

1½ cups chopped bell pepper, carrot, eggplant, broccoli, or sweet potato

½ cup + 1 to 2 tablespoons water

2 tablespoons garam masala

½ teaspoon ground turmeric

1 teaspoon ground cumin

1 teaspoon salt

½ cup raw sunflower seeds or cashews, soaked in water overnight or boiled for 10 minutes, or 1 cup full-fat coconut milk

1 (28-ounce) can crushed tomatoes, or 2 cups Scratch Tomato Sauce (page 164)

2 tablespoons pure maple syrup

1 cup green peas

FOR SERVING

Handful of fresh cilantro

1. Cook the rice according to the package directions.

2. Preheat the oven to 400°F, and line a baking sheet.

3. Make the tofu: Tear the tofu into 1-inch chunks, place in a bowl, and toss with the vegetable broth, cornstarch, salt, and black pepper. Pour evenly onto the prepared baking sheet and bake for 15 to 20 minutes, or until slightly crispy.

4. Make the curry: In a large skillet over medium heat, combine the onion, garlic, ginger, and your veggie of choice with 1 to 2 tablespoons of water, and sauté until the onion is translucent, for 2 to 3 minutes. If using a heartier vegetable, such as sweet potato or squash, cook for 5 to 10 minutes, or until softened.

5. Add the garam masala, turmeric, cumin, and salt and stir for an additional 2 minutes.

6. Meanwhile, in a blender, combine the sunflower seeds and remaining ½ cup of water and blend until a smooth cream is formed.

7. Add the crushed tomatoes, maple syrup, and sunflower cream to the pan and stir. Pour in the cooked tofu, mix, and simmer, uncovered, for 10 minutes.

8. Add the green peas and stir until thawed. Serve with rice, garnished with cilantro.

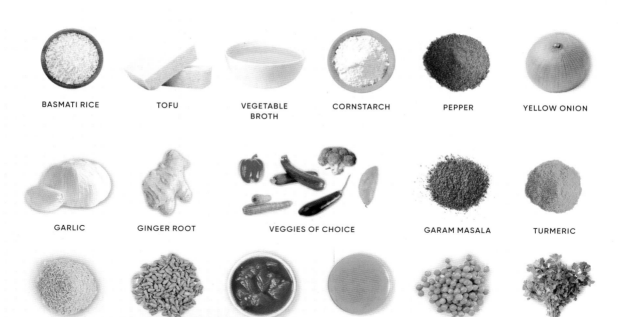

BASMATI RICE

TOFU

VEGETABLE BROTH

CORNSTARCH

PEPPER

YELLOW ONION

GARLIC

GINGER ROOT

VEGGIES OF CHOICE

GARAM MASALA

TURMERIC

CUMIN

SUNFLOWER SEEDS

CRUSHED TOMATOES

MAPLE SYRUP

GREEN PEAS

CILANTRO

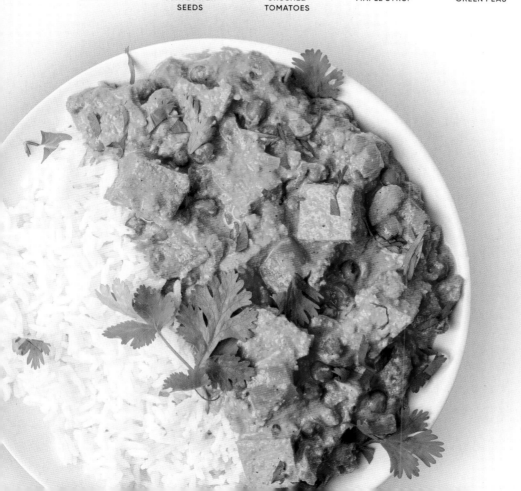

Storage: Store in a sealed container in the fridge for up to 4 days, or freeze for up to 2 months.

Save the Scraps: Onion peels for Onion Peel Powder (page 336), Scrappy Broth (page 102), or Bouilliant Bouillon Powder (page 336).

Perfect Peanut Butter Curry

One pot, bold flavors, and a seriously creamy curry. This recipe is a great excuse to use up the last of the peanut butter jar (or any nut butter you happen to have on hand). **Pro tip:** To get the last bits of PB out of your jar, add warm vegetable broth or coconut milk, pop the lid back on, and shake vigorously. You can then use a spoon or knife to scrape the remainder off the sides of the jar. Also, check out my Peanut Butter Jar Latte (page 294).

MAKES 6 servings ✦ **START TO FINISH:** 25 minutes

1 red bell pepper, seeded and sliced

1 red onion, diced finely

4 garlic cloves, minced

1 (1-inch) piece fresh ginger, minced

1½ cups vegetable broth

2 tablespoons Thai red curry paste

¼ teaspoon ground turmeric

2 tablespoons soy sauce

1 (15-ounce) can chickpeas, drained and rinsed, or 1½ cups homemade

1 (13.5-ounce) can full-fat coconut milk

3 tablespoons peanut butter, tahini, almond butter, or Wowbutter

1½ cups green peas

Juice of 1 lime

2 handfuls of spinach

FOR SERVING

Cooked rice or the Knead for Flatbread (page 68) or other vegan flatbread

Crushed peanuts and minced fresh cilantro, for garnish

1. In a large saucepan over medium heat, combine the red pepper, red onion, garlic, ginger, and 2 tablespoons of the vegetable broth. Sauté until the onion becomes translucent, about 3 minutes.

2. Stir in the red curry paste, turmeric, and soy sauce. Toss until fragrant, about 2 minutes.

3. Add the chickpeas, remaining vegetable broth, coconut milk, and peanut butter. Stir, bring to a boil, and then simmer for 5 minutes. Add the green peas, lime juice, and spinach. Stir until the peas have thawed and the spinach has wilted, about 2 minutes.

4. Serve with rice, garnished with crushed peanuts and cilantro.

Storage: Store in the fridge for up to 4 days, or freeze for up to 2 months.

Save the Scraps: Onion peels for Onion Peel Powder (page 336), Scrappy Broth (page 102), or Bouilliant Bouillon Powder (page 336). Aquafaba (chickpea water) for Mousse on the Loose (page 264) or Mini Aquafaba Pavlovas (page 266). Leftover coconut milk for Coo-Coo for Coconut Caramel (page 260) or Firecracker Tofu with Coconut Rice (page 184).

RED BELL PEPPER

RED ONION

GARLIC

GINGER ROOT

VEGETABLE BROTH

RED CURRY PASTE

TURMERIC

SOY SAUCE

CHICKPEAS

COCONUT MILK

PEANUT BUTTER

GREEN PEAS

LIME

SPINACH

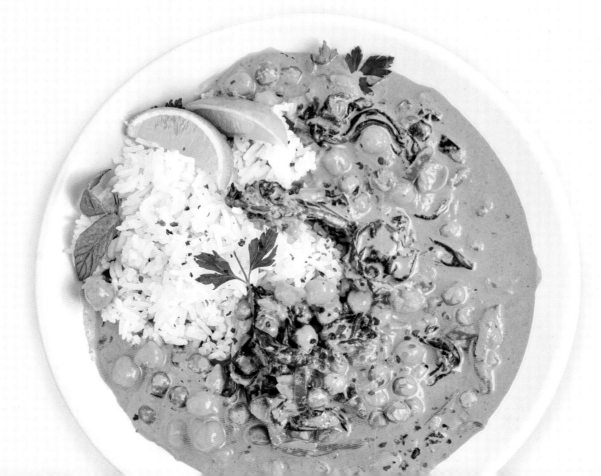

Palak "Paneer"

Oops, you did it again. That spinach you bought at the grocery store on Monday sits neglected, sobbing and wilting in the back of your fridge. And now it's the weekend! Time to give it a little love—and yourself, too—with this fragrant palak "paneer" inspired by the traditional Indian curry. We'll use the entire package of spinach (no neglect there!), along with the pulp (optional) from my Juicer-Free Green Juice. Too much flavor and nutrition? Nah . . . is that even possible?!

MAKES 4 servings ◆ **START TO FINISH:** 30 minutes

1 (14-ounce) block extra-firm tofu

Salt and freshly ground black pepper

1 yellow onion, diced

1 (1-inch) piece fresh ginger, minced

1 tomato, diced finely

3 garlic cloves, diced

1 teaspoon ground cumin

1½ tablespoons garam masala

¼ teaspoon ground turmeric

¼ teaspoon cayenne pepper (optional, for an extra kick)

¾ cup water

6 cups spinach (a scant 6 ounces)

1 cup green juice pulp from my Juicer-Free Green Juice (page 52; optional)

½ cup full-fat coconut milk or Sunflower Cream Sauce (page 272)

FOR SERVING

Cooked rice or the Knead for Flatbread (page 68) or other vegan flatbread

1. Preheat the oven to 400°F, and line a baking sheet with a reusable baking mat or parchment paper.

2. Slice the tofu into 1-inch cubes, transfer to the prepared baking sheet, and sprinkle with salt and black pepper. Bake for 20 minutes, flipping halfway through.

3. In a large skillet over medium heat, combine the onion, ginger, and tomato. Cook until the tomatoes are softened, and mash with the back of a spatula until smooth.

4. Add the garlic, cumin, garam masala, turmeric, and cayenne (if using), and sauté until fragrant, about 2 minutes. Add the water and bring to a boil.

5. Add the spinach and juice pulp to the pan, and simmer. Cover with the lid and steam for 3 to 4 minutes, or until the spinach is wilted and bright green.

6. When safe to handle, transfer the contents of the skillet into a high-speed blender and blend until smooth. Once smooth, pour back into the pan. Stir in the coconut milk and tofu.

7. Serve over rice or with vegan flatbread.

Storage: Store in a sealed container in the fridge for up to 5 days, or in the freezer for 3 months.

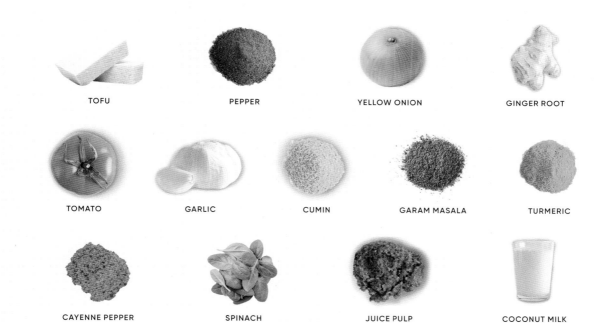

TOFU

PEPPER

YELLOW ONION

GINGER ROOT

TOMATO

GARLIC

CUMIN

GARAM MASALA

TURMERIC

CAYENNE PEPPER

SPINACH

JUICE PULP

COCONUT MILK

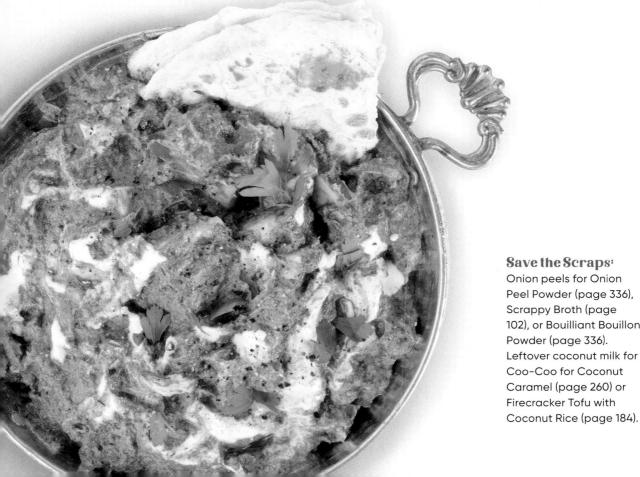

Save the Scraps:
Onion peels for Onion Peel Powder (page 336), Scrappy Broth (page 102), or Bouilliant Bouillon Powder (page 336). Leftover coconut milk for Coo-Coo for Coconut Caramel (page 260) or Firecracker Tofu with Coconut Rice (page 184).

Golden Immunity Stew

This wonder will have you glowing from the inside out. It's packed to the brim with such anti-inflammatory ingredients as turmeric, ginger, and cayenne pepper, along with fiber and protein from wild rice and lentils, for a rich, aromatic broth. So grab your favorite pot and let's simmer up a stew that's as comforting as it is nutritious.

MAKES 4 servings ✦ **START TO FINISH:** 40 minutes

1 medium-size yellow onion, diced

2 medium-size sweet potatoes, diced

1 medium-size carrot, diced

2 tablespoons water

½ teaspoon salt

½ teaspoon ground turmeric

¼ teaspoon cayenne pepper

½ teaspoon ground cumin

1 (1-inch) piece fresh ginger, minced

½ cup uncooked wild rice blend, brown rice, or quinoa, rinsed

¼ cup dried brown lentils

5 cups vegetable broth

1½ cups soy milk or 1 (13.5-ounce) can full-fat coconut milk

2 garlic cloves, minced

Juice of 1 lemon

2 cups roughly chopped kale

FOR SERVING

Red pepper flakes, fresh cilantro, black pepper, and more lemon juice, as desired

1. In a large pot over medium heat, combine the onion, sweet potato, carrot, and water. Sauté until slightly softened, about 5 minutes.

2. Add the salt, turmeric, cayenne, cumin, and ginger. Stir until the vegetables are coated, and then pour in the wild rice blend and lentils. Cook for 2 to 3 more minutes.

3. Now, add the vegetable broth and milk. Stir, then bring the soup to a boil. Cover and simmer for 35 minutes, or until the rice, lentils, and vegetables are fully cooked.

4. Stir in the garlic and lemon juice, then the kale, and simmer until the kale is wilted, about 4 minutes. Taste and adjust the seasonings as needed.

5. Serve with red pepper flakes, cilantro, black pepper, and more lemon juice, as desired.

Storage: Store in the fridge for up to 4 days, or freeze for up to 2 months.

Save the Scraps: Onion peels for Onion Peel Powder (page 336), Scrappy Broth (page 102), or Bouilliant Bouillon Powder (page 336). Carrot tops for the Carrot Top Chimichurri (page 272). Extra quinoa for Leftover Quinoa Truffles (page 248). Leftover coconut milk for Coo-Coo for Coconut Caramel (page 260) or Firecracker Tofu with Coconut Rice (page 184). Lemon peels for Candied Citrus Peels (page 254) or Citrus Peel Powder (page 332).

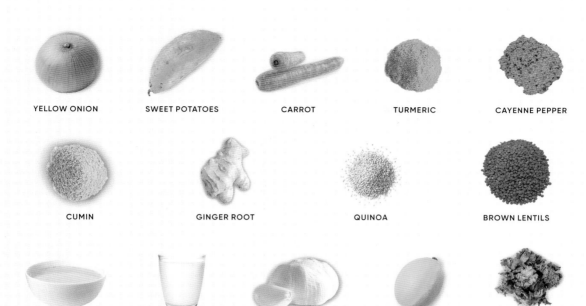

YELLOW ONION   SWEET POTATOES   CARROT   TURMERIC   CAYENNE PEPPER

CUMIN   GINGER ROOT   QUINOA   BROWN LENTILS

VEGETABLE BROTH   SOY MILK   GARLIC   LEMON   KALE

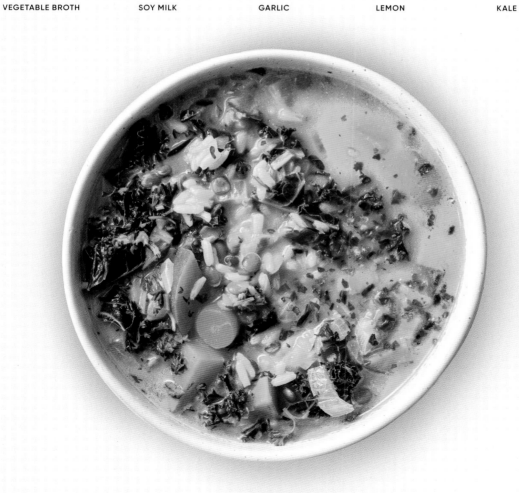

Spicy Eggplant & White Bean Stew

Like most great recipes, inspiration for this stew came from my fridge and pantry. It was the end of the week, and I had a single eggplant, a package of bell peppers, harissa paste, and a can of crushed tomatoes waiting to be used up before my next grocery excursion. I threw everything in a pot and hoped for the best. The result was—well—spectacular!

MAKES 6 servings ✦ **START TO FINISH:** 35 minutes

2 cups + 1 tablespoon vegetable broth or extra-virgin olive oil

3 garlic cloves, minced

1 red onion, minced

2 red bell peppers, seeded and chopped

2½ cups chopped eggplant (from ½ large eggplant or 1 small)

¼ teaspoon salt

1 tablespoon tomato paste

2½ tablespoons harissa paste, sriracha, or chili paste

½ teaspoon paprika

2 cups cherry tomatoes

1 (15-ounce) can white beans, drained and rinsed

1 (28-ounce) can crushed tomatoes

1 tablespoon pure maple syrup

Handful of kale, spinach, or chard, chopped

Juice of ½ lemon

FOR SERVING

Unsweetened Cultured Vegan Yogurt (page 48) or store-bought vegan yogurt, and crusty vegan bread, as desired

1. In a large skillet over medium heat, combine the tablespoon of vegetable broth, garlic, red onion, bell peppers, eggplant, and salt. Sauté until softened, about 8 minutes. Stir in the tomato paste, harissa paste, and paprika. Toss to coat the vegetables.

2. Add the cherry tomatoes and white beans. Stir until coated, then sauté for 3 minutes, or until the cherry tomatoes are soft.

3. Add the remaining 2 cups of vegetable broth, crushed tomatoes, and maple syrup. Bring the stew to a boil, then simmer for 15 minutes, or until everything is cooked through and combined.

4. Finish with the handful of chopped leafy greens and a squeeze of lemon. Serve with vegan yogurt and crusty vegan bread, as desired.

Storage: Store in a sealed container in the fridge for up to 4 days or freeze for up to 2 months.

Save the Scraps: Onion peels for Onion Peel Powder (page 336), Scrappy Broth (page 102), or Bouilliant Bouillon Powder (page 336). Lemon peels for Candied Citrus Peels (page 254) or Citrus Peel Powder (page 332).

VEGETABLE BROTH

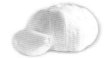

GARLIC

RED ONION

RED BELL PEPPER

EGGPLANT

TOMATO PASTE

HARISSA PASTE

PAPRIKA

CHERRY TOMATOES

WHITE BEANS

CRUSHED TOMATOES

MAPLE SYRUP

KALE

LEMON

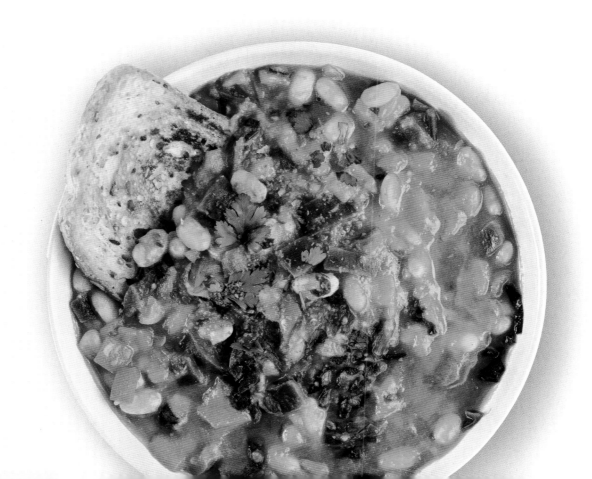

What a Dahl!

Lentils are fantastic not only for our health but Planet Earth as well. They improve soil quality by pulling life-giving nitrogen from the air and returning it to the earth. Lentils are also a drought-resistant crop because they require less water to grow compared to other protein sources and need no chemical fertilizers. There's no better way to celebrate the humble lentil than with an Indian-inspired dahl. Ready in one pot, this quick-and-easy red lentil dahl is a favorite weeknight meal that can utilize just about any vegetable from your fridge or pantry.

MAKES 4 servings ◆ **START TO FINISH:** 35 minutes

1 onion, chopped

1 large sweet potato, chopped (about 3 cups)

2 tablespoons tomato paste

4 Roma tomatoes, chopped

½ teaspoon salt

1 to 2 tablespoons water or extra-virgin olive oil

1 (1-inch) piece fresh ginger, minced

3 garlic cloves, minced

1 tablespoon garam masala

2 teaspoons ground cumin

1 teaspoon ground turmeric

2 teaspoons vegan granulated sugar or pure maple syrup

1 cup dried red lentils

3 cups vegetable broth

1 (13.5-ounce) can full-fat coconut milk or soy milk (about 1½ cups)

2 cups chopped kale

Juice of ½ lemon

FOR SERVING

Rice or vegan flatbread, such as the Knead for Flatbread (page 68)

Red pepper flakes, fresh cilantro, Spicy Pickled Red Onions (page 342), unsweetened Cultured Vegan Yogurt (page 48) or store-bought unsweetened vegan yogurt, for garnish

1. In a large saucepan over medium heat, combine the onion, sweet potato, tomato paste, chopped tomatoes, salt, and water. Sauté until softened, about 10 minutes.

2. Add the ginger, garlic, garam masala, cumin, turmeric, sugar, and red lentils to the pan, and stir until everything is evenly coated in the spices.

3. Add the vegetable broth, coconut milk, kale, and lemon juice. Bring to a boil, then simmer, covered, for 40 minutes, or until the red lentils are cooked and the mixture is thick.

4. Enjoy with rice or vegan flatbread, garnished with red pepper flakes, cilantro, pickled onions, and vegan yogurt, as desired.

Storage: Store in a sealed container in the fridge for up to 4 days, or freeze for up to 2 months.

Save the Scraps: Onion peels for Onion Peel Powder (page 336), Scrappy Broth (page 102), or Bouilliant Bouillon Powder (page 336). Lemon peels for Candied Citrus Peels (page 254) or Citrus Peel Powder (page 332). Leftover coconut milk for Coo-Coo for Coconut Caramel (page 260) or Firecracker Tofu with Coconut Rice (page 184).

YELLOW ONION

SWEET POTATOES

TOMATO PASTE

ROMA TOMATOES

GINGER ROOT

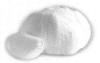

GARLIC

GARAM MASALA

CUMIN

TURMERIC

BROWN SUGAR

RED LENTILS

VEGETABLE BROTH

COCONUT MILK

KALE

LEMON

Eco Entrées

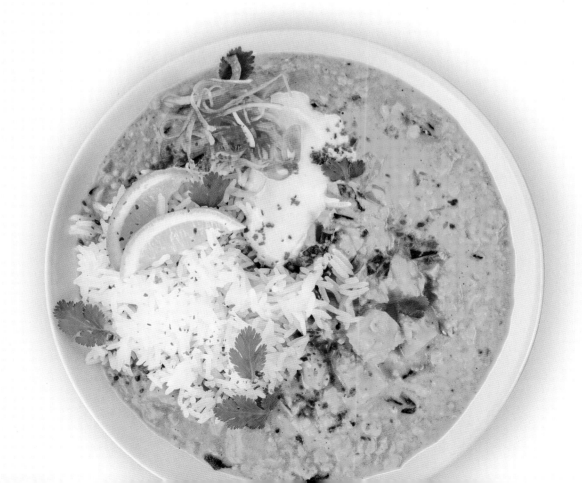

Jackfruit Bourguignon

If you've never tried cooked jackfruit before, you'll be shocked by its similarity in texture and flavor to meat. The key to preparing a great jackfruit recipe is purchasing canned, young green jackfruit in water or brine (not syrup); I recommend using canned here rather than the massive fruit you might have come across at Asian grocers. If you can't track down jackfruit, this delicious meatless bourguignon can easily be made with oyster mushrooms or even a can of drained and rinsed lentils!

MAKES 6 servings ✦ **START TO FINISH:** 60 minutes

1 yellow onion, sliced into chunks

4 garlic cloves, diced

2 tablespoons water

1 (13-ounce) can jackfruit, drained, rinsed, and shredded with a fork; 1½ cups oyster mushrooms, shredded; or 1½ cups cooked brown lentils, drained and rinsed

1 teaspoon freshly ground black pepper

2 tablespoons balsamic vinegar

1½ tablespoons tomato paste

1 tablespoon soy sauce or gluten-free tamari

1 teaspoon paprika

2 tablespoons nutritional yeast

2 medium-size carrots, chopped

3 Yukon Gold potatoes, chopped into 1-inch chunks

1 celery rib, diced

¼ cup all-purpose or gluten-free flour

3 cups vegetable broth

1 cup red wine (or an additional cup vegetable broth)

1 cup green peas

2 cups chopped spinach

Leaves from 1 thyme sprig

1 teaspoon vegan granulated sugar (optional)

FOR SERVING (OPTIONAL)

Vegan mashed potatoes

1. In a large pot over medium heat, combine the onion, garlic, and water. Sauté until the onion is translucent, for 3 to 5 minutes.

2. Add the shredded jackfruit to the pot, along with the pepper, balsamic vinegar, tomato paste, soy sauce, paprika, and nutritional yeast. Stir until the jackfruit, onion, and garlic are completely coated in the mixture.

3. Add the carrots, potatoes, and celery. Stir, then sauté for 5 minutes, or until slightly cooked. Add the flour and stir again until evenly dispersed.

4. Pour in the vegetable broth and red wine. Bring the mixture to a boil, then simmer for 30 minutes, or until the potatoes and carrots are cooked and the mixture has reduced to a slightly thick stew.

5. Stir in the green peas, spinach, thyme, and sugar, if using. Taste and adjust the salt and sweetness as needed.

6. Serve over vegan mashed potatoes or on its own, as desired.

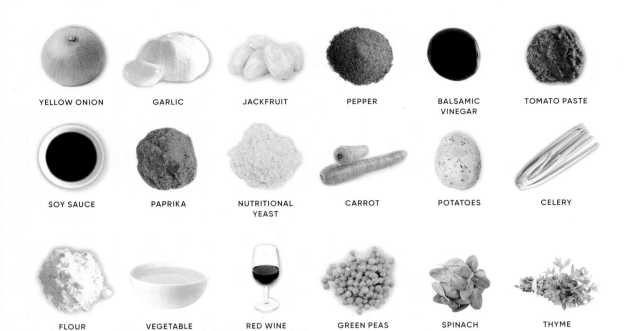

YELLOW ONION

GARLIC

JACKFRUIT

PEPPER

BALSAMIC VINEGAR

TOMATO PASTE

SOY SAUCE

PAPRIKA

NUTRITIONAL YEAST

CARROT

POTATOES

CELERY

FLOUR

VEGETABLE BROTH

RED WINE

GREEN PEAS

SPINACH

THYME

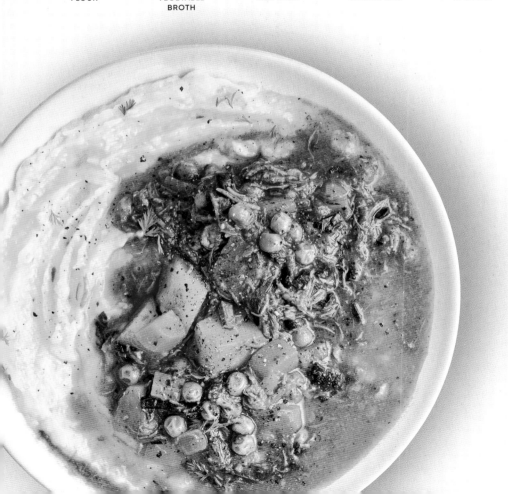

Storage: Store in a sealed container in the fridge for up to 4 days or freeze for up to 2 months.

Save the Scraps: Onion peels for Onion Peel Powder (page 336), Scrappy Broth (page 102), or Bouilliant Bouillon Powder (page 336). Carrot tops for the Carrot Top Chimichurri (page 272).

Stuffed Cabbage Dumplings

Got a cabbage playing hide-and-seek in the back of the fridge? No prob. A cross between a cabbage roll and a dumpling, this recipe is an excellent way to use up the tired leaves of that elusive cabbage. Here, carrot, tofu, ginger, and rice are tightly nestled and steamed in the leaves of a napa cabbage, then smothered in a sweet chili sauce. Yes, it tastes as good as it sounds.

MAKES 4 servings ✦ **START TO FINISH:** 40 minutes

8 leaves napa, purple, or green cabbage *(napa is easiest to roll)*

FILLING

1 carrot, grated

½ (14-ounce) block tofu, grated; ½ (14-ounce) block tempeh, crumbled; or ½ cup additional cooked rice

1 (1-inch) piece fresh ginger, minced

2 garlic cloves, minced

2 green onions, chopped

½ cup chopped cremini mushrooms or ½ cup chopped yellow onion

1 cup cooked white rice

2 tablespoons soy sauce

1 teaspoon rice vinegar

1 tablespoon extra-virgin olive oil, for panfrying

DIPPING SAUCE

¼ cup soy sauce

2 tablespoons sweet chili sauce

1 tablespoon hoisin sauce

1. In a large skillet over medium heat, combine all the filling ingredients and sauté until the carrot and mushrooms are cooked, about 5 minutes.

2. Blanch the cabbage leaves in boiling water until they begin to wilt, about 20 seconds. Remove and set on a cutting board.

3. Place one-eighth of the filling into each cabbage leaf. Wrap as you would a burrito, folding in the sides and then rolling over itself. Steam for 10 minutes, or alternatively panfry in oil on each side over medium heat, for 1 to 2 minutes, or until slightly browned.

4. Make the dipping sauce: In a jar or other container, mix together the dipping sauce ingredients until combined.

Storage: Store in a sealed container in the fridge for up to 3 days.

Save the Scraps: Onion peels for Onion Peel Powder (page 336), Scrappy Broth (page 102), or Bouilliant Bouillon Powder (page 336). Carrot tops for the Carrot Top Chimichurri (page 272).

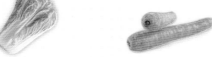

NAPA CABBAGE

CARROT

TOFU

GINGER ROOT

GARLIC

GREEN ONIONS

CREMINI MUSHROOMS

JASMINE RICE

SOY SAUCE

RICE VINEGAR

SWEET CHILI SAUCE

HOISIN SAUCE

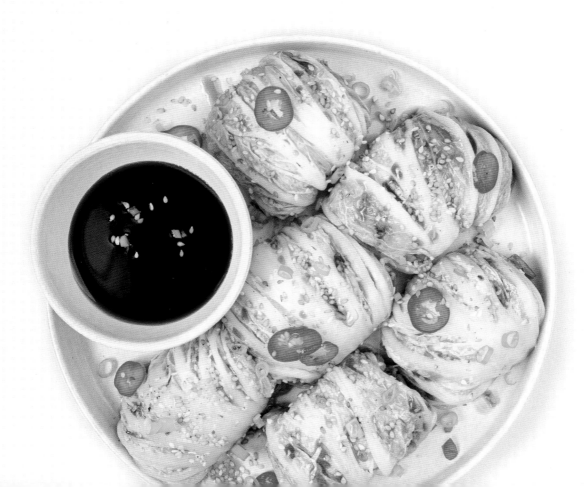

Can't-Miss Miso Cabbage Steaks

Move over cauliflower, there's a new plant steak in town. Whenever I buy cabbage, I'm never able to use the whole thing in one go—and this recipe is the perfect solution. Thick slices of cabbage are smothered in a tahini miso sauce, then roasted until they melt in your mouth.

MAKES 4 servings ✦ **START TO FINISH:** 45 minutes

½ cup uncooked quinoa, rice, or grain of choice

CABBAGE STEAKS

½ to 1 whole medium-size green or red cabbage

2 tablespoons vegetable broth or extra-virgin olive oil, for baking steaks

Salt and freshly ground black pepper

SAUCE

¼ cup tahini, almond butter, or peanut butter

2 teaspoons chili garlic sauce

2 tablespoons yellow or red miso paste, or soy sauce

1 tablespoon pure maple syrup

2 to 4 tablespoons vegetable broth

BUTTER BEANS (OPTIONAL)

1 (15-ounce) can butter beans, drained and rinsed, or 1½ cups homemade

1 tablespoon yellow or red miso paste, or soy sauce

1 teaspoon chili garlic sauce

1 tablespoon pure maple syrup

1½ teaspoons paprika

FOR SERVING

1 tablespoon Balsamic Glaze (page 290)

½ cup chopped fresh parsley

¼ cup peanuts, crushed (optional)

1. Cook the quinoa according to the package directions, then set aside.

2. Make the cabbage steaks: Preheat the oven to 400°F, and line two baking sheets with reusable baking mats or parchment paper.

3. Slice the cabbage into 1-inch steaks or quarters, and place on one of the prepared baking sheets. Spritz with 2 tablespoons of vegetable broth so the surface of the steaks is slightly moist. Season with salt and black pepper. Bake for 20 minutes.

4. While the steaks bake, make the sauce: In a small bowl, combine the tahini, chili garlic sauce, miso paste, maple syrup, plus vegetable broth to thin. Set aside.

5. Prepare the butter beans now (if using): Place the butter beans in a bowl. Add the miso paste, chili garlic sauce, maple syrup, and paprika. Toss, then transfer to the second prepared baking sheet; don't place in the oven yet.

6. Once the cabbage steaks are baked and out of the oven, use a barbecue brush or spoon to cover both sides with the tahini-miso sauce. Place them back in the oven for another 20 minutes, along with the baking sheet of butter beans.

7. Once the cabbage and butter beans are cooked, plate over the cooked quinoa, garnished with Balsamic Glaze, parsley, and crushed peanuts, as desired.

QUINOA

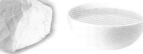
CABBAGE

VEGETABLE
BROTH

TAHINI

GARLIC CHILI
SAUCE

MISO PASTE

MAPLE SYRUP

BUTTER BEANS (OPTIONAL): BUTTER BEANS, MISO PASTE,
CHILI GARLIC SAUCE, MAPLE SYRUP, PAPRIKA

  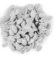

FOR SERVING: BALSAMIC GLAZE, PARSLEY, PEANUTS

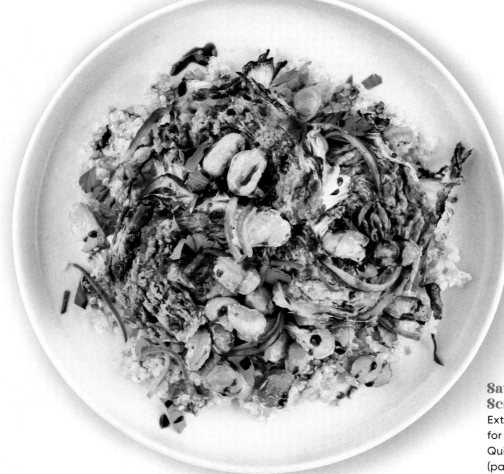

**Save the
Scraps:**
Extra quinoa
for Leftover
Quinoa Truffles
(page 248).

Bang-Bang Broccoli-cious Steaks

This dish takes broccoli to new heights. Crispy on the outside, tender on the inside, drizzled with the most incredible tahini bang-bang sauce. You'll want to lick the plate!

MAKES 6 servings ✦ START TO FINISH: 45 minutes

BROCCOLI

3 whole heads broccoli, stems intact

1½ cups Herbed Bread Crumbs (page 330) or store-bought vegan seasoned bread crumbs, regular or gluten-free

Sea salt

BANG-BANG SAUCE

½ cup tahini

2 tablespoons soy sauce or gluten-free tamari

2 tablespoons rice vinegar

2 tablespoons chili garlic sauce or sriracha

2 tablespoons pure maple syrup

3 tablespoons water, or more to thin

FOR SERVING

Red pepper flakes and more vegan bread crumbs, as desired

1. Make the broccoli: Preheat the oven to 400°F, and line a baking sheet with a reusable baking mat or parchment paper.

2. Bring a large pot of water to a boil. Peel the stems off the broccoli until the tender inner layer remains, then slice the broccoli in half carefully to create two steaks for each head.

3. Add the broccoli steaks to the boiling water and boil for 7 minutes, or until half cooked. Safely remove with a pair of tongs. Spread half the bread crumbs on a plate and dip the boiled broccoli into the crumbs until lightly coated on each side. Lay the broccoli steaks on the prepared baking sheet and sprinkle with the salt. Bake the broccoli in the oven for 20 minutes, flipping halfway through.

4. Meanwhile, prepare the bang-bang sauce: In a jar, combine the tahini, soy sauce, rice vinegar, red chili garlic sauce, maple syrup, and water and mix until smooth. Plate ¼ cup of the sauce, followed by the broccoli steaks, red pepper flakes, more bread crumbs, and a drizzle more of the sauce.

5. Serve as a side dish or with rice and lentils or pasta for a full meal.

Storage: Store in an airtight container in the fridge for up to 3 days.

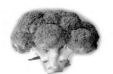

BROCCOLI

HERBED BREAD CRUMBS

TAHINI

SOY SAUCE

RICE VINEGAR

CHILI GARLIC SAUCE

MAPLE SYRUP

RED PEPPER FLAKES

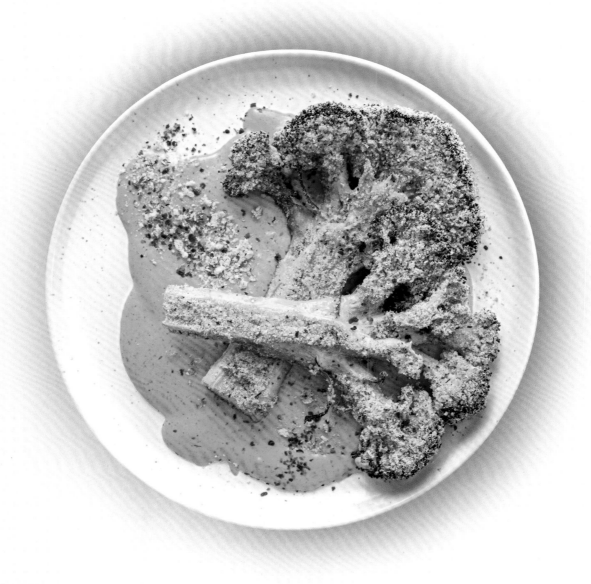

Whole Roasted Cauliflower

Place this whole roasted cauliflower in the center of your table and watch as your guests' eyes widen with anticipation. Not only is it a visual showstopper, this cauliflower tastes out-of-this-world delicious with an herby golden crust and tender juicy florets on the inside. Enjoy it with rice and brown lentils for a well-rounded plant-based culinary affair.

MAKES 4 servings   ✦   **START TO FINISH:** 45 minutes

1 cup uncooked jasmine rice

½ cup dried brown lentils

3 cups water

1 medium cauliflower head

RUB

¾ cup unsweetened Cultured Vegan Yogurt (page 48) or store-bought plant-based yogurt

¼ cup vegetable broth

1 tablespoon ground dried parsley

1½ teaspoons paprika

1 teaspoon salt

¼ teaspoon ground turmeric

FOR SERVING

1½ cups Roasted Red Pepper Sauce (page 276) or Everything Tahini Dressing (page 278)

Fresh parsley or cilantro, for garnish

1. Make the rice and lentils: Rinse the rice and lentils until the water is clear. Place in a large pot with the fresh water. Bring to a boil, then simmer, covered, for 30 to 40 minutes, or until cooked.

2. Preheat the oven to 400°F.

3. Remove the stems from the cauliflower head and set them aside. Fill a large pot with water, bring to a boil, and place the entire cauliflower head in the boiling water for 12 minutes, until tender.

4. Meanwhile, combine the rub ingredients in a bowl and mix until smooth.

5. Drain the cauliflower water. Place the cauliflower, along with the stems, in a casserole or roasting pan and pour the rub ingredients over all, using a barbecue brush to ensure it covers the surface of the cauliflower. Roast in the oven for 30 minutes, or until cooked through.

6. While the cauliflower is roasting, prepare your serving of choice, either Roasted Red Pepper Sauce (page 276) or Everything Tahini Dressing (page 278).

7. Once cooked, remove the cauliflower and stems from the oven and place on a serving platter with the cooked rice and lentils underneath. Pour the sauce over the top and serve immediately, garnished with parsley.

JASMINE RICE

BROWN LENTILS

CAULIFLOWER

YOGURT

VEGETABLE BROTH

DRIED PARSLEY

PAPRIKA

TURMERIC

ROASTED RED PEPPER
SAUCE

Eco Entrées

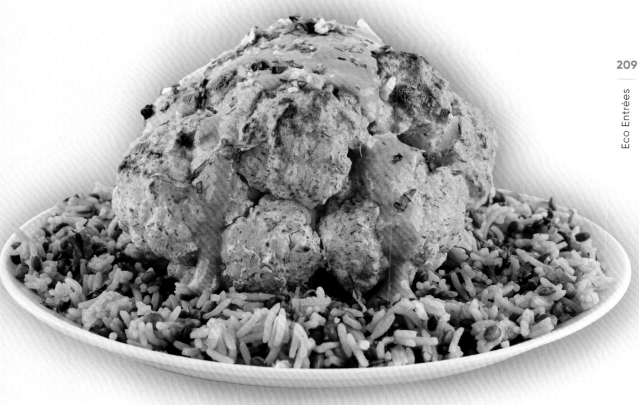

Confetti Sheet-Pan Tacos

Bright and bursting with flavor, these confetti sheet-pan tacos are a weeknight showstopper. Sweet potato, corn, bell pepper, and cauliflower (*or, seriously, whatever veggie you have kicking around in your fridge*) are thrown onto a baking sheet with a bold taco seasoning and roasted to perfection. While you wait, you can whip up a batch of Carrot Top Chimichurri to take these tacos to the next level.

MAKES 4 to 6 servings, 12 tacos ✦ **START TO FINISH:** 45 minutes

TACOS

2 medium-size sweet potatoes, cubed, or potato of choice

1½ cups corn, frozen and thawed or fresh

1 bell pepper, seeded and sliced into strips

1 small head cauliflower, broken into florets, leaves sliced into ½-inch bites, or broccoli florets

2 teaspoons chili powder

2 teaspoons paprika

1 teaspoon ground cumin

1 teaspoon garlic powder

½ teaspoon salt

12 tortillas, It's a (Flax) Wrap (page 70) or pita bread, to serve as tacos

1½ cups Carrot Top Chimichurri (page 272; optional)

½ cup Sunflower Cream Sauce (page 272) or store-bought vegan sour cream

TACO TOPPINGS (OPTIONAL)

Tomatoes

Red cabbage

Fresh cilantro

Red onion

Eco Entrées

1. Preheat the oven to 425°F, and line a baking sheet with a reusable baking mat or parchment paper.

2. Place the sweet potatoes, corn, bell pepper, cauliflower, and leaves in a bowl, along with the chili powder, paprika, cumin, garlic powder, and salt. Toss until coated.

3. Transfer to the prepared baking sheet and bake for 35 minutes until the corn, cauliflower, and sweet potatoes are starting to char, tossing halfway through.

4. While the vegetables bake, prepare your sauces, if using, including the Carrot Top Chimichurri and Sunflower Cream Sauce.

5. Assemble the tacos: Place the vegetable mixture in the center of each wrap, followed by 2 teaspoons of chimichurri sauce (if using), and a tablespoon of the Sunflower Cream Sauce. Finish with your desired toppings.

Storage: Store the taco filling in a sealed container in the fridge for up to 4 days, or freeze for up to 2 months.

Save the Scraps: Onion peels for Onion Peel Powder (page 336), Scrappy Broth (page 102), or Bouilliant Bouillon Powder (page 336).

SWEET POTATOES

CORN KERNELS

RED BELL PEPPER

CAULIFLOWER

CHILI POWDER

PAPRIKA

CUMIN

GARLIC POWDER

TORTILLAS

CARROT TOP
CHIMICHURRI

SUNFLOWER
CREAM SAUCE

FOR SERVING: TOMATOES. RED CABBAGE, CILANTRO, RED ONION

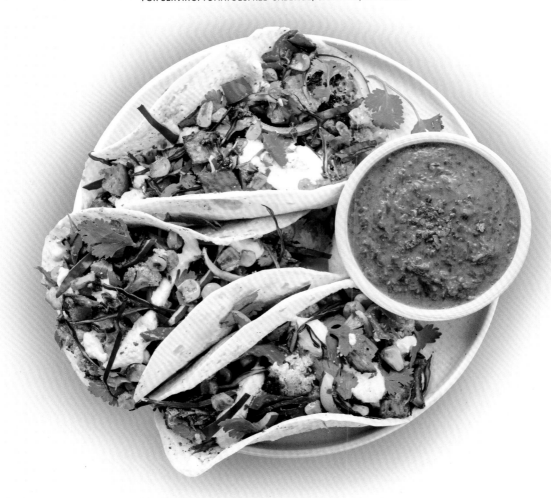

Chickpea Potpie

Time to break out those stretchy pants. Comfort food just got a plant-based upgrade with this mouthwatering potpie recipe, stacked with cornmeal drop dumplings.

MAKES 6 servings ✦ **START TO FINISH:** 60 minutes

1 yellow onion, diced

2 garlic cloves, minced

1 tablespoon water

1 thyme sprig

½ teaspoon dried sage

½ teaspoon ground turmeric

1 tablespoon nutritional yeast

½ teaspoon salt

1 Yukon Gold potato, chopped

2 celery ribs, diced

1 medium-size carrot, diced

¼ cup all-purpose or gluten-free flour

3½ cups vegetable broth

¼ cup unsweetened plant-based milk (soy, almond, cashew, or oat)

1 (15-ounce) can chickpeas, drained

½ cup peas, frozen and thawed

1 tablespoon cornstarch or arrowroot

2 tablespoons water

CORNMEAL DROP DUMPLINGS (YOU CAN MAKE SEPARATE FROM THE PIE; SEE PAGE 74)

1 cup cornmeal or all-purpose flour

1 cup all-purpose flour or gluten-free flour

3 tablespoons nutritional yeast

2 teaspoons dried parsley

¼ teaspoon garlic powder

2½ teaspoons baking powder

½ teaspoon salt

2 teaspoons Apple Scrap Vinegar (page 350) or store-bought apple cider vinegar

1 cup + 1 tablespoon full-fat coconut milk

1. Preheat the oven to 375°F.

2. In a large, oven-safe skillet (such as cast iron or Dutch oven) over medium heat, combine the onion, garlic, and water. Sauté until the onion is translucent, about 3 minutes. Add the thyme, sage, turmeric, nutritional yeast, salt, potato, celery, and carrot, and sauté for an additional 5 to 7 minutes, or until softened slightly.

3. Add the flour and ½ cup of the vegetable broth, and stir until everything is coated. Now, add the remaining 3 cups of the broth and the plant-based milk. Bring to a boil, then simmer, uncovered, until the vegetables are cooked through, about 20 minutes. Stir in the chickpeas and peas. To thicken your potpie base, combine the cornstarch and water in a small bowl to create a slurry. Pour into the potpie mixture, bring to a boil, then simmer for an additional 2 minutes.

4. Make your dumplings: In a large bowl, combine the dry ingredients. Then pour in the apple scrap vinegar and coconut milk. Gently stir until a dough is formed. Once the potpie filling has finished simmering, drop the dumpling dough 2 tablespoons at a time on top, about 1 inch apart.

5. Transfer to the oven and bake for 20 minutes, or until the dumplings are cooked.

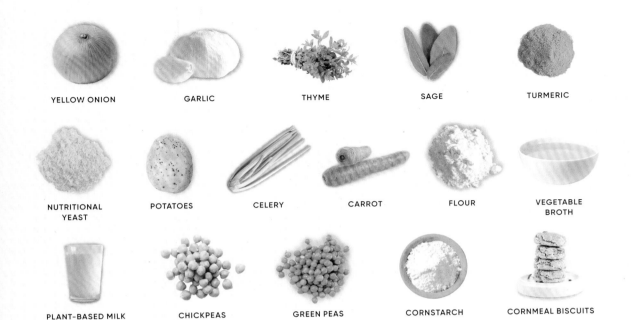

YELLOW ONION

GARLIC

THYME

SAGE

TURMERIC

NUTRITIONAL YEAST

POTATOES

CELERY

CARROT

FLOUR

VEGETABLE BROTH

PLANT-BASED MILK

CHICKPEAS

GREEN PEAS

CORNSTARCH

CORNMEAL BISCUITS

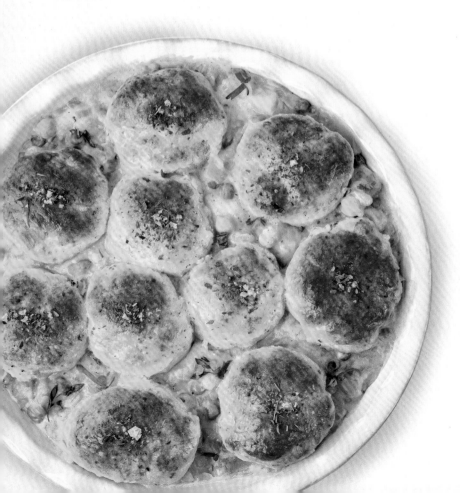

Storage: Store in a sealed container in the fridge for up to 4 days, or freeze for up to 2 months.

Save the Scraps: Onion peels for Onion Peel Powder (page 336), Scrappy Broth (page 102), or Bouilliant Bouillon Powder (page 336). Carrot tops for the Carrot Top Chimichurri (page 272). Leftover coconut milk for Coo-Coo for Coconut Caramel (page 260) or Firecracker Tofu with Coconut Rice (page 184). Aquafaba (chickpea water) for Mousse on the Loose (page 264) or Mini Aquafaba Pavlovas (page 266). Celery leaves in Celery Leaf "Tabbouleh" (page 106) or Scrappy Broth (page 102).

Orange Peel Chick'n

Tender tofu is panfried in a bold and zesty citrus sauce for a recipe that gives takeout a run for its money. To uplevel this dish, make Candied Citrus Peels and dice them up in the sauce for a mouthwatering sweet-and-sour addition.

MAKES 4 servings ✦ **START TO FINISH:** 25 minutes

1 cup uncooked jasmine rice

TOFU

1 (14-ounce) block extra-firm tofu, pressed and torn into 1-inch chunks, or 1 (8-ounce) block tempeh, torn into 1-inch chunks

¼ cup cornstarch or arrowroot powder

¼ teaspoon salt

SAUCE

½ cup freshly squeezed orange juice

2 garlic cloves, minced

1 teaspoon orange zest

½ teaspoon red pepper flakes

1 tablespoon brown sugar

⅓ cup vegetable broth

1½ teaspoons soy sauce

1 tablespoon rice vinegar

1 tablespoon cornstarch or arrowroot powder

¼ cup Candied Citrus Peels (page 254), chopped (optional)

FOR SERVING

Chopped green onions

Sesame seeds

1. Cook the rice according to the package directions.

2. Make the tofu: Preheat the oven to 400°F, and line a baking sheet with a reusable baking mat or parchment paper.

3. In a bowl, combine the tofu chunks with the cornstarch and salt. Arrange in a single layer on the prepared baking sheet and bake for 20 to 25 minutes, or until the tofu is crispy.

4. Meanwhile, combine all the sauce ingredients in a small bowl. Transfer the sauce to a large skillet over medium heat. Bring to a boil and then simmer, stirring often, for 4 to 5 minutes, or until thickened, adding the citrus peels (if using) halfway through.

5. Transfer the baked tofu to the skillet and stir until coated.

6. Serve over rice with chopped green onions and sesame seeds for garnish, as desired.

Storage: Store in a sealed container in the fridge for up to 4 days, or freeze for up to 2 months.

JASMINE RICE

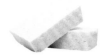
TOFU

CORNSTARCH

ORANGE JUICE

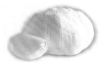
GARLIC

ORANGE ZEST

RED PEPPER FLAKES

BROWN SUGAR

VEGETABLE BROTH

SOY SAUCE

RICE VINEGAR

CANDIED CITRUS PEELS

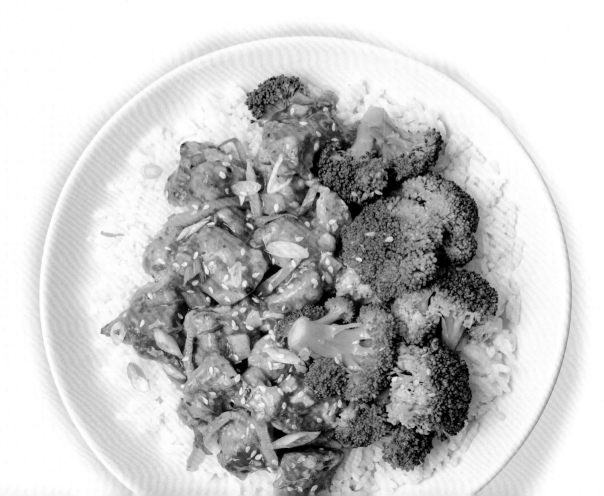

Celeriac Corned "Beef" Sandwich

Celeriac, also known as celery root, ain't much to look at. But when thinly sliced and slow-roasted in a savory sauce, this humble, often overlooked vegetable is transformed into meaty layers of goodness, perfect for a vegan-stacked corned beef sandwich. Try it with my Turmeric Sauerkraut, and don't forget, you can also use those celery leaves with my Celery Leaf "Tabbouleh" (page 106).

MAKES 4 sandwiches ✦ **START TO FINISH:** 2 hours

2 medium-size celeriac roots

MARINADE

1½ cups vegetable broth

¼ cup balsamic vinegar

1 tablespoon Dijon mustard

2 teaspoons smoked paprika

2 teaspoons garlic powder

2 teaspoons onion powder

1 teaspoon freshly ground black pepper

3 tablespoons soy sauce or gluten-free tamari

2 teaspoons tomato paste

FOR SERVING

8 slices vegan rye or gluten-free bread, toasted

¼ cup Turmeric Sauerkraut (page 340)

¼ cup Sunflower Cream Sauce (page 272) or vegan mayonnaise

Quick 'n' Easy Homemade Pickles (page 344) or other pickles of choice

1. Preheat the oven to 350°F.

2. First, prepare the celeriac. Because it's a root vegetable, it tends to be dirty, so give it a good scrub, then slice in half. Then, using a mandoline, if possible, slice the celeriac root into thin ⅛-inch rounds. If you do not have a mandoline, use a sharp knife to slice as thinly as possible.

3. Make the marinade: In a bowl or measuring cup, whisk together the vegetable broth, balsamic vinegar, Dijon mustard, smoked paprika, garlic powder, onion powder, black pepper, soy sauce, and tomato paste. Place the celeriac slices in a 9 x 13–inch casserole dish and pour the sauce over them. Toss until coated entirely.

4. Bake, covered, for 45 minutes, then toss again to ensure the celeriac root is coated. Bake, uncovered, for an additional 45 minutes, or until completely tender.

5. Serve between toasted slices of rye bread with Turmeric Sauerkraut, Sunflower Cream Sauce, and pickles, as desired.

Storage: Store the prepared celeriac root in a sealed container in the fridge for up to 4 days, or freeze for up to 2 months.

CELERIAC

VEGETABLE BROTH

BALSAMIC VINEGAR

DIJON MUSTARD

SMOKED PAPRIKA

GARLIC POWDER

ONION POWDER

SOY SAUCE

TOMATO PASTE

FOR SERVING: RYE BREAD, TURMERIC SAUERKRAUT, SUNFLOWER CREAM SAUCE, PICKLES

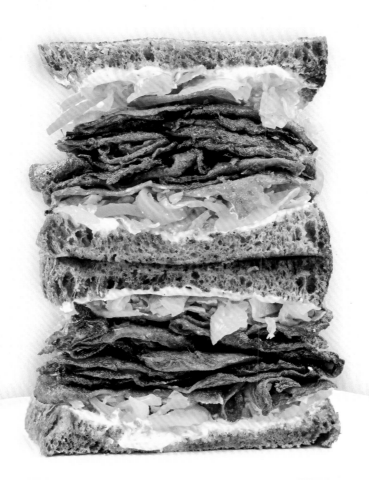

Cuppa Joe Chili

If you have a leftover cup of coffee sitting in the carafe on your countertop, don't toss it—make this delish chili. Java may just be the most secret ingredient for a bold and flavorful bowl of chili. Interestingly, you won't be able to taste the coffee itself when done, but it intensifies the chili flavor beautifully.

MAKES 4 servings ✦ **START TO FINISH:** 45 minutes

1 (5.5-ounce) can tomato paste

1 yellow onion, minced

2 tablespoons water or extra-virgin olive oil

1 (14-ounce) block extra-firm tofu, pressed, or 1½ cups Vegan Ground Beef (page 222)

4 jalapeño peppers or 1 bell pepper, seeded and diced

2½ tablespoons chili powder

2 tablespoons soy sauce or gluten-free tamari

3 tablespoons nutritional yeast

1 teaspoon paprika

½ teaspoon salt

1 tablespoon pure maple syrup, or light or dark brown sugar

4 garlic cloves, minced

1 (15-ounce) can red kidney beans, pinto beans, or black beans, drained and rinsed, or 1½ cups homemade

1 (28-ounce) can crushed tomatoes, or 2 cups tomato sauce

½ to ¾ cup prepared strong black coffee or vegetable broth

1. In a large pot over medium heat, combine the tomato paste and onion with the water. Sauté until the onion is fragrant, about 3 minutes.

2. Meanwhile, grate the tofu or crumble it with the back of a fork.

3. Add the tofu, jalapeño, chili powder, soy sauce, nutritional yeast, paprika, salt, and maple syrup to the pot. Stir until the tofu is covered and browned slightly, about 8 minutes.

4. Add the garlic, beans, crushed tomatoes, and coffee. Bring the mixture to a boil, then simmer, covered, for 15 to 20 minutes. Taste and adjust the seasonings as needed.

Storage: Store in a sealed container in the fridge for up to 4 days, or freeze for up to 2 months.

Save the Scraps: Onion peels for Onion Peel Powder (page 336), Scrappy Broth (page 102), or Bouilliant Bouillon Powder (page 336). Coffee grounds for Common Ground Granola (page 28).

TOMATO PASTE

YELLOW ONION

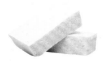

TOFU

JALAPEÑO

CHILI POWDER

SOY SAUCE

NUTRITIONAL YEAST

PAPRIKA

MAPLE SYRUP

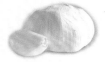

GARLIC

BEAN OF CHOICE

CRUSHED TOMATOES

COFFEE

Eco Entrées

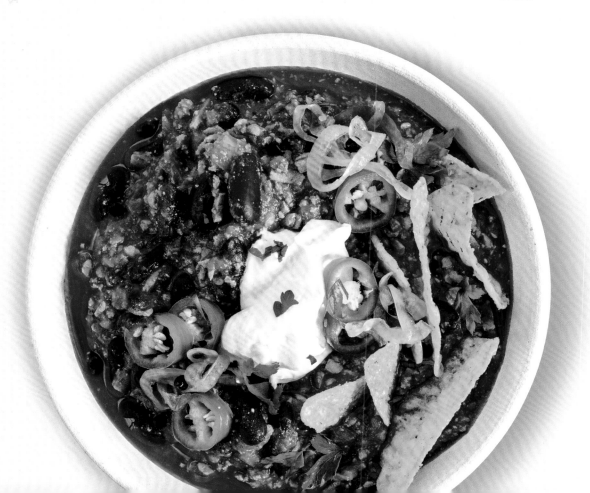

PlantYou Pizza Party

Grab your friends and get ready to chow down on this scrumptious pie. (No cows were harmed in the making of this pizza!) It starts with a two-ingredient pizza dough that takes just 5 minutes to prepare. Top with your favorites, and let's raise a slice to plant-based goodness.

MAKES 4 small pizzas ✦ **START TO FINISH:** 30 minutes

DOUGH

2 cups self-rising flour, or gluten-free self-rising flour, plus more for dusting

1 cup unsweetened Cultured Vegan Yogurt (page 48) or store-bought soy or coconut yogurt

VEGETABLES

1½ cups diced vegetables, such as cherry tomatoes, sun-dried tomatoes, zucchini, bell pepper, onion, and eggplant (I used: ½ cup cherry tomatoes; ½ cup sun-dried tomatoes; 1 red bell pepper, sliced; and ½ yellow onion, sliced)

1 tablespoon water

½ teaspoon dried parsley

½ teaspoon garlic powder

½ teaspoon salt

FOR ASSEMBLY AND SERVING

1 cup Scratch Tomato Sauce (page 164), or store-bought pizza sauce

¼ cup Vegan Nutty "Parm" (page 290)

1 cup fresh basil, chopped finely

1. Preheat the oven to 400°F, and line two baking sheets with reusable baking mats or parchment paper.

2. Make the dough: In a bowl, combine the flour and vegan yogurt with a spoon. It will be clumpy at this point. Transfer to a floured surface and knead with your hands until a dough is formed, about 5 minutes.

3. Slice the dough into four equal pieces. Roll each portion into a 10-inch round for your pizzas.

4. Prepare the vegetables: In a large skillet over medium heat, combine the diced vegetables, water, parsley, garlic powder, and salt. Sauté until the vegetables are softened, about 5 minutes.

5. Top the pizza dough with the tomato sauce, followed by the sautéed vegetables and vegan "Parm."

6. Bake for 15 to 17 minutes, or until the dough is cooked. Serve garnished with the fresh basil, as desired.

Storage: Store in the fridge for up to 4 days.

FLOUR

YOGURT

VEGETABLES OF CHOICE: CHERRY TOMATOES, SUN-DRIED TOMATOES, ZUCCHINI, RED BELL PEPPER, YELLOW ONION, EGGPLANT

DRIED PARSLEY

GARLIC POWDER

TOMATO SAUCE

VEGAN PARM

BASIL

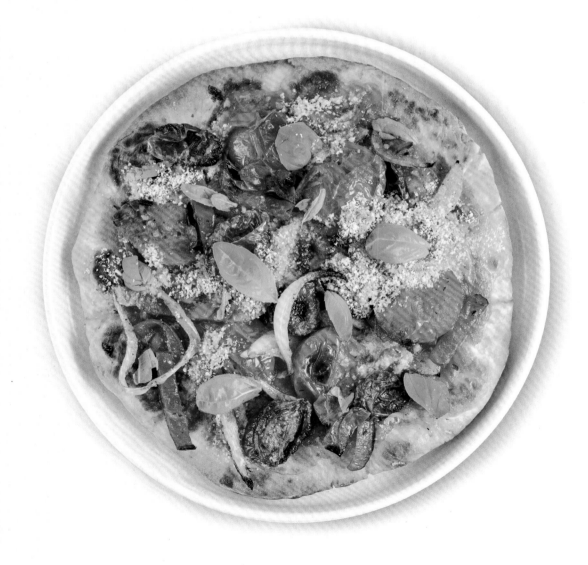

Vegan Ground Beef (Allergy-Friendly)

Move over, meat, there's a new sheriff in town. This vegan ground beef recipe is soy-free, nut-free, gluten-free, and yet unbelievably delicious. As it's made entirely of whole foods, including oats, eggplant, and carrot, you can load this "meat" into wraps. (Check out my A-Better-Burger Wrap, page 114; Fiesta Fries, page 60; or Cuppa Joe Chili, page 218.)

MAKES 8 servings, about 4 cups ✦ **START TO FINISH:** 60 minutes

1 cup raw sunflower seeds

¼ cup water for seed puree

2 tablespoons tomato paste

2 tablespoons ground flaxseed

5 tablespoons warm water for "flax egg"

1 yellow onion, diced

3 garlic cloves, minced

1 cup gluten-free rolled oats

1 cup diced eggplant

1 cup diced carrot

1 tablespoon dried parsley

1 tablespoon chili powder

2 teaspoons paprika

2 tablespoons soy sauce or gluten-free tamari

1. Boil the sunflower seeds in a pot of water for 20 minutes, drain, and transfer to a food processor along with ¼ cup of fresh water and the tomato paste. Puree until the sunflower seeds are broken up. Leave the seeds in the food processor while you prepare your other ingredients.

2. In a small bowl, make a "flax egg" by mixing the ground flaxseed with the warm water. Set aside to gel.

3. Preheat the oven to 375°F, and line a baking sheet with a reusable baking mat or parchment paper.

4. Add the onion, garlic, oats, eggplant, carrot, parsley, chili powder, paprika, and soy sauce to the processor and process (ideally on a "chop" setting) until combined with a ground consistency. Add the flax egg and process again until evenly dispersed.

5. Transfer the mixture to the prepared baking sheet and bake for 25 minutes, tossing halfway. You can broil for an additional 2 minutes if more crispiness is desired.

6. Enjoy straight from the oven.

Storage: Store in a sealed container in the fridge for up to 4 days or freezer for 3 months.

Save the Scraps: Onion peels for Onion Peel Powder (page 336), Scrappy Broth (page 102), or Bouilliant Bouillon Powder (page 336). Carrot tops for the Carrot Top Chimichurri (page 272).

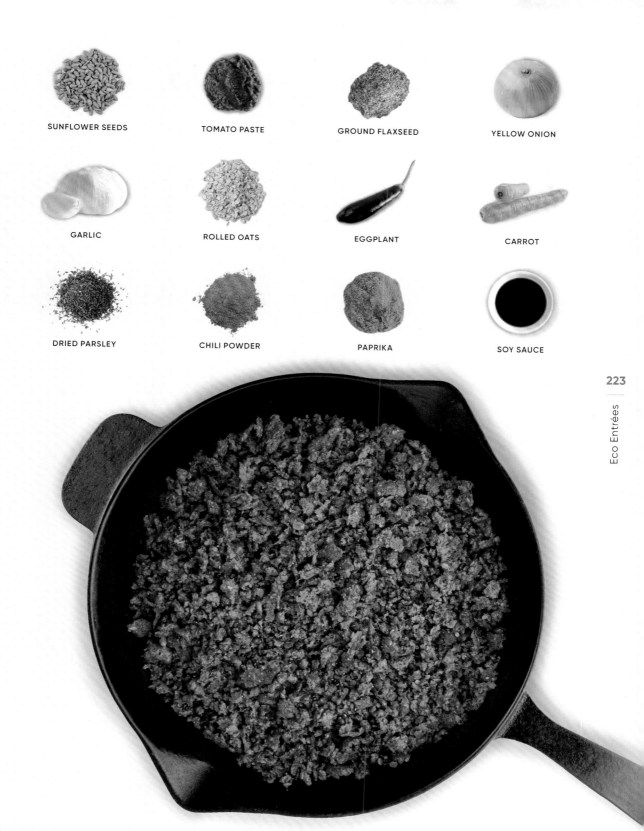

SUNFLOWER SEEDS

TOMATO PASTE

GROUND FLAXSEED

YELLOW ONION

GARLIC

ROLLED OATS

EGGPLANT

CARROT

DRIED PARSLEY

CHILI POWDER

PAPRIKA

SOY SAUCE

Vegan Sticky "Ribs" & Seitan Chick'n

Hold on to your bibs, folks, because these vegan sticky ribs are a full-blown meat rebellion—using vital wheat gluten to create a realistic plant-based substitute that packs a big punch in flavor and protein. My favorite way to eat these? With steamed asparagus and a baked potato for a full, no-meat hearty meal. If you're not into sticky ribs, check out the recipe instructions for how to make these into chick'n bites.

MAKES 12 ribs ◆ **START TO FINISH:** 75 minutes (+ overnight)

1 (15-ounce) can chickpeas or white beans, drained (reserve the liquid) and rinsed

1 cup vegetable broth

2 tablespoons olive oil

2 tablespoons soy sauce or tamari

2 tablespoons nutritional yeast

1 teaspoon garlic powder

1 teaspoon dried thyme

1½ cups vital wheat gluten

All-purpose flour, for dusting

½ cup barbecue sauce

1. In a blender, combine all the ingredients, except the vital wheat gluten, flour, and barbecue sauce. Blend until a liquid is formed.

2. Pour into a bowl, add half the vital wheat gluten, and mix. Pour in the remaining vital wheat gluten and mix again until you have a thick dough.

3. Transfer to a floured surface and knead for a few minutes, forming the mixture into a 1-inch thick rectangle, about the length and width of a small loaf of bread.

4. Place in a steamer basket and steam for 50 minutes. Remove from the steamer and, when cool, wrap in tinfoil and chill in the fridge overnight (you can use it as is, but it's better after chilling overnight).

5. Slice into "rib" shapes and coat with your favorite barbecue sauce. Alternatively, you can tear this seitan into chick'n bites (the possibilities are almost endless with this recipe).

6. Preheat the oven to 400°F, and line a baking sheet with a reusable baking mat or parchment paper. Bake for 15 minutes, or until heated through and sticky. Enjoy immediately.

Storage: Store in a sealed container in the fridge for up to 5 days.

Gluten-Free Substitute: Use tempeh in place of this rib recipe: Simply steam the tempeh for 5 minutes, coat with barbecue sauce, and then bake for 15 minutes as instructed.

Save the Scraps: Aquafaba (chickpea water) for Mousse on the Loose (page 264) or Mini Aquafaba Pavlovas (page 266).

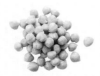

CHICKPEAS

VEGETABLE BROTH

OLIVE OIL

SOY SAUCE

NUTRITIONAL YEAST

GARLIC POWDER

THYME

VITAL WHEAT GLUTEN

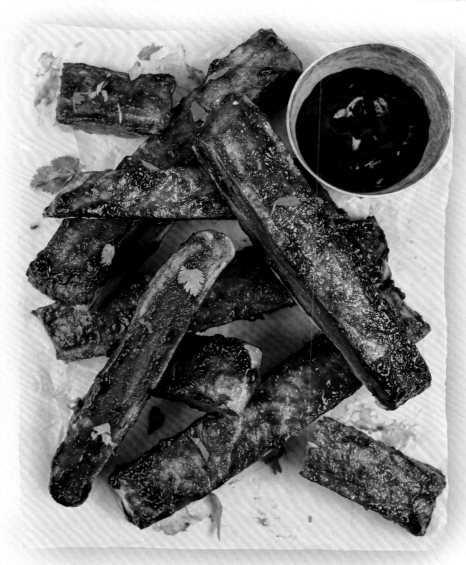

Pickled Tennessee Tenders

Pickle juice is a seriously underappreciated taste bud tantalizer—and perfect for these vegan chick'n tenders, marinated to perfection, then breaded and sauced for a dish that even the toughest carnivore will rave about.

MAKES 2 servings ✦ **START TO FINISH:** 45 minutes

1 (14-ounce) block extra-firm tofu

MARINADE

1 cup pickle juice, or 1 cup Apple Scrap Vinegar (page 350) or store-bought apple cider vinegar + a handful of fresh dill

1 tablespoon dried dill

1 tablespoon garlic powder

BREADING MIXTURE

½ cup Herbed Bread Crumbs (page 330) or store-bought vegan seasoned bread crumbs, gluten-free if needed

1 tablespoon dried dill

1 tablespoon garlic powder

1 teaspoon paprika

½ teaspoon salt

FOR SERVING

Hot sauce of choice

Creamy Hummus Caesar (page 278), for dipping

1. Freeze the tofu overnight. You can skip this step, but it lends a "meatier" texture. Thaw in the fridge or the microwave and drain the liquid. Now, wrap the tofu in a clean cloth and place something heavy on top (such as a stack of books) to press for 20 minutes, until as much liquid as possible is drained out.

2. Once pressed, tear the tofu into eight to ten "tender"-shaped slices. You can also slice the tofu, but it won't have that "chicken tender" look.

3. Make the marinade: In a bowl, combine the pickle juice with the dill and garlic powder. Add the tenders to the marinade and allow to soak for 15 minutes, or as long as an hour.

4. Meanwhile, preheat the oven to 400°F and line a baking sheet with a reusable baking mat or parchment paper.

5. Make the breading mixture: In a bowl, combine the bread crumbs with the dill, garlic powder, paprika, and salt. One at a time, take the tofu tenders from the marinade, toss in the bread crumbs until coated, and place on the prepared baking sheet. Bake for 25 minutes, or until crispy, flipping halfway through.

6. Once cooked, toss in your favorite hot sauce and maybe give it a dip in the hummus Caesar.

Storage: Store in a sealed container in the fridge for up to 4 days, or in the freezer for up to 2 months.

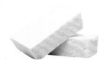

TOFU

PICKLE JUICE

DRIED DILL

GARLIC POWDER

BREAD CRUMBS

PAPRIKA

HOT SAUCE

CREAMY HUMMUS CAESAR

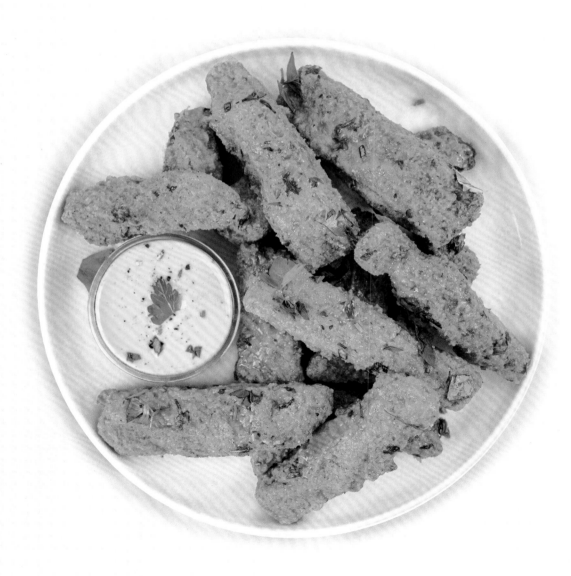

Broccoli 'n' "Beef" Stir-Fry

Beef requires twenty times more land and emits twenty times more greenhouse gas emissions per gram of edible protein than most common plant proteins, such as tempeh. Tempeh is an incredible fermented soy product with a nutty and earthy flavor that lends itself perfectly to a swap in meaty dishes, like this simple stir-fry. With bold flavors and a tender meaty texture, you won't miss the beef (and, seriously, Mother Earth will thank you).

MAKES 4 servings ✦ **START TO FINISH:** 25 minutes

1 cup uncooked jasmine rice

STIR-FRY

1 (8-ounce) package tempeh, sliced into ¼-inch chunks

2 cups broccoli florets (from about 2 heads broccoli), stems removed

2 red bell peppers, seeded and sliced

1 yellow onion, sliced

½ cup water

SAUCE

1 (1-inch-long) piece fresh ginger, minced

4 garlic cloves, minced

1 cup vegetable broth

¼ cup soy sauce or gluten-free tamari

2 tablespoons coconut or dark brown sugar

1 teaspoon red pepper flakes

1½ tablespoons cornstarch or arrowroot powder

FOR SERVING

¼ cup sesame seeds

1. Cook the rice according to the package directions.

2. Make the stir-fry: In a large skillet over medium heat, combine the tempeh, broccoli florets, bell pepper, and onion with the water. Increase the heat to medium-high, then steam, covered, for 3 to 4 minutes, or until the broccoli is bright green. This will also remove any bitterness from the tempeh.

3. Lower the heat to medium and sauté the mixture for about 5 minutes, or until the tempeh begins to brown.

4. Meanwhile, make the sauce: Whisk together the sauce ingredients in a bowl until fully combined and then add to the skillet. Stir until completely incorporated, then simmer for 3 to 5 minutes, or until thick.

5. Serve over the cooked rice, garnished with sesame seeds.

Storage: Store in a sealed container in the fridge for up to 5 days, or freeze for up to 2 months.

Save the Scraps: Broccoli stems for Broccoli Stem Summer Rolls (page 108) or Citrus Cabbage Slaw (page 122). Onion peels for Onion Peel Powder (page 336), Scrappy Broth (page 102), or Bouilliant Bouillon Powder (page 336).

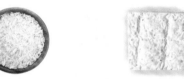

JASMINE RICE

TEMPEH

BROCCOLI

RED BELL PEPPER

YELLOW ONION

GINGER ROOT

GARLIC

VEGETABLE BROTH

SOY SAUCE

COCONUT SUGAR

RED PEPPER FLAKES

CORNSTARCH

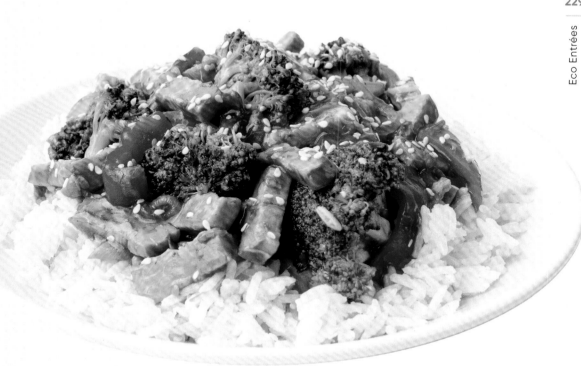

Kitchen Raid Recipe

Second Chance Sheet-Pan "Fried" Rice

Have leftover rice? This one-pan wonder is the ideal opportunity to turn a "has-been" into a "must-have." Toss it in an irresistible sauce with your veggies of choice, and roast in the oven to perfection.

MAKES 4 servings ◆ **START TO FINISH:** 40 minutes

¼ cup soy sauce or gluten-free tamari

3 tablespoons drippy almond butter, peanut butter, tahini, or sunflower seed butter

1½ tablespoons pure maple syrup

1½ tablespoons rice vinegar

1½ teaspoons red pepper flakes

3 cups leftover cooked rice

2 cups diced vegetables, such as onion, carrot, broccoli, cauliflower, peas, corn, bell pepper

½ cup almonds (optional)

1. Preheat the oven to 375°F, and line a baking sheet with a reusable baking mat or parchment paper.

2. In a bowl, combine the soy sauce, almond butter, maple syrup, rice vinegar, and red pepper flakes. Add the leftover rice and diced vegetables, and toss until evenly coated in the sauce mixture.

3. Arrange in a single layer on the prepared sheet. Roast for 30 minutes, or until the rice is slightly crispy and the vegetables are cooked, tossing halfway through. If using the almonds, add them to the sheet pan 10 minutes before the dish is cooked completely.

Storage: Store in a sealed container in the fridge for up to 4 days.

Eco Entrées

SOY SAUCE

NUT BUTTER

MAPLE SYRUP

RICE VINEGAR

RED PEPPER FLAKES

JASMINE RICE

VEGGIES OF CHOICE: YELLOW ONION, CARROT, BROCCOLI, CAULIFLOWER, GREEN PEAS, CORN KERNELS, RED BELL PEPPER

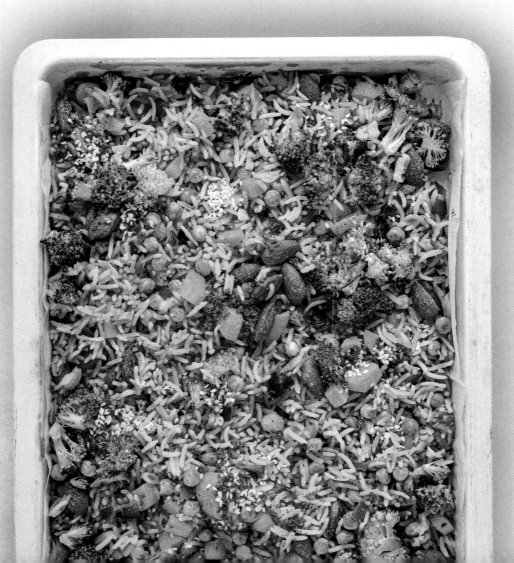

Veggie Masala Burgers

These vegetable masala burgers are as if a samosa and burger got it on. They can be eaten like a veggie burger patty or with a knife and fork, fritter style. The best part? Just about any vegetable works in these for a versatile, low-waste recipe that packs in the spice and flavor. My favorite is a blend of cauliflower, onion, carrot, and green peas for a perfect workable patty.

MAKES 4 servings, 4 to 6 burgers ✦ **START TO FINISH:** 75 minutes

2 medium-size Yukon Gold potatoes, diced

3 cups diced mixed vegetables (cauliflower, onion, carrot, peas, corn, bell pepper, green beans)

¼ cup Herbed Bread Crumbs (page 330) or store-bought vegan seasoned bread crumbs, gluten-free if needed

1 teaspoon garam masala

½ teaspoon ground turmeric

½ teaspoon garlic powder

½ teaspoon paprika

½ teaspoon ground ginger

¾ teaspoon salt

FOR SERVING (OPTIONAL)

4 vegan burger buns, regular or gluten-free

Everything Tahini Dressing, spicy version (page 278)

Green Goddess Dressing (page 280)

Citrus Cabbage Slaw (page 122)

1. Preheat the oven to 400°F, and line a baking sheet with a reusable baking mat or parchment paper.

2. In a large bowl, toss the diced potatoes and vegetables with the bread crumbs, garam masala, turmeric, garlic powder, paprika, ground ginger, and salt, then transfer to the prepared baking sheet. Roast in the oven for 40 minutes, tossing halfway through.

3. Remove from the oven and allow to cool. Mash into a moldable consistency but not completely blended (you should be able to see some vegetable chunks). Form into patties about ¾ inch thick.

4. Bake the patties for 25 minutes, or until crispy on the outside, flipping halfway through.

5. Assemble your burgers: Place on a vegan bun and top with your favorite toppings, as desired. Alternatively, serve on a salad, in a wrap, or as a side.

Storage: Store patties in a sealed container in the fridge for up to 5 days or in the freezer for 3 months.

POTATOES

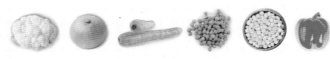

VEGGIES OF CHOICE: CAULIFLOWER, YELLOW ONION, CARROT, GREEN PEAS, CORN KERNELS, RED BELL PEPPER, GREEN BEANS

BREAD CRUMBS

GARAM MASALA

TURMERIC

GARLIC POWDER

PAPRIKA

GROUND GINGER

FOR SERVING: BURGER BUNS, EVERYTHING TAHINI DRESSING, GREEN GODDESS DRESSING, CITRUS CABBAGE SLAW

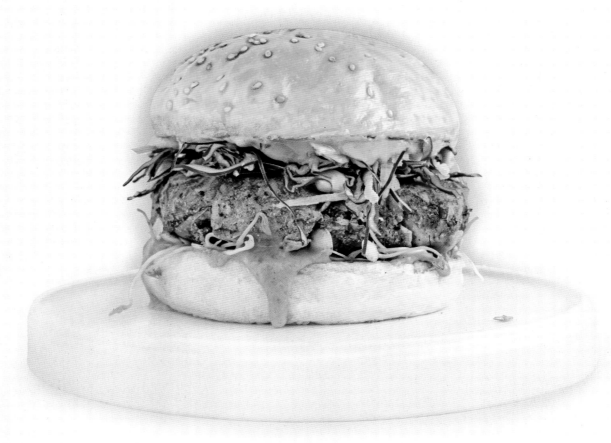

Vegan Meaty Hand Pies

I brought these to my extended family's Christmas dinner, and they flew off the plates faster than kids open presents—with everyone asking for seconds. These easy, veggie-loaded hand pies can stand out as the main dish at your holiday dinner table, as a portable party food, or a weeknight or lunchtime staple. So grab one or two and get ready for a meatless masterpiece.

MAKES 6 pockets ✦ **START TO FINISH:** 60 minutes

1 yellow onion, diced

3 garlic cloves, minced

1 tablespoon tomato paste

¼ teaspoon salt

2 cups diced cremini mushrooms or diced eggplant (about 1 small eggplant)

½ cup ground raw sunflower seeds

1 (15-ounce) can brown lentils, drained and rinsed, or 1½ cups homemade

2 tablespoons ground flaxseed

3 tablespoons water

Leaves from 3 thyme sprigs

1 tablespoon soy sauce

½ teaspoon paprika

½ teaspoon mustard powder

2 tablespoons balsamic vinegar

¼ cup red wine or vegetable broth

All-purpose flour, for dusting

1 (1-pound) package vegan puff pastry, gluten-free if needed

1. In a large skillet over medium heat, combine the onion, garlic, tomato paste, and salt, sautéing until translucent, about 5 minutes.

2. Add the mushrooms and cook for 8 to 10 minutes, or until soft and brown.

3. While the mushrooms cook, combine the sunflower seeds, lentils, ground flaxseed, and water in a food processor or blender. Pulse/blend until a thick puree is achieved (it doesn't have to be smooth).

4. Add the blended mixture to the pan, along with the thyme sprigs, soy sauce, paprika, mustard powder, balsamic vinegar, and red wine or vegetable broth. Stir until coated, then sauté for 8 to 10 minutes, or until everything is cooked through.

5. Preheat the oven to 400°F, and line a baking sheet with a reusable baking mat or parchment paper.

6. On a lightly floured surface, roll out the puff pastry sheets slightly. Slice each individual sheet into six equal rectangles, for twelve rectangles in total.

7. Place ¼ cup of the vegan filling in the center of six of the rectangles, leaving space around the edges. Top each piece with a remaining rectangle of puff pastry to create six pies, and use a fork to seal the edges. Transfer the pies to a baking sheet, and bake for about 35 minutes, or until the pastry is flaky and golden brown. Remove from the oven and allow to cool before eating.

YELLOW ONION

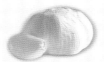

GARLIC

TOMATO PASTE

CREMINI MUSHROOMS

SUNFLOWER SEEDS

BROWN LENTILS

GROUND FLAXSEED

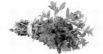

THYME

SOY SAUCE

PAPRIKA

MUSTARD POWDER

BALSAMIC VINEGAR

VEGETABLE BROTH

PUFF PASTRY

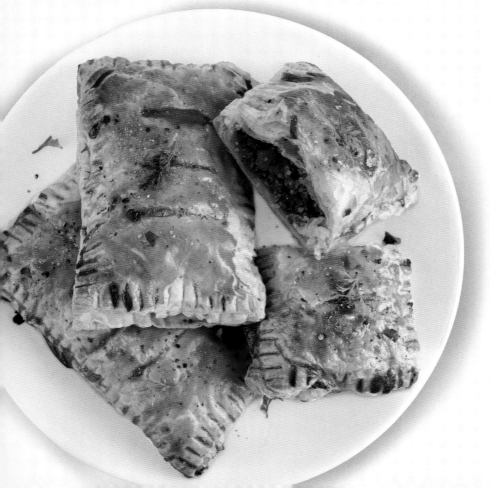

Storage: Store in a sealed container in the fridge for up to 4 days, or in the freezer for 3 months. If you have leftover filling, serve it in pasta sauce, or as a "ground beef" replacement.

Save the Scraps: Onion peels for Onion Peel Powder (page 336), Scrappy Broth (page 102), or Bouilliant Bouillon Powder (page 336).

Soy-Free Tofu

When you think of tofu, the soy-based variety may first come to mind. But you can make delicious tofu with a range of beans. This recipe is inspired by Burmese tofu, a traditional dish of Myanmar, which is made from a mixture of chickpea flour and water. With a little experimentation, I learned that tofu can be made with just about any bean, including dried lima beans, white beans, and chickpeas!

MAKES 8 to 12 servings ✦ **START TO FINISH:** 1 hour (after overnight soaking)

¾ cup dried lima beans, white beans, or chickpeas, soaked in water overnight

2 cups water

½ teaspoon salt

½ teaspoon garlic powder

1. Drain and rinse the soaked beans, then transfer to a blender along with the water. Blend until completely smooth.

2. Drain the mixture through a fine-mesh sieve or nut milk bag into a bowl. You will be using the drained liquid in the bowl to make the "tofu." Save the leftover bean pulp to thicken stews or soups.

3. Place the liquid, salt, and garlic powder in a saucepan over medium heat. Bring to a boil, whisking constantly, until you achieve a thick, velvety consistency that sticks to the whisk.

4. Transfer to a 6 x 8-inch rectangular container. Refrigerate, uncovered, for at least 4 hours. The tofu should be completely set.

5. Slice and prepare as you would regular tofu. This is going to be a bit softer than the traditional kind, but by carefully slicing and handling, it can be baked and stir-fried as normal.

Storage: Store in a sealed container in the fridge for up to 4 days.

WHITE BEANS

GARLIC POWDER

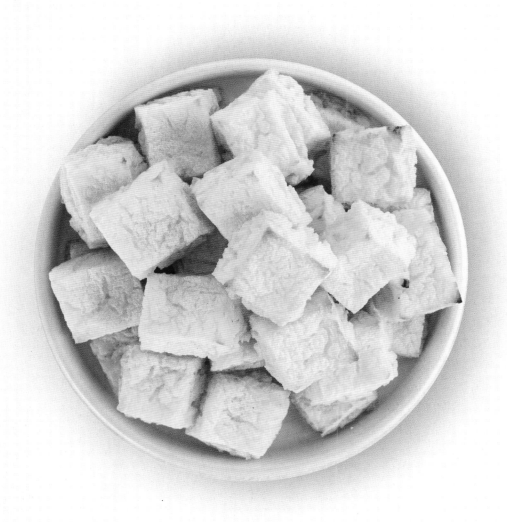

Eco Entrées

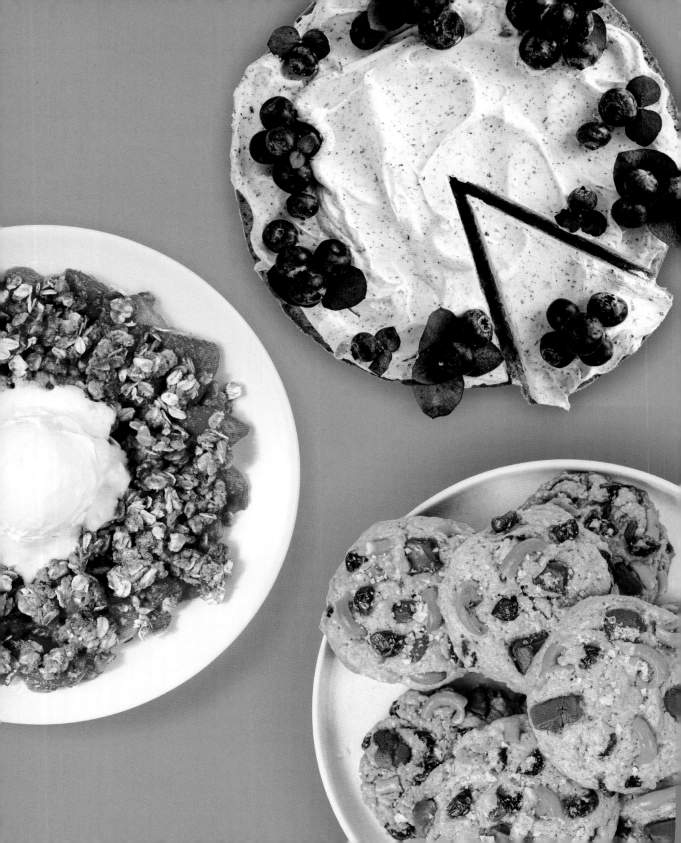

CHAPTER 8

Sustainable Sweets

Who says dessert can't be sweet and sustainable at the same time?

Wacky Cake

Have you ever heard of a wacky cake?! Also referred to as a crazy cake and Great Depression cake, this amazing recipe dates back to the Great Depression, when there was a shortage of eggs, milk, and butter. It turns out that the historic recipe is naturally vegan and really delicious. I've made a few small tweaks for an oil-free version, with an incredible chocolate peanut butter icing. You'll be obsessed with how easy this is to whip up.

MAKES 8 servings ✦ **FROM START TO FINISH:** 45 minutes

DRY INGREDIENTS

1½ cups all-purpose flour

¾ cup light or dark brown sugar

½ cup unsweetened cocoa powder

2 teaspoons baking soda

¼ teaspoon salt

WET INGREDIENTS

⅓ cup aquafaba or extra-virgin olive oil

1 tablespoon Apple Scrap Vinegar (page 350) or store-bought apple cider vinegar

2 teaspoons Homemade Vanilla Extract (page 324) or store-bought pure vanilla extract

1 cup water

ICING (OR USE STORE-BOUGHT VEGAN ICING)

⅓ cup pure maple syrup or liquid sweetener of choice

¼ cup unsweetened cocoa powder

1½ teaspoons Homemade Vanilla Extract (page 324) or store-bought pure vanilla extract

Pinch of salt

½ cup smooth nut butter (I use peanut butter)

1. Preheat the oven to 350°F, and line an 8 x 8–inch baking dish with parchment paper, or spray it with nonstick oil.

2. Combine the dry ingredients: Place the flour, sugar, cocoa powder, baking soda, and salt in the prepared baking dish and stir until completely mixed. Alternatively, you can make the batter in a bowl before pouring it into the dish.

3. Now, add the wet ingredients: Make two wells in the flour. Into one, pour in the aquafaba; into the second, add the apple scrap vinegar and vanilla. Pour the water over all, and then gently stir until a cake batter is formed.

4. Bake for about 28 minutes, or until a toothpick poked in the center comes out clean.

5. While the cake is baking, make the icing (if using homemade). In a small bowl, combine the maple syrup, cocoa powder, vanilla, and salt. Whisk until combined, then stir in the nut butter. Mix until an icing consistency is formed.

6. Allow the cake to cool completely before coating with the icing.

FLOUR

BROWN SUGAR

COCOA POWDER

BAKING SODA

AQUAFABA

APPLE CIDER VINEGAR

VANILLA EXTRACT

PEANUT BUTTER

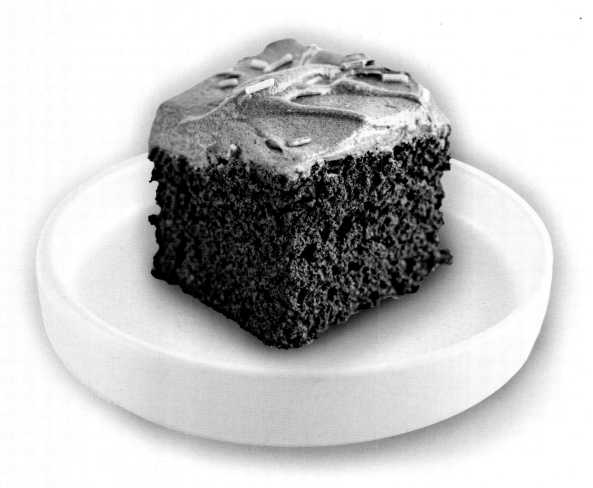

Storage: Store in a sealed container on the counter for up to 3 days.

The Scrappy Cookie

Say bye-bye to boring cookies and hello to the ultimate waste-free treat—the Scrappy Cookie! This recipe makes use of those random odds and ends in your pantry (such as the crumbs at the bottom of your potato chip bag) to make a wondrously eclectic dessert.

MAKES 12 to 14 extra-large cookies ✦ **FROM START TO FINISH:** 20 minutes

1 cup runny peanut butter or tahini, almond butter, sunflower seed butter, or another favorite

⅓ cup unsweetened plant-based milk

1 teaspoon Homemade Vanilla Extract (page 324) or store-bought pure vanilla extract

⅔ cup coconut sugar, or light or dark brown sugar

1 cup all-purpose flour or gluten-free oat flour

1 teaspoon baking soda

Pinch of salt

1 cup chopped mix-ins (potato chips, vegan pretzels, dried cranberries, vegan chocolate chips, vegan graham crackers, etc.)

1. Preheat the oven to 400°F, and line two baking sheets with reusable baking mats or parchment paper.

2. In a medium-size bowl, combine the nut butter, plant-based milk, vanilla, and sugar and stir until smooth. Next, add the flour, baking soda, and salt. Mix until a very thick cookie dough is formed. If needed, and an additional 1 to 2 tablespoons of plant-based milk to make a moldable batter.

3. Fold in your mix-ins of choice.

4. Scoop 3 tablespoons balls of dough, placed at least 2 inches apart, onto the prepared baking sheets, around six cookies per pan. Using your hands or a fork, squish down each cookie into a ½-inch-thick disk.

5. Bake for 9 to 12 minutes, or until cooked through. They will be slightly soft coming out of the oven. Allow to set for at least 10 to 15 minutes before serving.

   Storage: Store in an airtight container on the counter for up to 5 days.

PEANUT BUTTER   PLANT-BASED MILK   COCONUT SUGAR   FLOUR   BAKING SODA   COOKIE MIX

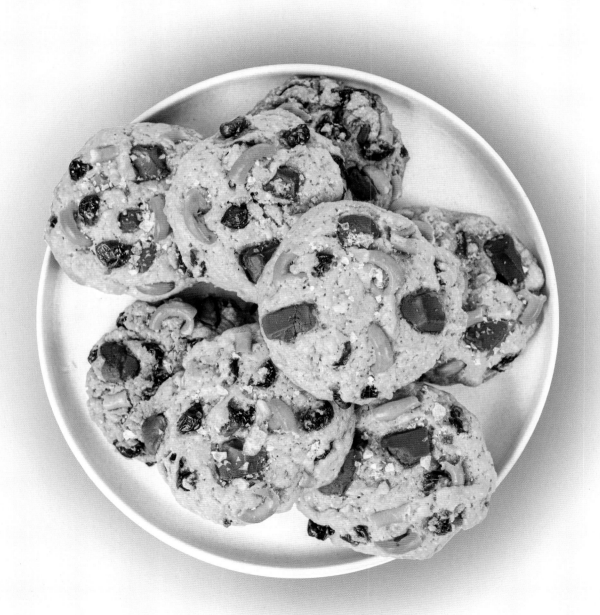

Hot-Chocolate Cookies

Like a warm hug in cookie form, these spicy specialties are going to be your new obsession. Perfect, rich chocolaty cookies are infused with a hint of cayenne and cinnamon for an irresistible experience that's like drinking a hot chocolate, *in cookie form*!

MAKES 12 to 14 extra-large cookies ✦ **FROM START TO FINISH:** 20 minutes

1 cup gluten-free oat flour or all-purpose flour

⅔ cup unsweetened cocoa powder

½ cup coconut sugar, or light or dark brown sugar

¼ teaspoon cayenne pepper (optional)

½ teaspoon ground cinnamon

½ cup unsweetened plant-based milk (soy, oat, or almond)

½ cup runny peanut butter or tahini, almond butter, sunflower seed butter, or another favorite

¼ cup pure maple syrup

1 tablespoon miso paste

1 teaspoon Homemade Vanilla Extract (page 324) or store-bought pure vanilla extract

½ cup chopped vegan dark chocolate

1. Preheat the oven to 375°F, and line two baking sheets with reusable baking mats or parchment paper.

2. Get two bowls. In the first, combine the oat flour, cocoa powder, coconut sugar, cayenne, and cinnamon.

3. In the second bowl, combine the plant-based milk, peanut butter, maple syrup, miso paste, and vanilla.

4. Pour the dry mixture into the wet mixture and stir until a dough is formed. Fold in the dark chocolate chunks.

5. Scoop ¼-cup balls of dough, placed at least 2 inches apart, onto the prepared baking sheets, around six cookies per pan. Using your hands or a fork, squish down each cookie into a ½-thick disk.

6. Bake for 12 to 13 minutes. They will be slightly soft. Allow to set for at least 10 to 15 minutes before serving.

Storage: Store in an airtight container on the counter for up to 5 days.

OAT FLOUR

COCOA POWDER

COCONUT SUGAR

CAYENNE PEPPER

CINNAMON

PLANT-BASED
MILK

PEANUT BUTTER

MAPLE SYRUP

MISO PASTE

VANILLA
EXTRACT

CHOPPED DARK
CHOCOLATE

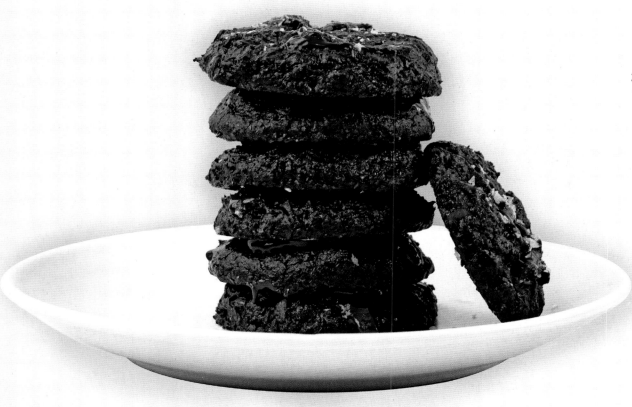

Not-Picky Fruit Crisp

Brace yourself for a fruity experience. Give us your tired, your poor, and your huddled masses of apples, peaches, berries, or cherries wasting away in your freezer or fridge. Serve this yummy treat with vegan yogurt or ice cream scooped on top for breakfast or dessert!

MAKES 8 servings ✦ **START TO FINISH:** 40 to 50 minutes

6 cups chopped of fruit of choice (cherries, berries, diced apples, peaches, or a combination)

¼ cup coconut sugar, or light or dark brown sugar

Juice of ½ lemon

1 teaspoon Homemade Vanilla Extract (page 324) or store-bought pure vanilla extract

2 tablespoons cornstarch

CRISP

1 cup gluten-free oat flour

2 cups gluten-free rolled oats

½ cup pure maple syrup

2 tablespoons ground flaxseed

¼ teaspoon baking powder

½ teaspoon ground cinnamon

¼ cup drippy tahini, peanut butter, almond butter, or sunflower seed butter

1 teaspoon Homemade Vanilla Extract (page 324) or store-bought pure vanilla extract

Juice of ½ lemon

Pinch of salt

FOR SERVING

Vegan yogurt or ice cream

1. Preheat the oven to 400°F.

2. In a large bowl, combine the fruit with brown sugar, lemon juice, vanilla, and cornstarch. Pour into an 8 x 8–inch casserole dish and bake the mixture for 10 minutes (20 minutes if using frozen fruit).

3. Make the crisp: In a large bowl, combine the oat flour, rolled oats, maple syrup, ground flaxseed, baking powder, cinnamon, tahini, vanilla, lemon juice, and salt. Massage the mixture until it turns into small clumps.

4. Remove the fruit from the oven and pour the oat mixture over the top. Bake for 30 minutes, or until golden brown.

5. Serve warm with vegan yogurt, as desired.

Storage: Store in an airtight container in the fridge for up to 4 days.

Save the Scraps: Lemon peel for Citrus Peel Powder (page 332).

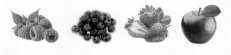

FRUIT OF CHOICE: CHERRIES, BERRIES, APPLE, PEACHES

COCONUT SUGAR

LEMON

VANILLA EXTRACT

CORNSTARCH

OAT FLOUR

ROLLED OATS

MAPLE SYRUP

GROUND FLAXSEED

BAKING POWDER

CINNAMON

TAHINI

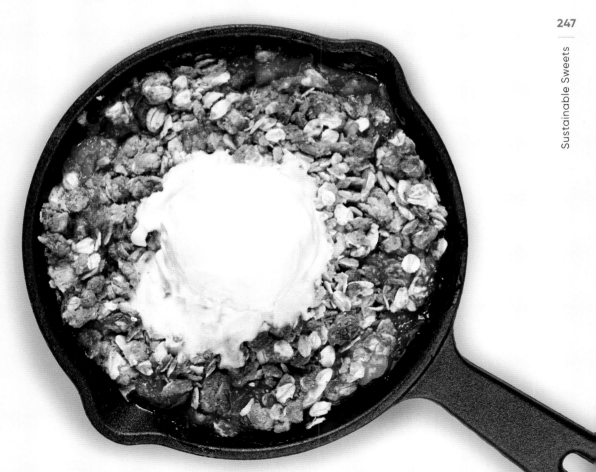

Leftover Quinoa Truffles

I don't know why, but every time I make quinoa, I seem to overestimate the amount needed for a recipe. If you're anything like me and have a sad pot of quinoa destined for the compost bin, use it up in this incredible truffle recipe. These decadent delicacies are packed with fiber and protein.

MAKES 8 to 12 truffles ✦ **START TO FINISH:** 10 minutes

¼ cup pitted dates, or 5 Medjool dates, pitted

¾ cup cooked and cooled quinoa

½ cup ground flaxseed

¼ cup unsweetened cocoa powder

3 tablespoons drippy almond butter, tahini, peanut butter, or sunflower seed butter

2½ tablespoons pure maple syrup

1 teaspoon Homemade Vanilla Extract (page 324) or store-bought pure vanilla extract

1 tablespoon brewed coffee, for depth of flavor (optional)

COATING (OPTIONAL)

¼ cup unsweetened cocoa powder

1. Place the dates in a bowl of hot water and allow them to soften, about 5 minutes. Drain.

2. In a food processor, combine the dates, quinoa, ground flaxseed, cocoa powder, almond butter, maple syrup, vanilla, and coffee (if using), and process until a smooth batter is formed.

3. Using your hands, form eight to twelve truffles, each about 1½ inches in diameter. Roll them in additional cocoa powder, if desired.

Storage: Store the truffles in an airtight container in the fridge for up to 5 days.

Save the Scraps: Date seeds for Date Seed Coffee (page 300).

DATES

QUINOA

GROUND FLAXSEED

COCOA POWDER

TAHINI

MAPLE SYRUP

VANILLA EXTRACT

COFFEE

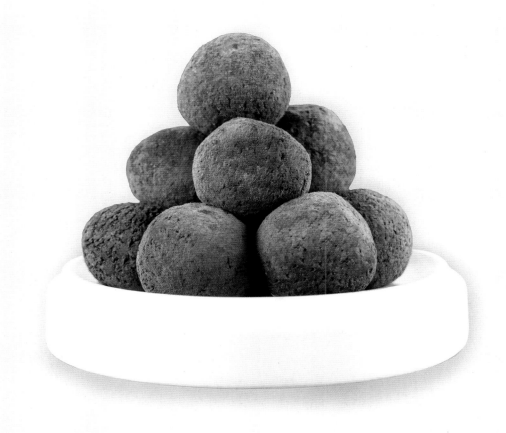

PB&J Chickpea Blondies

These are no basic blondies. Whether you have leftover oat pulp or just want a delicious healthy dessert, these blondies are sure to satisfy any sweet tooth. With a soft peanut butter–flavored center topped with a jammy swirl, they're like a PB&J party in your mouth!

MAKES 8 to 12 servings ✦ **START TO FINISH:** 30 minutes

1¼ cups gluten-free rolled oats

½ cup oat pulp (page 314), or ½ cup additional oats

1 (15-ounce) can chickpeas, drained and rinsed

1 tablespoon ground flaxseed

½ cup peanut butter, or another nut or seed butter of your choice

½ cup pure maple syrup or another liquid sweetener

1 teaspoon baking powder

¼ teaspoon baking soda

½ teaspoon salt

1 cup Mushy Berry Jam (page 252) or jam of choice

1. Preheat the oven to 375°F, and line an 8-inch square baking pan with parchment.

2. In a food processor, process the rolled oats until you achieve a fine oat flour.

3. Add all the remaining ingredients, except the jam, and process until a smooth batter is formed.

4. Transfer the batter to the prepared baking pan. Drop teaspoon-size spoonfuls of jam all around the top of the blondie mixture, working from the outside inward. Then drag the end of a knife or spoon through the jam drops, to create swirls.

5. Bake for 20 to 25 minutes until the center is set.

Storage: Store in an airtight container on the counter for up to 4 days.

ROLLED OATS

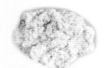
OAT PULP (OPTIONAL)

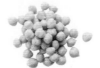
CHICKPEAS

GROUND FLAXSEED

PEANUT BUTTER

MAPLE SYRUP

BAKING POWDER

BAKING SODA

BERRY JAM

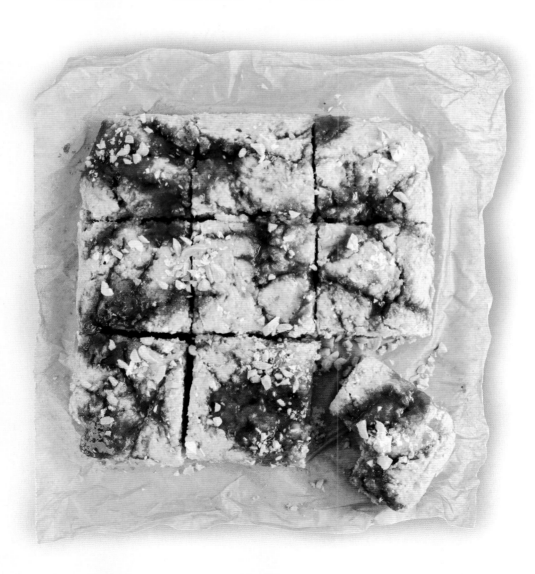

Sustainable Sweets

Mushy Berry Jam

You'll never buy store-bought jam after seeing how easy it is to make your own. Take any of the mushy berries in your fridge (blueberry is my personal favorite), and mash them in a pot with lemon juice and a small amount of your sweetener of choice. You can add chia seeds for some extra gel-like action, if desired, but it's not even necessary. Perfect on toast, on yogurt, or straight off the spoon.

MAKES 2 cups ✦ **START TO FINISH:** 15 minutes

2 cups fresh strawberries, blueberries, raspberries, or blackberries

1½ tablespoons pure maple syrup or coconut sugar (optional)

1½ teaspoons lemon zest

1 tablespoon freshly squeezed lemon juice

1 tablespoon chia seeds, for firmness (optional)

1. Preheat the oven to 375°F, and line an 8-inch square baking pan with parchment.

2. In a large skillet over medium heat, combine the berries, maple syrup (if using), and lemon zest and juice. Toss to mix.

3. Cook, covered, for 8 to 10 minutes, or until the berries are soft. Using the back of a wooden spoon or a potato masher, mash until the berries are broken down into a jam. Stir in the chia seeds (if using).

4. Remove from the heat and allow to cool. Transfer to clean jars.

Storage: Store in the fridge for up to 5 days.

Save the Scraps: Lemon peels for Candied Citrus Peels (page 254).

Note: Lemon seeds contain pectin. You can collect them in your fridge or freezer, then place them in a tea canister to simmer with your jam as a natural "scrappy" thickener. Compost when done.

STRAWBERRIES, BLUEBERRIES, RASPBERRIES

MAPLE SYRUP

LEMON

LEMON ZEST

CHIA SEEDS

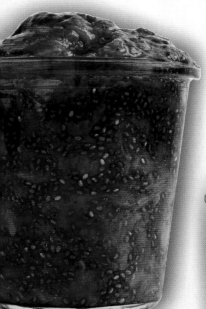

RASPBERRY JAM

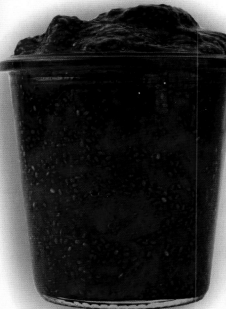

BLACKBERRY JAM

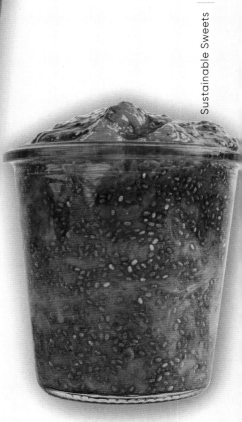

STRAWBERRY JAM

Candied Citrus Peels

Get ready for a sweet-and-tangy explosion of flavor that will make your taste buds dance like they're at a citrus-themed rave. Seriously, though, citrus peels are extremely nutritious and perfectly safe to eat, but they can be a little bitter on their own. By simmering and then candying them, they're transformed into a delicious sweet snack reminiscent of a gummy worm.

MAKES 4 servings ✦ **START TO FINISH:** 5 hours

2 cups citrus peels—lemon, orange, or lime, around 8 peels

2 cups water, for simple syrup

1 cup vegan granulated sugar or monk fruit sweetener

OPTIONAL

½ cup vegan dark chocolate, chopped and melted (optional)

Flaky salt

1. Line a baking sheet with parchment paper or a reusable baking mat and set aside.

2. To help remove any residue from your citrus peels, soak them in a half-water, half-vinegar mixture, and scrub vigorously with your hands. Drain, then dry, using a clean cloth.

3. Slice the citrus peels into thin strips. Remove as much of the pith as you can to make the citrus peel less bitter.

4. Bring a pot of water to a boil, then simmer the citrus peels for about 15 minutes. Drain and rinse with cold water.

5. Now, in the same pot, bring the fresh water and sugar to a boil to make a simple syrup. Whisk until combined. Add the citrus peels and simmer for 30 minutes, stirring intermittently, until the peels have candied.

6. Transfer to the prepared baking sheet, and allow to cool for 4 hours.

7. If desired, coat some of the slices in chocolate by dipping half of each peel in the melted chocolate and drying on a parchment-lined baking sheet. Finish with flaky salt.

Storage: Store in a sealed container on the counter for up to 1 week.

ORANGE

VEGAN SUGAR OR
MONK FRUIT

CHOPPED DARK
CHOCOLATE

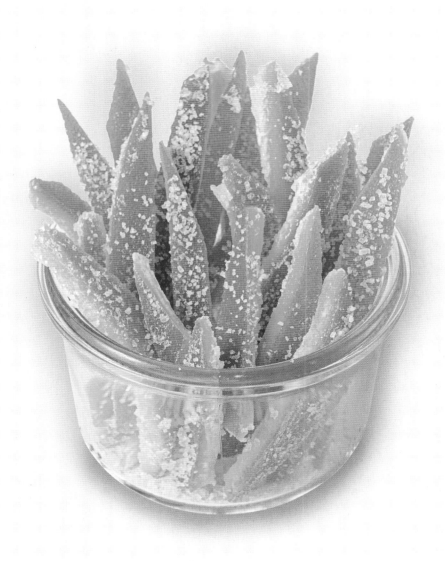

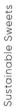

Apple Scrap Honey

This *Scrappy* cook doesn't toss her apple scraps. When boiled down, they provide the most incredible flavor infusion for something I call Apple Scrap Honey. This is a sweet and floral nectar reminiscent of traditional bee honey. Drizzle it on yogurt, use it as a liquid sweetener, or stir it into tea.

MAKES 4 to 6 cups ✦ **START TO FINISH:** 2 hours

Peels and cores from 15 apples, saved in a reusable freezer bag

Vegan granulated sugar (measured per cup of liquid) or monk fruit sweetener

Freshly squeezed lemon juice (measured per cup of liquid)

1. In a pot, add the apple peels and cores and enough water to cover. Boil until the apple scraps are soft and mushy, about 30 minutes.

2. Strain out the apple scraps and measure the remaining liquid. Add the liquid back to the pot along with ¾ cup of sugar and 1½ teaspoons of lemon juice per every cup of liquid.

3. Bring back to a boil, then simmer, stirring often, for 45 minutes or until a slightly thickened mixture has been achieved. It will thicken even more once it sets. Ladle into a container and enjoy. This is a very sweet treat and should be used sparingly in place of honey, maple syrup, or simple syrup.

Storage: Store in a sealed jar in your fridge for up to 1 month.

APPLE SCRAPS

VEGAN SUGAR

LEMON

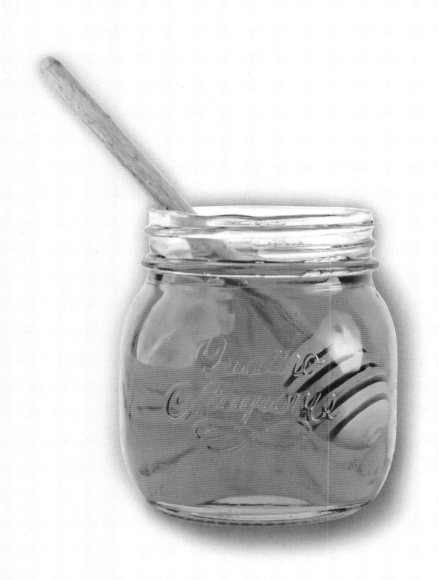

Berry Fruit Leather

Step aside, store-bought fruit snacks. Here, you're using up the leftover berries in your kitchen to make a tasty snack that is healthy and environmentally friendly. Simply take any combination of berries and blend them with chia seeds and maple syrup, then dehydrate into a fruit-roll-up-esque portable snack. This recipe is inspired by a popular Persian snack called *lavashak*, which is traditionally made by drying fruit outside in the sun.

MAKES 10 servings ✦ **START TO FINISH:** 5 hours

3 cups blueberries, strawberries, raspberries, plums, etc. (mixed berries work)

1 tablespoon chia seeds

2 tablespoons pure maple syrup (optional)

1. Preheat the oven to 175°F, and line a baking sheet with a reusable baking mat. Parchment paper can also work, but it must lie completely flat on your baking sheet. Alternatively, if you're in a warm climate, you can dry this fruit leather in the sun for several days.

2. In a high-speed blender, combine the fruit, chia seeds, and maple syrup (if using), and blend until smooth.

3. Pour onto the prepared baking sheet, and using a flat spatula, spread out into a rectangle around ⅛ inch thick. Ensure the edges are thicker than the center because they will dry faster.

4. Bake for 2½ hours and then rotate the baking sheet. Bake for another 2 hours and check the consistency—the water content of the fruit. The fruit leather is ready when it effortlessly lifts off the reusable baking mat or parchment paper. If it is dry around the edges, you can rehydrate those areas with a clean, wet cloth. The fruit leather is ready when you touch it with your fingers and it does not stick.

5. Remove from the oven, slice into six to ten equal strips, and roll with parchment or waxed paper for a homemade fruit-roll-up experience.

   Storage: Store rolled in waxed paper or parchment in a sealed container on your counter for up to 5 days.

BLUEBERRIES

CHIA SEEDS

MAPLE SYRUP

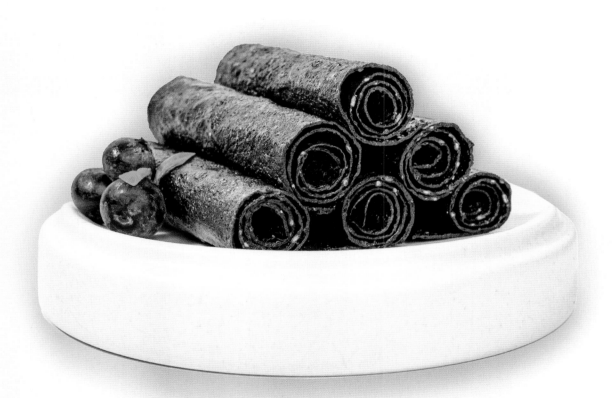

Coo-Coo for Coconut Caramel (Sauce)

I seem to always have a half can of coconut milk ensconced in the depths of my fridge. This mouthwatering recipe will gobble it up. This caramel sauce goes great with my Sticky Date Pudding (page 262) or as a delicious dip for apple slices.

MAKES 4 to 6 servings (about ¼ cup per serving) ✦ **START TO FINISH:** 5 minutes

1 tablespoon cornstarch or arrowroot powder

2 tablespoons water

¾ cup coconut milk or coconut cream

½ cup coconut sugar, or light or dark brown sugar

½ teaspoon salt

1 teaspoon Homemade Vanilla Extract (page 324) or store-bought pure vanilla extract

1. In a small bowl, combine the cornstarch with the water until a slurry is formed.

2. In a small pot, combine the slurry with the remaining sauce ingredients and bring to boil over medium-high heat, stirring continuously, until lots of bubbles form. Then simmer for 5 minutes, stirring often to prevent burning. Remove from the heat and allow to cool for 5 minutes.

Storage: Store in a sealed container in the fridge for up to 3 days. It might solidify slightly, and it can be reheated on the stove or in a microwave.

CORNSTARCH

COCONUT MILK

COCONUT SUGAR

VANILLA EXTRACT

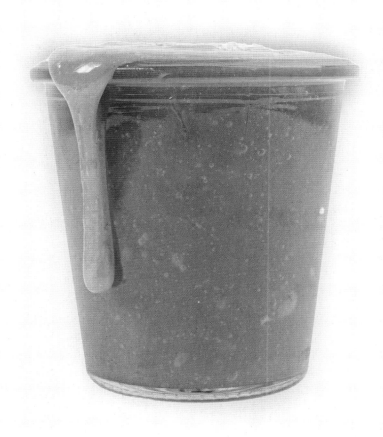

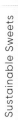

Sticky Date Pudding

I was thirteen and in the basement of an old Scottish pub when I tried sticky toffee pudding for the first time. I can still feel the warmth and sweetness of that pudding hitting my taste buds. Ever since, I've been trying to re-create that experience with a vegan healthier version of the beloved Scottish dessert. I present to you my Sticky Date Pudding. Enjoy!

MAKES 6 to 8 servings ✦ **START TO FINISH:** 30 minutes

1 cup Medjool dates, pitted

1 cup unsweetened Homemade Oat Milk (page 314) or store-bought plant-based milk of choice

1 teaspoon baking soda

¼ cup applesauce

¼ cup Cultured Vegan Yogurt (page 48) or store-bought coconut or soy yogurt

1 teaspoon Homemade Vanilla Extract (page 324) or store-bought pure vanilla extract

1½ cups all-purpose flour or all-purpose gluten-free flour

1 teaspoon baking powder

2 tablespoons coconut sugar or brown sugar

1 batch Coo-Coo for Coconut Caramel (Sauce) (page 260)

FOR SERVING (OPTIONAL)

Vegan whipped cream or vegan ice cream

1. Preheat the oven to 375°F, and line an 8 x 8–inch baking dish with parchment or spray with nonstick spray.

2. In a medium-size saucepan over medium heat, combine the dates, oat milk, and ½ teaspoon of the baking soda. Bring to a boil and then simmer until most of the dates dissolve, about 15 minutes.

3. Get two bowls. In the first, combine the date mixture with the applesauce, vegan yogurt, and vanilla until smooth. In the second, combine the flour, baking powder, coconut sugar, and remaining ½ teaspoon of baking soda. Fold the dry mixture into the wet mixture until a smooth batter is formed.

4. Pour into the prepared pan and bake for 15 minutes.

5. Remove the pudding from the oven and allow to set for 5 minutes. Poke holes about 2 inches apart along the entire surface of the pudding base, using a fork. Pour about half the caramel sauce over the top of the pudding, starting near the edges and working your way inward. Place the pudding back in the oven to bake for an additional 5 minutes.

6. Remove from the oven and allow to stand for 5 minutes. Slice and serve upside down, with vegan whipped cream or vegan ice cream, as desired, along with the remaining caramel sauce.

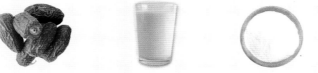

DATES

UNSWEETENED OAT MILK

BAKING SODA

APPLE SAUCE

YOGURT

VANILLA EXTRACT

FLOUR

BAKING POWDER

COCONUT SUGAR

CARAMEL SAUCE

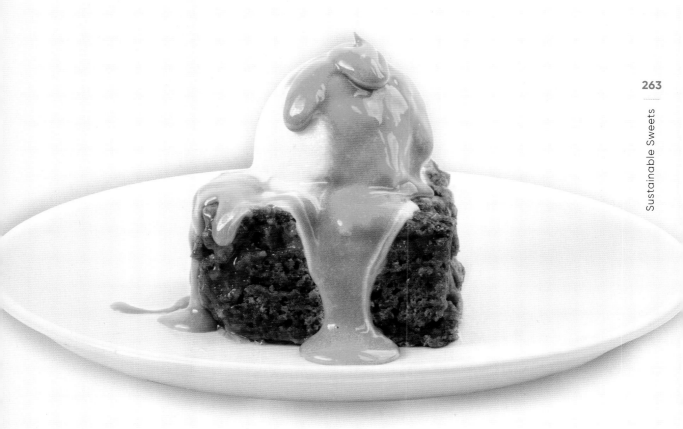

Storage: Store in an airtight container in the fridge for up to 3 days.

Save the Scraps: Date seeds for Date Seed Coffee (page 300).

Mousse on the Loose

You know the liquid from a can of chickpeas? Well, it is pure *magic*. Beat it up with a hand mixer and some cream of tartar, and aquafaba will transform into a beautiful glossy meringue. Add chocolate to it, and you're left with a decadent rich chocolate mousse that is off the chain—on the loose! Now you just need to find a use for those chickpeas (check out my Life-Altering Mediterranean Wraps, page 110).

MAKES 4 servings ✦ **FROM START TO FINISH:** 25 minutes

5 ounces vegan dark chocolate, 75% or sweeter

1 (15-ounce) can chickpeas or ½ cup aquafaba

½ teaspoon cream of tartar

FOR SERVING

Cultured Vegan Yogurt (page 48) or store-bought vegan yogurt or whipped cream

Fruit of choice, such as raspberries

1. Using a double broiler, melt the chocolate until smooth. Alternatively, in a microwave-safe bowl, melt the chocolate in a microwave in 5-second increments. Once melted, set aside to cool.

2. Drain the can of chickpeas (setting them aside for another recipe), capturing the aquafaba in a large bowl.

3. In a bowl, combine ½ cup of the aquafaba and the cream of tartar. Using a handheld mixer or a stand mixer fitted with the whisk attachment, beat until the liquid begins to foam, for 5 to 6 minutes.

4. Keep mixing until the meringue has stiff peaks. You should be able to lift the whisk and have the meringue stick to it. This will take about 10 minutes.

5. Using a spatula, gently fold in the chocolate, a tablespoon at a time (do not overmix here, which could deflate the meringue) until it is completely mixed in. Transfer to jars and refrigerate overnight or until firm. Enjoy topped with vegan yogurt and fresh fruit.

Storage: Store in sealed containers in the fridge for up to 3 days.

Save the Scraps: Chickpeas for PB&J Chickpea Blondies (page 250).

Sustainable Sweets

**CHOPPED DARK
CHOCOLATE**

AQUAFABA

CREAM OF TARTAR

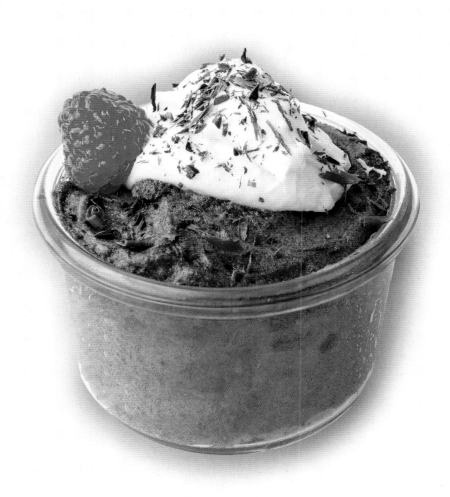

Mini Aquafaba Pavlovas

By now, you may know my love of chickpea water, a.k.a. aquafaba. Here, I use it to make adorable meringue nests with a creamy coconut milk icing. They're sweet, crispy, creamy, and fruity all wrapped into one zero-waste pavlova extravaganza.

MAKES 15 to 20 pavlova cookies ✦ **FROM START TO FINISH:** 1 hour 30 minutes

PAVLOVA

1 (15-ounce) can chickpeas

¼ teaspoon cream of tartar

⅓ cup vegan granulated sugar

½ teaspoon Homemade Vanilla Extract (page 324) or store-bought pure vanilla extract

ICING

1 (13.5-ounce) can full-fat coconut milk, chilled in the fridge for at least 24 hours

3 tablespoons pure maple syrup

1 teaspoon Homemade Vanilla Extract (page 324) or store-bought pure vanilla extract

FOR SERVING

Jam

Fresh berries

1. Make the pavlovas: Preheat the oven to 250°F, and line a baking sheet with a reusable baking mat or parchment paper.

2. Drain the can of chickpeas (setting the chickpeas aside for another recipe), capturing the aquafaba in a large bowl.

3. In a bowl, combine ½ cup of the aquafaba and the cream of tartar. Using either a handheld mixer or a stand mixer fitted with the whisk attachment, beat until the liquid begins to foam, for 2 to 3 minutes.

4. While continuing to mix, gradually add the sugar to the bowl, along with the vanilla. Keep mixing until the meringue has stiff peaks. You should be able to lift the whisk and have the meringue stick to it.

5. Scoop the meringue into a piping bag and pipe into 15 to 20 cookies, each about 3 inches in diameter and 1 inch high, on the prepared baking sheet. Alternatively, use a tablespoon to scoop the meringue into 3-inch mounds on the prepared baking sheet.

6. Bake until the cookies have set and are slightly browned, for 1 to 1½ hours. Using your oven light and keeping the oven door closed, keep an eye on the cookies to make sure they do not overbrown.

7. While the cookies bake, make the icing: In a bowl, combine the chilled coconut cream, maple syrup, and vanilla. Using a hand mixer, whisk until stiff peaks form and the mixture has an icing consistency.

8. Remove the meringues from the oven and allow them to cool. Spoon the icing over the top of the pavlovas, swirl in your jam of choice, and add berries on top. Love immediately.

AQUAFABA

CREAM OF TARTAR

VEGAN SUGAR

VANILLA EXTRACT

COCONUT MILK

MAPLE SYRUP

STRAWBERRY JAM

BLUEBERRIES

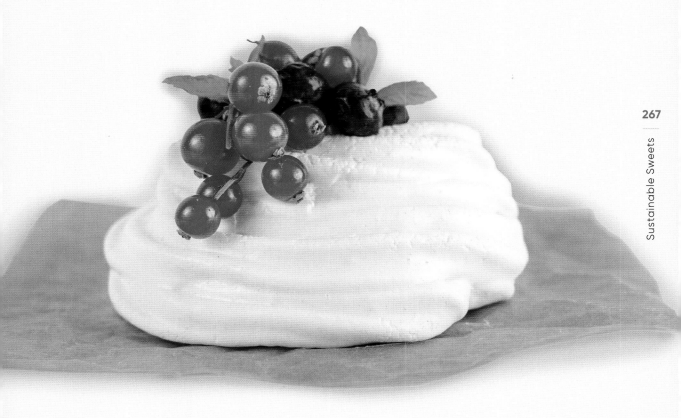

Storage: Store the pavlovas, without the coconut frosting or fruit, in an airtight container on your counter for up to 3 days.

Save the Scraps: Chickpeas for PB&J Chickpea Blondies (page 250).

All the Earl Grey Tea Cake

Creating a cake recipe that is low-waste, vegan, gluten-free, and oil-free is ONE tall order, and I had to call in the big guns. Hats off to my dear friend Alee LaPlaca of Alpaca Bakes for helping me develop a delicious cake infused with Earl Grey tea leaves from batter to icing.

MAKES 8 servings ✦ **START TO FINISH:** 60 minutes

CAKE BASE

1 cup unsweetened Homemade Oat Milk (page 314) or store-bought oat milk

6 Earl Grey tea bags

5½ cups gluten-free rolled oats

2 teaspoons baking powder

1 teaspoon baking soda

1 tablespoon cornstarch or arrowroot powder

½ cup Cultured Vegan Yogurt (page 48) or store-bought coconut or soy yogurt

¾ cup unsweetened applesauce

2 tablespoons vanilla extract

1 cup granulated coconut sugar, or light or dark brown sugar

EARL GREY ICING

1 cup unsalted cashews or raw sunflower seeds, soaked in water overnight

½ cup unsweetened Cultured Vegan Yogurt (page 48) or store-bought vegan yogurt

Zest and juice of ½ lemon

¼ cup pure maple syrup

FOR SERVING

Fresh fruit

1. Preheat the oven to 350°F, and line an 8-inch round cake pan, or spray it with oil.

2. In a pot over medium heat, bring the oat milk to a boil. Remove from heat and place all six tea bags in the pot, allowing them to steep for at least 10 minutes, then remove the tea bags and set aside.

3. Place the oats in a blender and blitz into a flour-like consistency. Transfer to a large bowl along with the baking powder, baking soda, and cornstarch.

4. In a second bowl, mix together the vegan yogurt, applesauce, vanilla, coconut sugar, and steeped oat milk. Cut the top off three of the used tea bags, and pour the leaves into the yogurt mixture. Stir until evenly dispersed. Reserve the other tea bags for later.

5. Mix together the wet and dry ingredients until a smooth batter is formed. Transfer to the cake pan, and bake for 35 minutes or until a fork inserted into the center comes out clean.

6. Make the icing: In a blender, combine the listed ingredients, as well as the leaves from the remaining three tea bags. Blend until a smooth, thick icing is formed, adding more liquid as needed.

7. Once the cake is cooled, pour the icing onto the center and spread over the top. Garnish with fresh fruit, as desired.

UNSWEETENED OAT MILK

EARL GREY TEA BAGS

ROLLED OATS

BAKING POWDER

BAKING SODA

CORNSTARCH

YOGURT

APPLE SAUCE

VANILLA EXTRACT

COCONUT SUGAR

CASHEWS

LEMON

MAPLE SYRUP

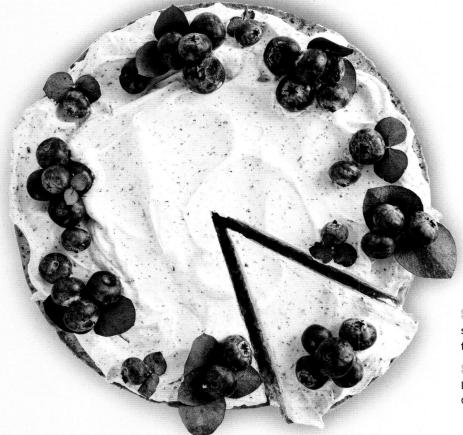

Storage: Store in a sealed container in the fridge for up to 3 days.

Save the Scraps: Lemon peels for Candied Citrus Peels (page 254).

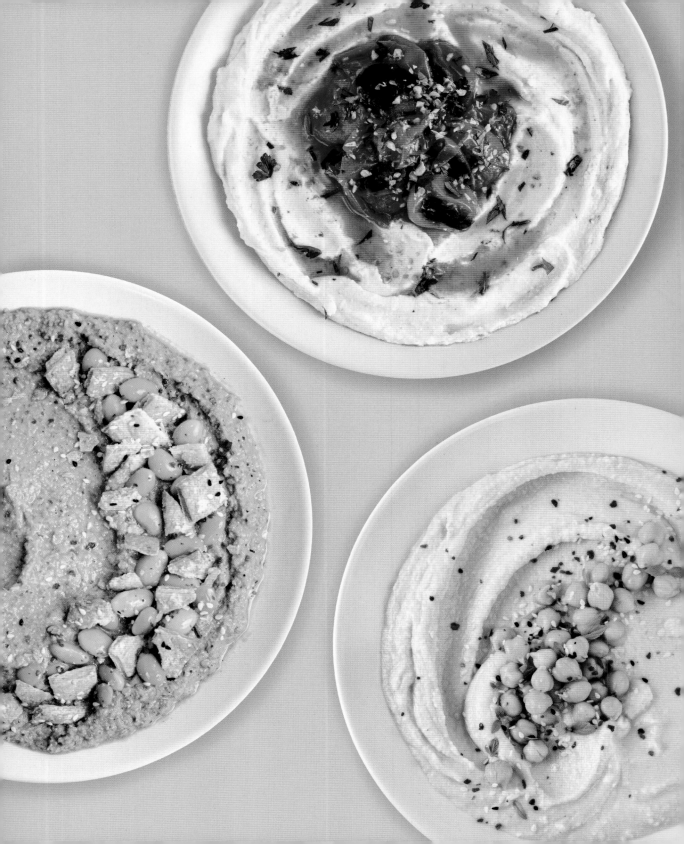

CHAPTER 9

Dressings, Dips & Saucy Things

Tired of wasting money on store-bought condiments you only use once? This chapter is for you.

Sunflower Cream Sauce

This is perhaps one of the most used sauces in the *Scrappy* kitchen, and it's for good reason! Raw sunflower seeds are affordable (when compared to other nuts, such as cashews or walnuts), they're generally allergy-friendly, and they're considered a sustainable crop, helping to detoxify soil and requiring a fraction of the resources to grow and harvest when compared to other nuts and seeds.

MAKES 4 to 6 servings (about 3 tablespoons per serving) ✦ **FROM START TO FINISH:** 5 minutes

⅓ cup raw hulled sunflower seeds or raw cashews, soaked in hot water for 10 minutes

½ cup water, plus more as needed

1 tablespoon freshly squeezed lemon juice

4 garlic cloves

½ teaspoon sea salt

¼ cup nutritional yeast, for "cheesy" version (optional)

1. In a high-speed blender, combine all the ingredients and blend until smooth. Add more water, as desired, to thin.

Carrot Top Chimichurri

Thought to originate in Uruguay and Argentina, chimichurri is an uncooked condiment that is typically served with grilled meat or as a marinade. In a *Scrappy* twist, I've added delicious carrot tops to my chimichurri for an unexpected fresh flavor. Best served with Confetti Sheet-Pan Tacos (page 210) and Sweet & Spicy Carrot Showstopper (page 76).

MAKES 4 to 6 servings (about ¼ cup per serving) ✦ **START TO FINISH:** 5 minutes

1 cup fresh parsley

1 cup carrot tops, or 1 cup fresh additional parsley if you don't have carrot tops

½ cup fresh cilantro

¼ cup red wine vinegar

1 tablespoon freshly squeezed lime juice

2 tablespoons extra-virgin olive oil (optional)

½ teaspoon red pepper flakes, for heat (optional)

½ teaspoon salt

1. In a blender or food processor, combine all the ingredients and blitz until a sauce is formed.

SUNFLOWER SEEDS

LEMON

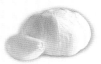

GARLIC

NUTRITIONAL YEAST

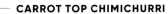

273

CARROT TOP CHIMICHURRI

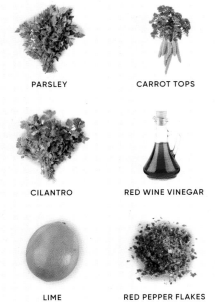

PARSLEY

CARROT TOPS

CILANTRO

RED WINE VINEGAR

LIME

RED PEPPER FLAKES

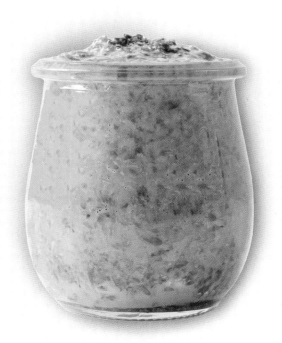

Storage: Store in a sealed container in the fridge for up to 4 days (or longer . . . just do the smell test).

Scrappy Pesto

Let's not toss out those much-maligned radish tops (or any greens hiding in the crisper), my friend. Instead, transform them into a pesto that's as delicious as it is environmentally conscious. Radish greens have an earthy, subtle, peppery tang that makes the perfect base for this bowl of plant-based goodness. This pesto is also fabulous with carrot tops, kale, chard, or other leafy greens. Best served with Pesto & Herb Vitality Bowl (page 174), White Bean "Tuna" Sandwich (page 118), and Stacked Veggie Sandwich (page 116).

MAKES 4 servings (about ¼ cup per serving)   **START TO FINISH:** 5 minutes

1 cup fresh basil

2 cups radish leaves, carrot tops, kale, chard, or other leafy green

3 garlic cloves

Juice of ½ lemon

¾ cup sunflower seeds or cashews, boiled for 10 minutes to soften

¾ cup warm water, plus more as needed to thin

½ teaspoon salt

1. In a blender, combine all the ingredients and blend until smooth.

Mango Peanut Sauce

This is the type of sauce I wish I could take a swim in. Sweet, savory, and so delicious—it's best served on everything. But seriously, try it with my Broccoli Stem Summer Rolls (page 108) and Nutty Noodle Bowl (page 180).

MAKES 4 servings (about 2 tablespoons per serving)   **START TO FINISH:** 5 minutes

1 ripe mango, peeled, pitted, and chopped roughly

3 tablespoons peanut butter

1 garlic clove

1 (1-inch) piece fresh ginger, minced

Juice of 1 lime

2 tablespoons soy sauce or gluten-free tamari

1 teaspoon pure maple syrup

1 to 3 tablespoons warm water, as needed to thin

FOR SERVING

Sesame seeds and red pepper flakes, for garnish

1. In a blender, combine all the ingredients, except the garnishes, and blend until smooth. Garnish with sesame seeds and red pepper flakes, as desired.

SCRAPPY PESTO

BASIL

GREENS OF CHOICE: RADISH LEAVES,
CARROT TOPS, SPINACH, KALE, OR CHARD

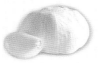

GARLIC

LEMON

SUNFLOWER SEEDS

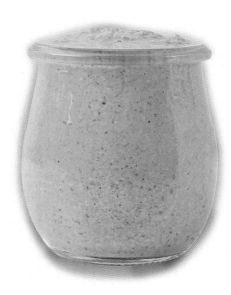

MANGO PEANUT SAUCE

MANGO

PEANUT BUTTER

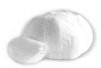

GARLIC

GINGER ROOT

LIME

SOY SAUCE

MAPLE SYRUP

SESAME SEEDS

RED PEPPER FLAKES

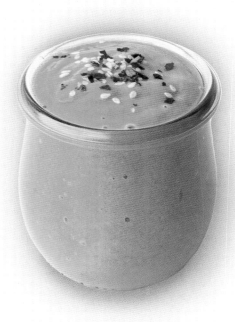

Storage: Store in a sealed container in the fridge for up to 4 days (or longer . . . just do the smell test).

Roasted Red Pepper Sauce

This sauce is reminiscent of both romesco and *muhammara*. It's bold, zippy, and simply unforgettable. Try it with my Whole Roasted Cauliflower (page 208) and Dill Pickle Chips (page 66).

MAKES 6 servings (about ¼ cup per serving) ✦ **START TO FINISH:** 5 minutes

1 (12-ounce) jar roasted red peppers, drained, or 2 red bell peppers, roasted at 400°F for 40 minutes

¾ cup walnuts or sunflower seeds, soaked in water overnight or boiled for 10 minutes

1 teaspoon salt

1 cup unsweetened Cultured Vegan Yogurt (page 48) or store-bought coconut or soy yogurt

½ teaspoon red pepper flakes, for heat (optional)

3 garlic cloves

1 tablespoon Apple Scrap Vinegar (page 350) or store-bought apple cider vinegar

1. In a blender, combine the roasted red peppers, walnuts, salt, vegan yogurt, red pepper flakes (if using), garlic, and Apple Scrap Vinegar and blend until smooth. In a skillet over medium heat, warm the sauce, as desired.

Creamy Vegan Tzatziki

Who doesn't love tzatziki? This vegan version is quick to whip up using an entire cucumber and fresh dill for some zing. Have it with my Zucchini "Falafel" Fritters (page 186) and Life-Altering Mediterranean Wraps (page 110).

MAKES 6 servings (about 3 tablespoons per serving) ✦ **START TO FINISH:** 5 minutes

1 medium-size cucumber, grated

1 cup unsweetened Cultured Vegan Yogurt (page 48) or store-bought coconut or soy yogurt

1 tablespoon Apple Scrap Vinegar (page 350) or store-bought apple cider vinegar

1 tablespoon freshly squeezed lemon juice

3 garlic cloves, minced

2 tablespoons minced fresh dill

½ teaspoon sea salt

Freshly ground black pepper

1. Place the grated cucumber in a clean dish towel or piece of cheesecloth, and squeeze out as much of the excess liquid as possible. Reserve the liquid for Tummy-Soothing Lemon, Ginger & Mint Ice Cubes (page 308).

2. In a bowl, combine the cucumber, vegan yogurt, Apple Scrap Vinegar, lemon juice, garlic, dill, salt, and pepper, to taste. Whisk together until fully mixed. Taste and adjust the salt and other seasonings as needed.

ROASTED RED PEPPER SAUCE

ROASTED RED PEPPERS

WALNUTS

YOGURT

RED PEPPER FLAKES

GARLIC

APPLE CIDER VINEGAR

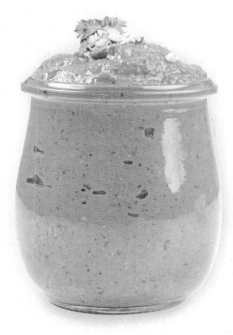

CREAMY VEGAN TZATZIKI

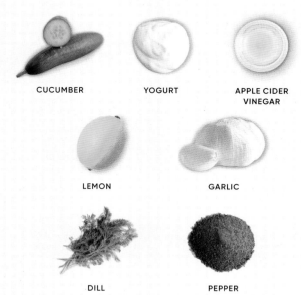

CUCUMBER

YOGURT

APPLE CIDER VINEGAR

LEMON

GARLIC

DILL

PEPPER

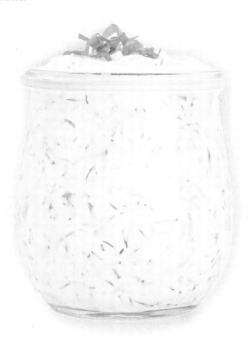

Dressings, Dips & Saucy Things

Storage: Store in a sealed container in the fridge for up to 4 days (or longer . . . just do the smell test).

Everything Tahini Dressing

Once I developed this tahini dressing, I had to stop myself from putting it on every recipe in this book. It immediately makes everything a million times better! Have it on the Saucy Kale (page 128) and my Super Loaded Harvest Bowl (page 170).

MAKES 4 to 6 servings (about 3 tablespoons per serving) ✦ **START TO FINISH:** 2 minutes

⅓ cup tahini

2 garlic cloves, minced

1 teaspoon soy sauce

2 teaspoons pure maple syrup

Pinch of salt

¼ to ½ cup warm water, to thin, plus more as needed

FOR SPICY VERSION (OPTIONAL)

1 to 2 tablespoons sriracha or chili garlic sauce

1. In a jar or other container, combine all the basic dressing ingredients, adding warm water, 1 tablespoon at a time, until it reaches your desired drippy consistency. For the spicy version, add the sriracha.

Creamy Hummus Caesar

This hummus Caesar would give any nonvegan version a run for its money, and it's ridiculously easy to make. Try it with my Brussels Sprouts Caesar Salad (page 130), Buffalo Chickpea Lettuce Cups (page 120), and Grilled Romaine Salad (page 124).

MAKES 4 to 6 servings (about 2 tablespoons per serving) ✦ **START TO FINISH:** 5 minutes

½ cup plain or garlic (Almost) the Whole Can Hummus (page 282)

1 teaspoon vegan Dijon mustard

2 garlic cloves, minced

1 teaspoon nutritional yeast

Juice of 1 lemon

½ teaspoon kosher salt

½ teaspoon pure maple syrup

1 teaspoon caper brine, Apple Scrap Vinegar (page 350), or store-bought apple cider vinegar

½ teaspoon freshly ground black pepper

¼ cup warm water, to thin

1. In a jar, combine all the ingredients, except the water, and whisk or shake until a smooth sauce is formed. Add warm water, 1 tablespoon at a time, as needed, to thin.

EVERYTHING TAHINI DRESSING

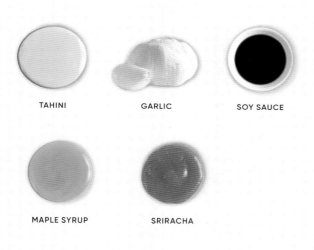

TAHINI

GARLIC

SOY SAUCE

MAPLE SYRUP

SRIRACHA

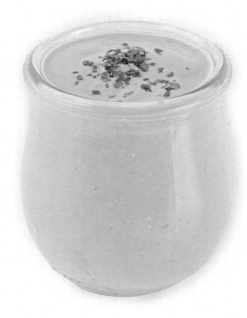

CREAMY HUMMUS CAESAR

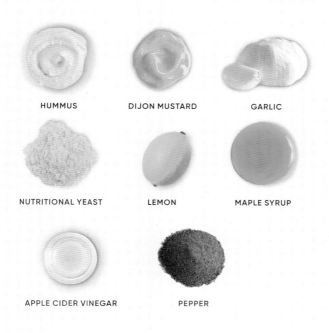

HUMMUS

DIJON MUSTARD

GARLIC

NUTRITIONAL YEAST

LEMON

MAPLE SYRUP

APPLE CIDER VINEGAR

PEPPER

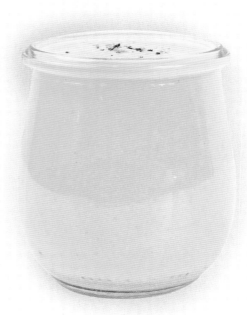

Storage: Store in a sealed container in the fridge for up to 4 days (or longer . . . just do the smell test).

Strawberry Top Vinaigrette

This gorgeous pink-hued salad dressing screams "summertime"! Sweet and a little tangy, it's amazing served with my Strawberry Farro Salad (page 136).

MAKES 6 servings (about 2 tablespoons per serving) ✦ **START TO FINISH:** 5 minutes

¼ cup Strawberry Top Vinegar (page 348) or white wine vinegar

¼ cup unsweetened Cultured Vegan Yogurt or store-bought coconut or soy yogurt

1 tablespoon pure maple syrup

¼ teaspoon salt

¼ teaspoon freshly ground black pepper

1 tablespoon vegan Dijon mustard

1 tablespoon poppy seeds

1. In a cup or jar, combine all the ingredients and mix until a smooth dressing is formed.

Green Goddess Dressing

True to its name, this glowing bright-green dressing is a true showstopper. Its flavor is unique, best described as herby, bright, and tangy. Best enjoyed with my Sproutichoke Wrap (page 112) and Microbiome Bowl (page 172).

MAKES 6 servings (about 3 tablespoons per servings) ✦ **START TO FINISH:** 5 minutes

Juice of ½ lemon

½ avocado, peeled, or ½ cup shelled edamame

½ cup fresh parsley or cilantro

½ cup sunflower seeds or cashews, soaked in water overnight or boiled for 10 minutes

1 garlic clove

1 tablespoon nutritional yeast

¾ cup water, plus more as needed

¼ teaspoon salt

1. In a blender, combine all the ingredients and blend until smooth.

Save the Scraps: Use up the remaining avocado half in Loaded Tortilla Bowls (page 178).

STRAWBERRY TOP VINAIGRETTE

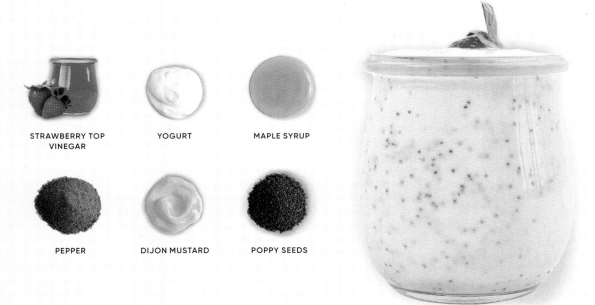

STRAWBERRY TOP VINEGAR

YOGURT

MAPLE SYRUP

PEPPER

DIJON MUSTARD

POPPY SEEDS

GREEN GODDESS DRESSING

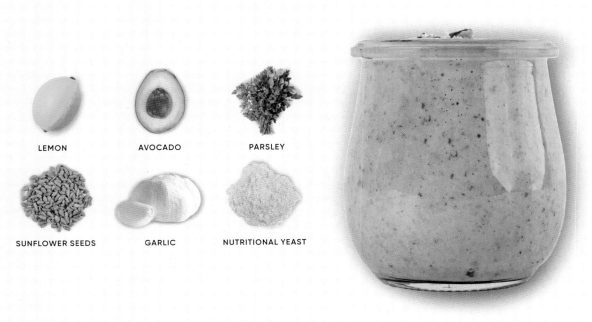

LEMON

AVOCADO

PARSLEY

SUNFLOWER SEEDS

GARLIC

NUTRITIONAL YEAST

Storage: Store in a sealed container in the fridge for up to 4 days (or longer . . . just do the smell test).

Luscious Lemon Dressing

This preserved lemon dressing is akin to bottling sunshine. Intensely bright, flavorful, and, of course . . . lemony. Serve it with my Pantry Bean Salad (page 134) and Beaming Lentil Lemon Salad (page 138).

MAKES 4 servings (about 2 tablespoons per serving) ✦ **START TO FINISH:** 5 minutes

¼ cup Perfect Preserved Lemons (page 326), chopped finely, seeds removed, or zest of ½ lemon

Juice of 1 lemon

1 tablespoon pure maple syrup

2 tablespoons vegan Dijon mustard

¼ teaspoon freshly ground black pepper

¼ teaspoon salt

½ teaspoon dried oregano

1 tablespoon extra-virgin olive oil (optional)

1. Put the preserved lemons on a cutting board or plate, and using the back of a fork, mash until a paste is formed, or chop finely. Combine the lemon paste with the remaining ingredients until a smooth dressing is formed.

(Almost) the Whole Can Hummus

This is the easiest, creamiest hummus you will ever make that uses an entire can of chickpeas AND the aquafaba. The secret to making it extra creamy is adding ice cubes to the food processor (don't ask me how that works)!

MAKES 8 servings ✦ **START TO FINISH:** 5 minutes

1 (15-ounce) can chickpeas, drained, ¼ cup aquafaba reserved

Juice of 1 lemon

¾ teaspoon salt

2 heaping tablespoons tahini

2 garlic cloves

2 ice cubes

1. In a food processor, combine the chickpeas, ¼ cup of their aquafaba, lemon juice, salt, tahini, and garlic. Process, adding the ice cubes halfway through, to achieve a creamy consistency.

LUSCIOUS LEMON DRESSING

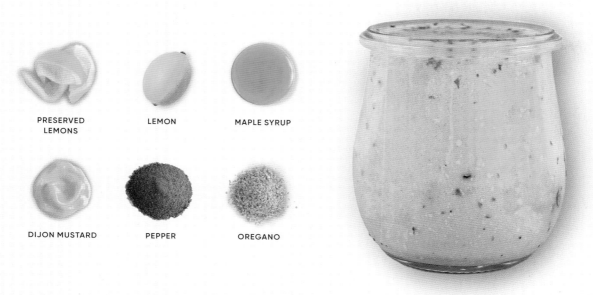

PRESERVED LEMONS

LEMON

MAPLE SYRUP

DIJON MUSTARD

PEPPER

OREGANO

(ALMOST) THE WHOLE CAN HUMMUS

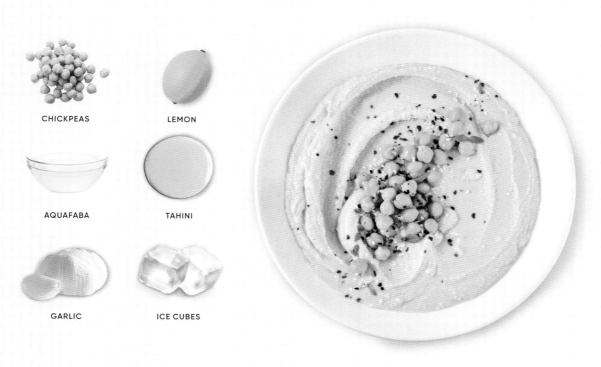

CHICKPEAS

LEMON

AQUAFABA

TAHINI

GARLIC

ICE CUBES

Storage: Store in a sealed container in the fridge for up to 4 days (or longer . . . just do the smell test).

High-Protein Kale, Asparagus & Edamame Spread

This dip is bonkers. It's spicy, creamy, and somehow reminiscent of guacamole, even though there's no avocado! It also has a wonderful kick of protein from the edamame and sunflower seeds. I love it spread on my morning toast for breakfast, or served as a dip with Sourdough Discard Crackers (page 322).

MAKES 4 to 6 servings ✦ **START TO FINISH:** 15 minutes

1½ cups frozen shelled edamame

½ cup woody asparagus ends (optional)

1 cup curly kale

Juice of ½ lemon

½ jalapeño pepper, deseed if you don't like heat

½ teaspoon freshly ground black pepper

¼ teaspoon red pepper flakes

1 teaspoon salt

¼ cup sunflower seeds, soaked in water overnight or boiled for 10 minutes

1. Bring a shallow pot of water to a boil. Place the edamame and asparagus ends in the water, and cook, covered, for 5 to 10 minutes, or until tender. Drain, reserving ½ cup of the cooking water.

2. In a high-speed blender, combine all the ingredients, including the ½ cup of reserved water, and blend until smooth. If you aren't a spice fan, omit the red pepper flakes and jalapeño.

3. Spread on toast for breakfast or use as a delicious dip.

Storage: Store in a sealed container in the fridge for up to 4 days (or longer . . . just do the smell test).

Save the Scraps: Reserve the remaining ½ jalapeño for my Spicy Pickled Red Onions (page 342).

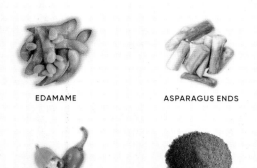

EDAMAME

ASPARAGUS ENDS

KALE

LEMON

JALAPEÑO

PEPPER

RED PEPPER FLAKES

SUNFLOWER SEEDS

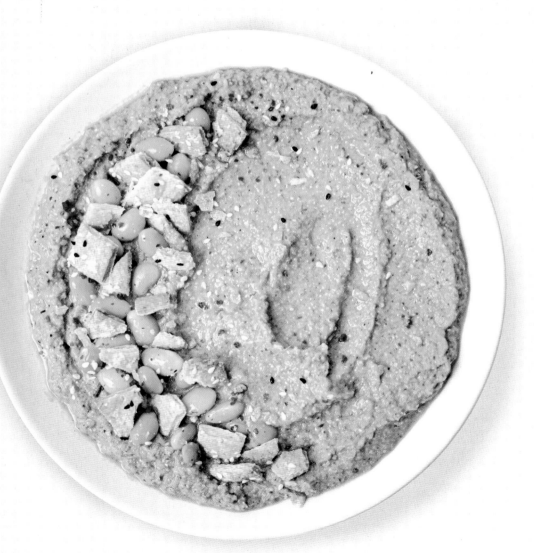

Whipped Feta Dip with Roasted Tomatoes

Shh! Not only does this feta dip contain NO CHEESE, it also has a whole cup of hidden white beans; can anyone say, "Cool beans!"? Give it a try and you'll be amazed at this creamy, cheezy dream.

MAKES 6 servings (about ¼ cup per serving) ✦ START TO FINISH: 25 minutes

ROASTED TOMATOES

1½ cups cherry tomatoes

½ teaspoon sea salt

WHIPPED FETA DIP

1 (15-ounce) can white beans, drained and rinsed

1¼ cups sunflower seeds or cashews, soaked in water overnight

3 garlic cloves

1 teaspoon dried parsley

½ teaspoon sea salt

¼ teaspoon garlic powder

Juice of ½ lemon

1 tablespoon nutritional yeast

3 tablespoons water or more, as needed, to thin

1 tablespoon fresh parsley, for garnish

FOR SERVING

The Knead for Flatbread (page 68) or Sourdough Discard Crackers (page 322)

1. Roast the tomatoes: Preheat the oven to 400°F. In a roasting pan, combine the tomatoes and salt and roast in the oven for 20 to 25 minutes, or until the tomatoes have burst.

2. Meanwhile, combine all the dip ingredients, except the water and fresh parsley, in a blender. Blend until smooth, adding warm water as needed to thin.

3. Transfer to a serving dish, and with the back of a spoon, create a swirl. Top with the roasted tomatoes, fresh parsley, and any tomato juices remaining in the roasting pan. Enjoy with flatbread.

Storage: Store in a sealed container in the fridge for up to 4 days (or longer . . . just do the smell test).

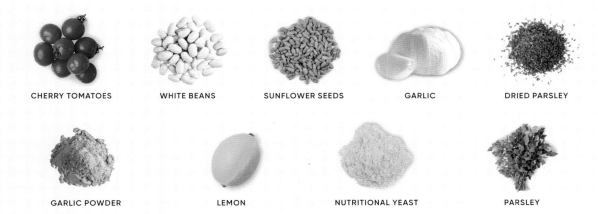

CHERRY TOMATOES   WHITE BEANS   SUNFLOWER SEEDS   GARLIC   DRIED PARSLEY

GARLIC POWDER   LEMON   NUTRITIONAL YEAST   PARSLEY

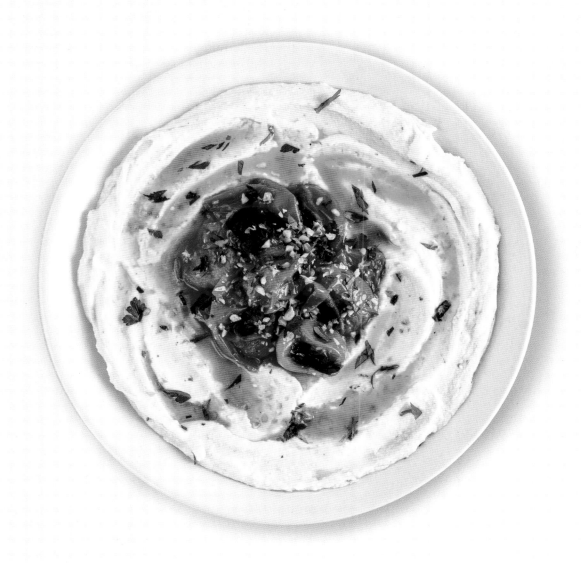

Dressings, Dips & Saucy Things

Tofu Feta

Get ready for a cheese experience like no other with this tangy, salty vegan feta. For this recipe, you're going to marinate cubes of extra-firm tofu in an herby mix of lemon juice and vinegar for the perfect protein accompaniment to any salad (check out my Street Corn Pasta Salad, page 132).

MAKES 16 ounces/16 servings (about 2 tablespoons per serving) ✦ **PREP TIME:** 10 minutes ✦
MARINATING TIME: 6 to 10 hours

1 (14-ounce) block extra-firm tofu

¼ cup vegetable broth or extra-virgin olive oil, for a more indulgent and realistic feta

2 tablespoons Apple Scrap Vinegar (page 350) or store-bought apple cider vinegar

2 tablespoons freshly squeezed lemon juice

½ lemon, sliced thinly

1 teaspoon dried oregano

1 teaspoon dried rosemary

1 teaspoon dried dill

1 teaspoon dried chives

½ teaspoon onion powder

½ teaspoon garlic powder

1 teaspoon salt

½ teaspoon freshly ground black pepper

1. Wrap the tofu in a clean cloth, and stack something heavy on top, such as a cast-iron pan. Allow to press for 15 to 20 minutes.

2. While the tofu is pressing, combine the vegetable broth, Apple Scrap Vinegar, lemon juice, lemon slices, oregano, rosemary, dill, chives, onion powder, garlic powder, salt, and pepper in a glass jar (I use a 16-ounce jar). Screw on the lid, and give the jar a shake to mix the ingredients.

3. Once the tofu is pressed, tear it into ½-inch chunks and stuff it into the jar as well. Close the jar and give it another shake to make sure the tofu is coated.

4. Place the jar in the fridge to marinate for 6 to 12 hours. During that period, shake the jar a few times.

5. This vegan feta can be enjoyed straight from the jar, or added to salads, sandwiches, wraps, and more!

Storage: Store in the fridge for up to 5 days.

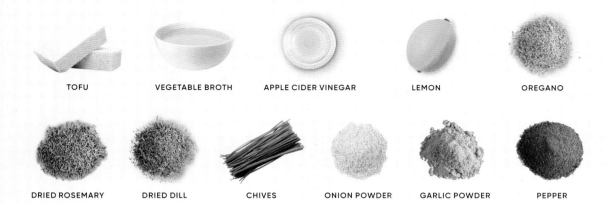

TOFU VEGETABLE BROTH APPLE CIDER VINEGAR LEMON OREGANO

DRIED ROSEMARY DRIED DILL CHIVES ONION POWDER GARLIC POWDER PEPPER

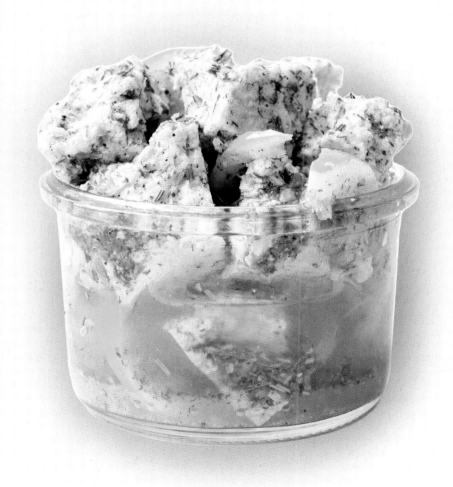

Dressings, Dips & Saucy Things

Vegan Nutty "Parm"

You'll want to sprinkle this ridiculously simple vegan "Parm" on *everything*. Nutty, salty, and just the right amount of umami, this "Parm" comes together in just 5 minutes. Try it on my Sunday Sauce (page 162) and Green with Envy Spaghetti (page 160).

MAKES 12 servings (about 1 tablespoon per serving) ✦ **START TO FINISH:** 5 minutes

¼ cup walnuts or raw sunflower seeds

½ cup nutritional yeast

½ teaspoon salt

2 garlic cloves, or ¼ teaspoon garlic powder

½ teaspoon onion powder

1. In a blender, combine all the ingredients and blend until a thick powder is formed. Alternatively, crush with a mortar and pestle, then transfer to a jar.

Storage: Store in the fridge for up to 2 weeks.

Balsamic Glaze

A drizzle of balsamic glaze elevates any ordinary recipe to restaurant quality in seconds, and you can make it yourself at home! The method couldn't be easier—you just simmer balsamic vinegar until it becomes a thick, syrup-like consistency. I love it on salads, my Can't-Miss Miso Cabbage Steaks (page 204) and Microbiome Bowl (page 172).

MAKES ½ cup ✦ **FROM START TO FINISH:** 30 minutes

2 cups balsamic vinegar

1. In a small saucepan over medium heat, bring the balsamic vinegar to a low boil, then simmer. Stir occasionally until the vinegar thickens and reduces to about ½ cup in about 20 minutes. It should be slightly thinner than maple syrup.

2. Remove from the heat and allow to cool. It will thicken slightly while it cools.

Storage: Store in a sealed jar in the fridge for up to 4 weeks.

VEGAN NUTTY "PARM"

WALNUTS

NUTRITIONAL YEAST

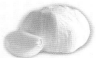

GARLIC

ONION POWDER

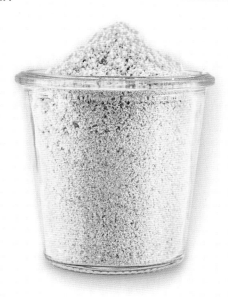

BALSAMIC GLAZE

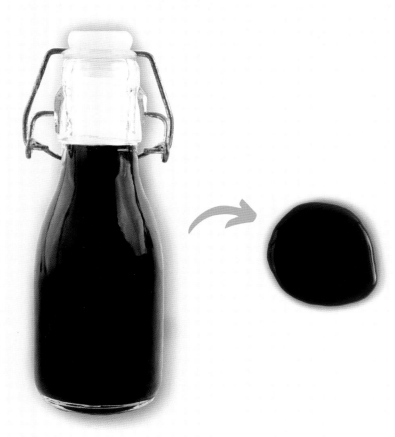

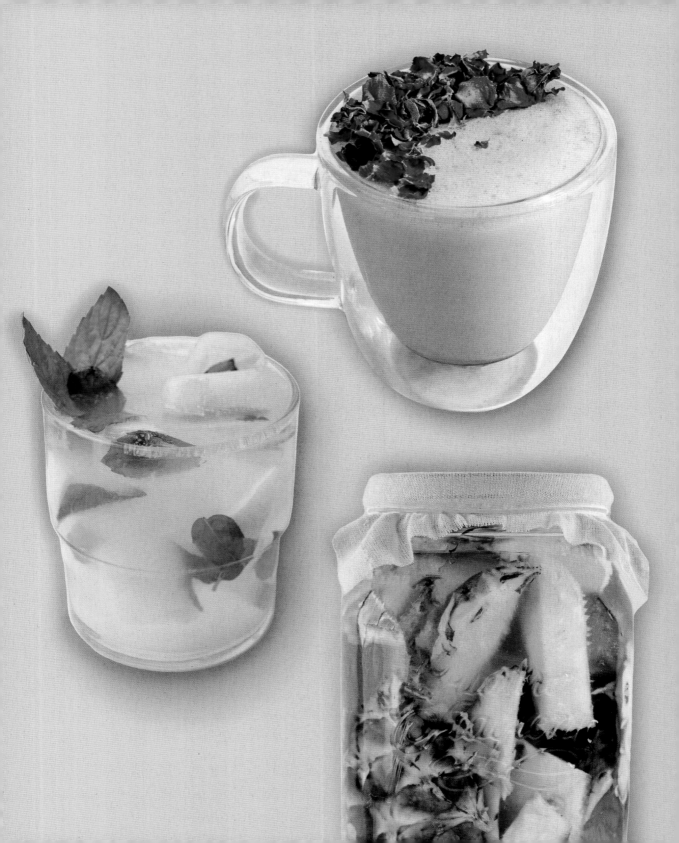

CHAPTER 10

Sip & Save

Eco-elixirs, conscious cocktails,
and sustainable sips are just
a page away.

Peanut Butter Jar Latte

It's time to embrace your nutty side. When you get to the end of your peanut butter jar, it's the perfect opportunity to make a delicious creamy latte by using up any remnants that you couldn't get at with a knife or spoon. The result is a rich and velvety latte that tastes like a warm hug.

MAKES 2 servings ✦ **START TO FINISH:** 5 minutes

1¾ cups unsweetened plant-based milk (soy, oat, almond, or cashew)

1 nut butter jar with some "butter" still left on the sides, or 2 tablespoons peanut butter

2 tablespoons pure maple syrup (optional; omit or use less for a less sweet drink)

½ teaspoon ground cinnamon, plus more for garnish

½ teaspoon Homemade Vanilla Extract (page 324) or store-bought pure vanilla extract

½ cup hot coffee, espresso, or orange pekoe tea

1. In a saucepan over medium heat, simmer the plant-based milk.

2. When the milk is hot, safely pour into the empty peanut butter jar (or a clean jar with 2 tablespoons of peanut butter) and add all the remaining ingredients, except the coffee.

3. Screw on the lid and shake until combined. You can also use a spoon to scrape any remaining peanut butter off the sides of the jar and into the drink.

4. Pour ¼ cup of the coffee into a cup, then pour the latte mixture from the peanut butter jar over the top. Stir and garnish with additional cinnamon. Enjoy immediately.

PLANT-BASED MILK

PEANUT BUTTER JAR

MAPLE SYRUP

CINNAMON

VANILLA EXTRACT

COFFEE

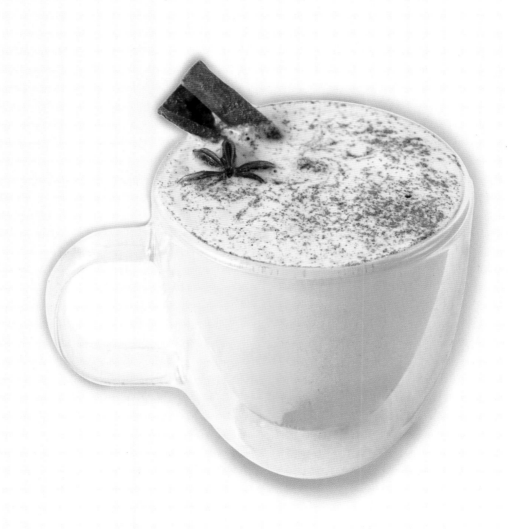

Rose Water

Who says roses are just for romance? Tune into your *Scrappy* side and put those roses to good use by whipping up a batch of rose water, which can be used to infuse dishes with a subtle flowery essence (I love to add a drop on fruit salad). Try it in my Rose-Water Latte (page 298). This recipe must be made with unsprayed organic rose petals if being used for culinary purposes.

MAKES 16 servings (about 1 tablespoon per serving) ✦ **START TO FINISH:** 45 minutes

1 cup unsprayed fresh organic rose petals, or ½ cup dried culinary rose petals

1½ to 2 cups water

1. In a pot or saucepan, add the clean rose petals and enough water to just cover the petals.

2. Over medium-low heat, simmer the water, then cover. Let simmer until the petals lose their color, for 30 to 45 minutes.

3. Remove from the heat and let the rose water cool completely. Strain into a sterilized bottle, composting the remaining rose petals.

Storage: Store in the refrigerator for several weeks, or on the counter for up to 1 week.

ROSE PETALS

WATER

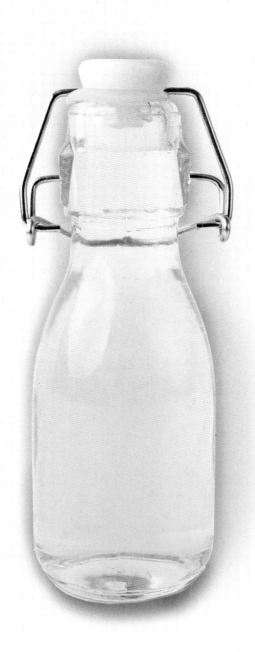

Rose-Water Latte

Here is a pick-me-up that's as sweet as it is sophisticated! The subtle sweetness of the Rose Water combines perfectly with the richness of coffee and creamy oat milk, creating a sip that's as dreamy as a love song. . . . Like drinking a bouquet of flowers, but in the best way possible.

MAKES 2 servings ✦ **START TO FINISH:** 10 minutes

1½ cups unsweetened Homemade Oat Milk (page 314) or store-bought oat milk

1 teaspoon pure maple syrup

1 teaspoon Rose Water (page 296)

½ teaspoon Homemade Vanilla Extract (page 324) or store-bought pure vanilla extract

¼ teaspoon ground cinnamon

1 cup strong brewed Earl Grey tea or coffee

1 teaspoon dried culinary rose petals

1. In a medium-size saucepan, combine the oat milk, maple syrup, Rose Water, vanilla, and cinnamon. Bring to a boil, then simmer for 5 minutes. Remove from the heat and, using a handheld foamer, foam the milk, as desired.

2. Divide the brewed tea between two mugs.

3. Pour the oat milk mixture over the top until full. Garnish with dried rose petals, as desired.

UNSWEETENED OAT MILK

MAPLE SYRUP

ROSE WATER

VANILLA EXTRACT

CINNAMON

COFFEE

DRIED ROSE PETALS

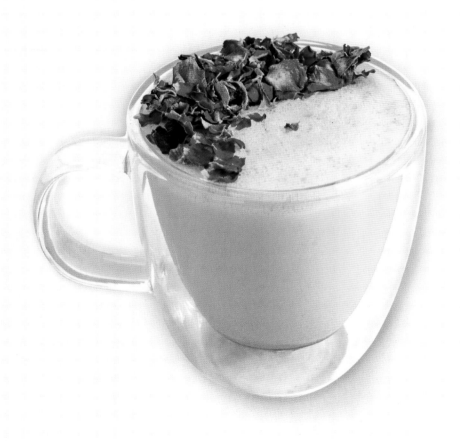

Date Seed Coffee

Who knew the pits of sweet, chewy dates could be transformed into the perfect coffee substitute? This date seed coffee is the ultimate zero-waste brew, making use of a seed that is often thrown away. Instead, save the seeds in a sealed container in your pantry, until ready to brew this drink. The result is a caffeine-free beverage with a subtle flavor profile that lies somewhere between a black coffee and tea.

MAKES 1 serving ✦ **START TO FINISH:** 40 minutes

**½ cup date seeds (15 to 20 seeds)
(I used the seeds from Medjool dates)**

1. Preheat the oven to 400°F, and line a baking sheet with a reusable baking mat or parchment paper.

2. Clean the seeds thoroughly, then spread them on the prepared baking sheet and roast for 25 to 35 minutes, or until browned, watching to ensure they do not burn.

3. After removing from the oven, use a food processor or spice grinder to grind date coffee grounds. Prepare as you would regular coffee, such as with a pour-over method or French press.

   Storage: Store ground date seeds in a sealed container in your pantry for up to a few weeks.

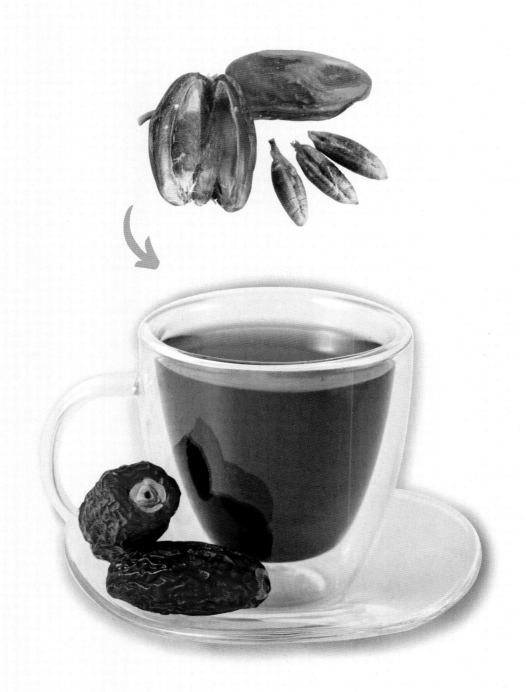

Pineapple Skin Tea

Originating in Jamaica, this tea is a fragrant drink served both hot and cold to aid with digestion. Loaded with the nutrient-dense pineapple core, ginger, turmeric, cinnamon, and maple syrup, it also contains anti-inflammatory properties. With sweet, citrusy notes and a refreshing aroma, it's like sipping on a summer breeze.

MAKES 6 servings (about ¾ cup per serving)   ✦   **START TO FINISH:** 40 minutes

1 organic pineapple, peel and core only
1 (1-inch) piece fresh ginger
¼ teaspoon ground turmeric
1 cinnamon stick
1 tablespoon pure maple syrup
8 cups water

FOR SERVING
Tajín
6 fresh pineapple slices

1. First, make sure to wash the pineapple skin thoroughly, using a scrub brush and vegetable wash if possible.

2. After thoroughly washing your pineapple skin, place it in a large pot along with the core, ginger, turmeric, cinnamon stick, and maple syrup. Add the water, or enough to cover the ingredients by 1 inch. Bring to a boil, then simmer, uncovered, for 30 minutes.

3. Strain, reserving the liquid for your tea. Enjoy hot or cold with Tajín sprinkled on top and a slice of pineapple.

   Storage: Store the cooled pineapple skin tea in the fridge for up to 3 days.

PINEAPPLE

GINGER ROOT

TURMERIC

CINNAMON

MAPLE SYRUP

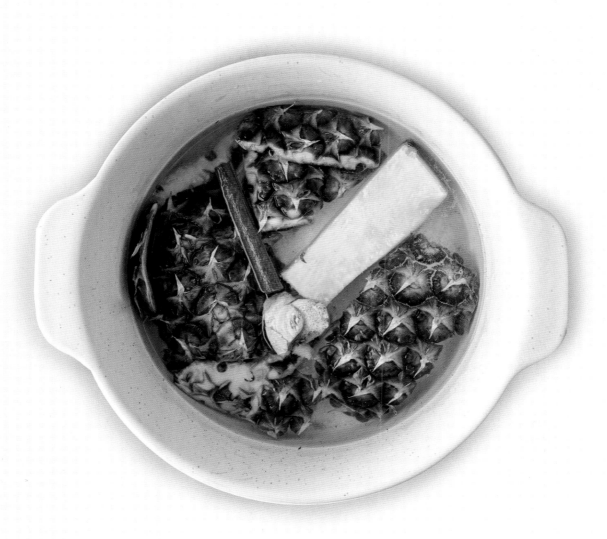

Tangy Tepache

Originating in Mexico, *tepache* is an incredible fermented beverage that utilizes the skin and core of pineapple. By fermenting the pineapple scraps with sugar, water, cinnamon, and cloves, you're left with a refreshing tangy drink having a low alcohol content. If you accidentally let this ferment for too many days, you'll have pineapple skin vinegar!

MAKES 10 cups ✦ **START TO FINISH:** 36 to 72 hours

1 organic pineapple, peel and core only

1 cup light or dark brown sugar

1 cinnamon stick

2 to 3 whole cloves

8 cups filtered water

1. First, make sure to wash the pineapple skin thoroughly, using a scrub brush and vegetable wash if possible.

2. Place the skin from the pineapple, its core, the sugar, cinnamon stick, and cloves in a large jar (I use a wide-mouthed gallon-size jar or two 64-ounce jars). Pour the filtered water into the jar until it covers the skins and other ingredients. Cover the mouth of the jar with a clean kitchen cloth and secure it with a rubber band.

3. Allow the mixture to ferment for 36 to 72 hours at room temperature. The fermentation time will vary depending on ripeness of the pineapple, room temperature, and other environmental factors.

4. When you see signs of carbonation (small bubbles forming at the top), you'll know the fermentation process has been successful. You can taste test by lowering the end of a clean straw into the jar and closing the top end with your finger to draw some liquid out. Taste the liquid. (If you need to test again, use a fresh, clean straw—no double-dipping.)

5. Once you achieve the desired balance of sweetness and tanginess, strain out the solids and pour your tepache into bottles or a pitcher. If there are signs of mold, compost and try again.

6. Place the mixture in the fridge to slow down the carbonation process and enjoy over ice.

Storage: Store in the fridge for up to 5 days.

PINEAPPLE

BROWN SUGAR

CINNAMON STICKS

CLOVES

Sip & Save

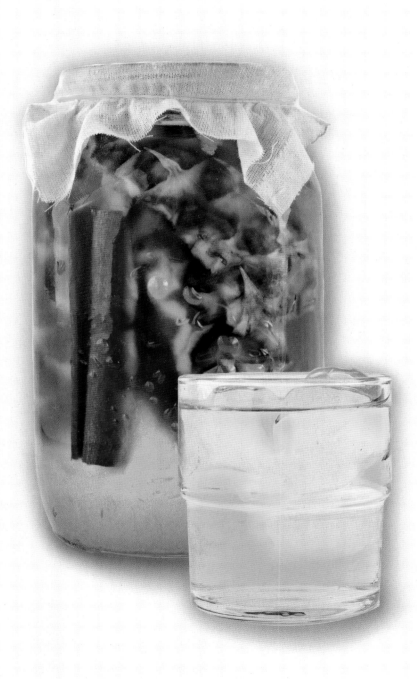

Ginger Turmeric Immunity Shots

These are nothing like the shots you took on your twenty-first birthday. Liquid gold for your health, these Ginger Turmeric Immunity Shots have strong anti-inflammatory and antioxidant properties. They pack a punch of flavor, combining spicy ginger and earthy turmeric for a sip that's healing and invigorating. I love to take a shot in the morning, or whenever I feel a scratchy throat coming on. A forewarning: These can burn on the way down, so proceed with caution!

MAKES 8 shots ✦ **START TO FINISH:** 5 minutes

1 (1-inch) piece fresh ginger, chopped

2 oranges, chopped, including rind

½ teaspoon ground turmeric

Pinch of freshly ground black pepper

Juice of 1 lime

2 cups filtered water

1. In a high-speed blender, combine all the ingredients and blend until smooth.

2. Pour the juice through a fine-mesh sieve into a bowl and separate the pulp from the liquid. You can reserve the pulp for stir-fries or curries, to add a spicy kick.

3. Once you have only liquid remaining, transfer to a sealable jar or container.

Storage: Store in the fridge for up to 4 days, and enjoy shots as you please.

GINGER ROOT

ORANGE

TURMERIC

PEPPER

LIME

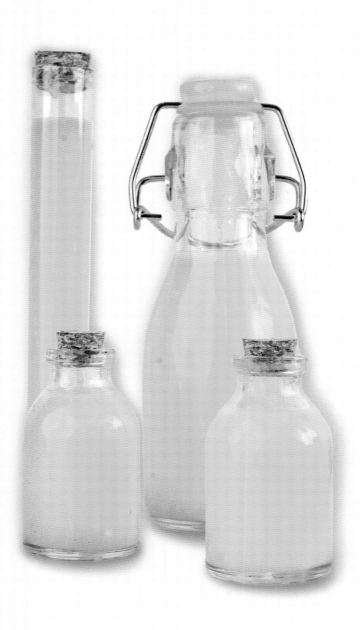

Tummy-Soothing
Lemon, Ginger & Mint Ice Cubes

Like a spa day for your digestive system, these lemon, ginger, and mint ice cubes are the perfect way to use up extra produce while giving your tummy a little love! Add them to a cup of peppermint tea for a refreshing drink or in your morning water for a nourishing start to your day.

MAKES 3 ice cube trays ✦ **START TO FINISH:** 3 hours

1 (1-inch) piece fresh ginger, unpeeled

Juice of 1 lemon

3 cups water or 2 cups water plus 1 cup reserved zucchini or cucumber water

¼ cup fresh mint leaves

½ lemon, sliced into ½-inch chunks

1. In a blender, combine the ginger, lemon juice, and water and blend until smooth.

2. To each well of three ice cube trays, add a chunk of the lemon and mint leaf. Pour in the liquid to fill the wells.

3. Freeze for at least 3 hours.

4. Serve in hot or cold water, or paired with chamomile tea.

Storage: Store in the freezer for up to 1 month.

GINGER ROOT

LEMON

MINT

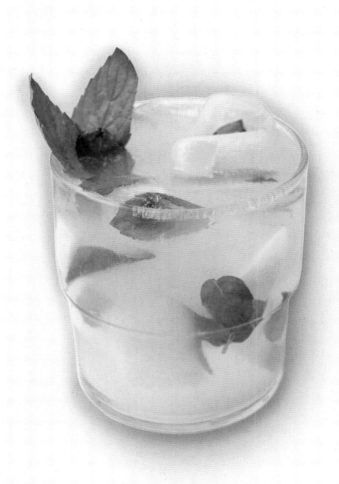

Sip & Save

DIY Ginger Ale

Whether you have extra ginger taking up space in your produce bin, or too many plastic bottles and cans cluttering up your recycling one, this homemade ginger ale recipe is about to be a staple in your low-waste repertoire. Ready in under half an hour, this homemade ale has a crisp, bubbly texture and zingy flavor in every sip!

MAKES 8 servings ✦ **START TO FINISH:** 30 minutes

4 cups water

2 (1-inch) pieces fresh ginger, grated or pulsed in a food processor

Juice of 1 lemon

1 tablespoon pure maple syrup or sweetener of choice

4 cups seltzer or sparkling water

1. In a saucepan, combine the water with the grated ginger. Bring to a boil, then simmer, uncovered, for 20 minutes.

2. Remove from the heat, and using a fine-mesh sieve or piece of cheesecloth, strain out the ginger pulp, reserving the remaining liquid. You can place the remaining ginger pulp in ice cube trays for ginger stir-fries or smoothies.

3. Combine the ginger liquid with the lemon juice and maple syrup. Per serving, to a large glass, add ice, then ½ to 1 cup of the ginger liquid, followed by ½ cup to 1 cup of the sparkling water, depending on how weak or strong you want your ginger ale. Stir and enjoy immediately.

Storage: Store the ginger liquid in the fridge for up to 4 days, or in an ice cube tray in the freezer for up to a month.

GINGER ROOT

LEMON

MAPLE SYRUP

SELTZER

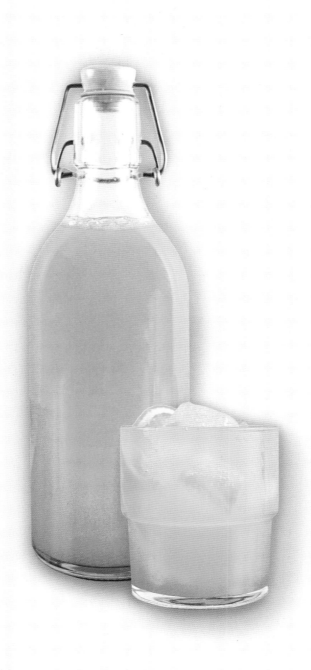

No-Waste Nut Milk

This creamy plant-based milk takes 30 seconds to make with just two ingredients. No straining, no messy nut milk bags, and no fillers or excess ingredients. Just delicious plant-based milk made from blending up your nut butter of choice with water! You'll never buy the store-bought stuff again.

MAKES: 4 servings ◆ **START TO FINISH:** 5 minutes

PLAIN MILK

¼ cup nut butter (cashew, almond), peanut butter, or tahini

3½ cups water

STRAWBERRY MILK

¼ cup nut butter (cashew, almond), peanut butter, or tahini

3½ cups water

1 cup fresh strawberries

2 tablespoons pure maple syrup or sweetener of choice

CHOCOLATE NUT MILK

¼ cup nut butter (cashew, almond), peanut butter, or tahini

3½ cups water

3 tablespoons unsweetened cocoa powder

1 teaspoon Homemade Vanilla Extract (page 324) or store-bought pure vanilla extract

3 Medjool dates, pitted

1. In a blender, combine all the ingredients for your desired nut milk until smooth.

Hot Tip: You can increase or decrease the amount of nut butter for your desired creaminess. You can also increase or decrease the dates or maple syrup for your desired sweetness.

Storage: Store in the fridge for up to 4 days. If separated, blend again or stir. Add maple syrup, vegan sugar, or vanilla extract to sweeten, if desired.

PLAIN MILK

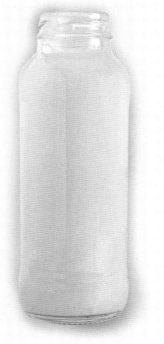

NUT BUTTER OF CHOICE

STRAWBERRY MILK

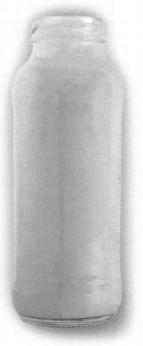

NUT BUTTER OF CHOICE

STRAWBERRIES

MAPLE SYRUP

CHOCOLATE NUT MILK

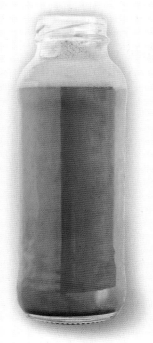

NUT BUTTER OF CHOICE

COCOA POWDER

VANILLA EXTRACT

DATES

Homemade Oat Milk

Ready for an udderly satisfying milk alternative? This delicious creamy homemade oat milk is perfect for your morning cereal or straight out of the jar. The issue with many homemade oat milks is that they can turn out very slimy because of the starchiness in oats. The keys to nonslimy oat milk are to avoid overblending your oats and to use ice-cold water to prevent gumminess.

MAKES 4 servings, about 4 cups ✦ **START TO FINISH:** 40 minutes

¾ cup old-fashioned rolled oats, gluten-free if needed

2 Medjool dates, pitted (optional, for sweetness)

¼ teaspoon sea salt

3 cups ice-cold water

1. In a blender, combine the oats, dates (if using), salt, and cold water and blend for 15 to 30 seconds. Make sure to not overblend. Pour the mixture through a piece of cheesecloth, nut milk bag, or strainer, allowing the excess milk to pour into a bowl below. Do not oversqueeze, as this could also cause sliminess. Strain a second time if you are using cheesecloth or a nut milk bag. This process will ensure the batch is as smooth as possible.

Storage: Store in a sealed container in the fridge for up to 4 days.

Save the Scraps: Reserve the Oat Pulp for PB&J Chickpea Blondies (page 250).

ROLLED OATS

MEDJOOL DATES

WATER

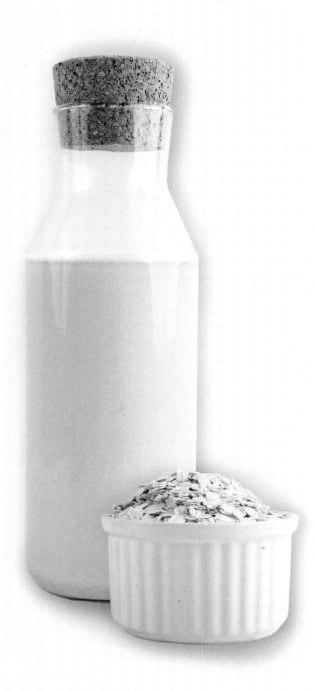

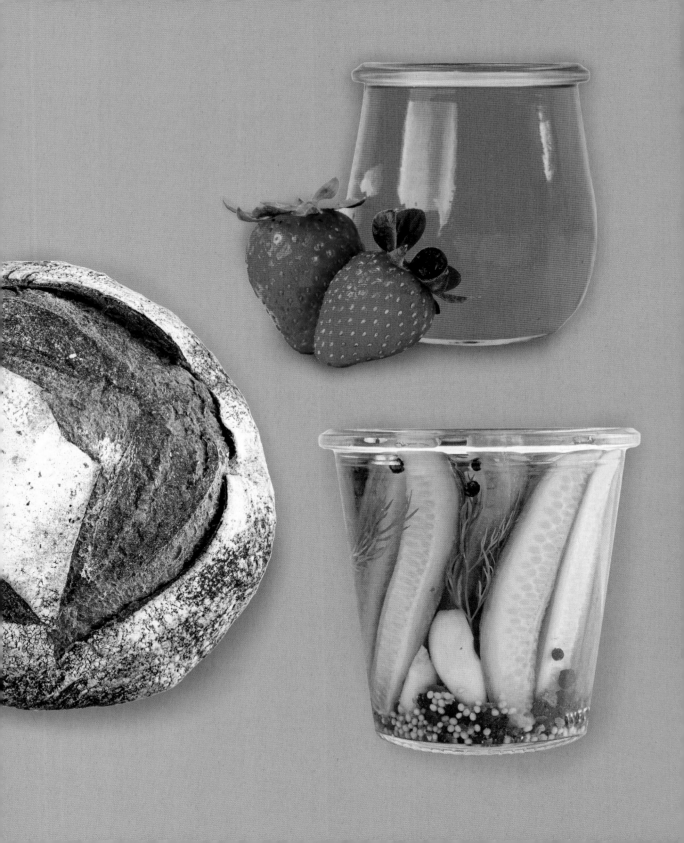

CHAPTER 11

Preserves, Powders, Ferments & Other Fun Stuff

Transform your produce into pantry staples.

Sourdough Starter

A sourdough starter is a live colony of active yeast and bacteria created by combining flour and water. It provides your loaves with a natural leavening agent and a healthy boost of probiotics! It also contains less gluten than your average store-bought bread, so many people with a sensitivity can enjoy it as well (unfortunately not those with celiac disease or a gluten allergy, though). The first essential step in starting your sourdough journey is to name your starter. You're about to begin a hopefully long-lasting, fruitful relationship, so the least you can do is give it a name. Mine is called Gertrude.

MAKES ½ cup ✦ **START TO FINISH:** 7 to 10 days

¼ cup all-purpose flour

¼ cup whole wheat or rye flour

⅓ cup lukewarm water

TO FEED THE STARTER (PER FEED)

¼ cup all-purpose flour

2 to 3 tablespoons room-temperature water

1. Before you start, make sure everything, from the kitchen surface to your hands and equipment, is clean.

2. In a clean glass jar, combine the flours and lukewarm water. Stir well until there are no flour streaks. The initial consistency will be like a thick paste. Cover the opening with a clean cloth and secure it in place with a rubber band. Let the mixture rest in a warm place (75°F to 80°F) for 24 hours.

3. The next day, check on your starter. A good sign of fermentation are small bubbles near the top—another reason why a glass jar is preferable. You might also detect a slightly sour smell. If no bubbles appear, leave your starter for another 24 hours.

4. Time to feed the starter! Add the ¼ cup of flour and the room-temperature water, and use a spoon to mix everything together. You will notice a change in consistency: the mixture will be more gooey and stretchy. Again, cover the starter with a cloth and leave it in a warm place for another 24 hours.

5. For the next 3 to 5 days, you will repeat the feeding process. However, to make space in the jar, you will need to discard half your starter before you add more flour and water. Don't worry; the starter will pick back up. (Also don't worry about wasting: use that discard for Sourdough Discard Crackers, page 322.)

6. The fermentation process may take longer depending on several factors, so don't give up. Generally speaking, after 7 to 10 days of feeding, your starter will be ready for use. You can check that it is ready by adding a spoonful of starter to a glass of room-temperature water. If it floats, it's good to go!

FLOUR

WHOLE WHEAT FLOUR

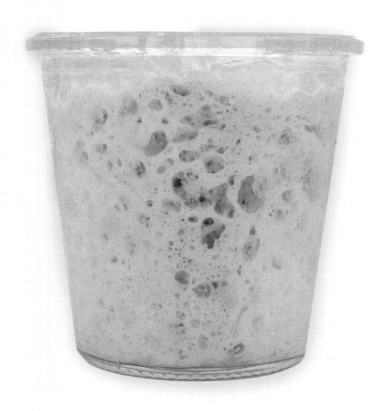

A note on maintaining a sourdough starter: If you are planning on using your starter every day, or nearly every day, continue as you are, feeding your starter and removing half of it (saving your discard for Sourdough Discard Crackers, page 322). If you're more likely to use sourdough starter once a week or even less frequently, store your jar in the fridge. Feed it once a week. After you feed your starter, allow it to rise before using.

Small Sourdough Loaf

There are few things more satisfying in life than breaking into a crusty loaf of bread you baked all by yourself. This small sourdough loaf is the perfect place to start. It takes a little bit of tender loving care, but the end result is an airy fermented loaf that will make the store-bought stuff pale in comparison. Making sourdough is a little like an experiment, so for accuracy I have used metric weight measurements for this recipe.

MAKES 1 loaf ✦ **START TO FINISH:** 15 hours

60 g Sourdough Starter (page 318)

300 g all-purpose flour, plus more for dusting

30 g whole wheat flour

220 ml lukewarm water

8 g salt

4 to 5 ice cubes

1. In a large bowl, mix everything but the salt and ice cubes. Cover with a damp, clean kitchen towel and let it rest for 1 hour. Fold in the salt. Cover and let rest for 30 more minutes.

2. Fold in the edges: Simply pinch the dough at the edges of the bowl and stretch it toward the middle. Cover and let rest for 30 minutes. Repeat this process two or three times.

3. Dust a clean kitchen surface with flour. Transfer the dough and, once again, fold the edges toward the center. Keep going until you struggle to stretch the dough. Flip it over and shape into a loaf. Transfer onto a parchment-lined baking sheet and dust generously with flour. Cover with a dry, clean kitchen towel.

4. Proof in a warm place for 3 hours, or rest in the fridge for 8 to 12 hours, or until about doubled in size.

5. Preheat the oven to 450°F, along with a Dutch oven placed on a second, unlined baking sheet. Score the loaf and transfer it into the Dutch oven together with its parchment paper. Cover with the lid and bake for 30 minutes.

6. Remove the lid and drop the ice cubes into the surrounding baking sheet. Bake for another 15 to 20 minutes, or until the crust is golden. The loaf should make a hollow sound when tapped.

Storage: Store in a sealed bread box or container on the counter for 3 to 4 days.

SOURDOUGH STARTER

FLOUR

WHOLE WHEAT FLOUR

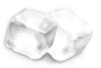

ICE CUBES

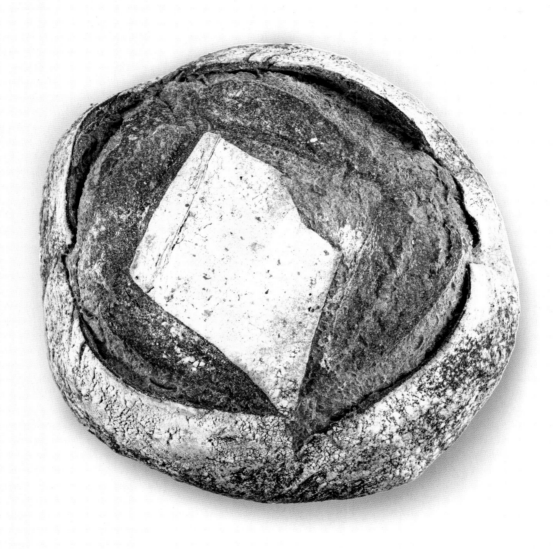

Preserves, Powders, Ferments & Other Fun Stuff

Sourdough Discard Crackers

Part of the process of keeping your sourdough starter alive is discarding some mother dough to make space for more flour and water. To avoid food waste, transform that excess sourdough starter into delicious crackers with a tangy aftertaste. Serve with my High-Protein Kale, Asparagus & Edamame Spread (page 284) or Whipped Feta Dip with Roasted Tomatoes (page 286).

MAKES 40 to 50 small crackers, or 25 large   **START TO FINISH:** 30 minutes

½ cup Sourdough Starter (page 318)

1 cup all-purpose or 1:1 gluten-free flour, plus more for dusting

2 tablespoons extra-virgin olive oil

½ teaspoon salt

½ teaspoon light or dark brown sugar

Sesame seeds

Flaky salt

1. Preheat the oven to 400°F, and line a baking sheet with parchment or a reusable baking mat.

2. In a large bowl, combine all the ingredients, except the sesame seeds and flaky salt, until you achieve an elastic dough. Dust a flat surface with flour, and roll out the dough to about ⅛ inch thick. Transfer to a sheet of parchment paper, the size of a baking sheet, or a reusable baking mat.

3. Sprinkle with sesame seeds and flaky salt. Go over the dough with a rolling pin (or a bottle of wine) to press them into the dough.

4. Use a pizza cutter to score the dough into future crackers. This can make 25 to 50 crackers, depending on size. Transfer to the baking sheet.

5. Bake for 15 to 20 minutes, or until golden. Break into crackers along the lines you scored earlier.

   Storage: Store in a sealed container on your counter for up to 1 week.

SOURDOUGH
STARTER

FLOUR

OLIVE OIL

BROWN SUGAR

SESAME SEEDS

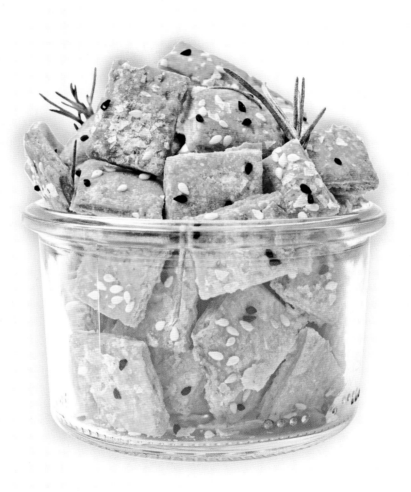

Homemade Vanilla Extract

If you're looking for the absolutely perfect zero-waste, edible gift for a loved one, make your own bottles of vanilla extract. It takes about 5 minutes of work, and you'll have a fragrant and flavorful extract that will elevate your culinary creations to new heights. You'll just want to plan in advance because the vanilla takes at least 8 weeks to brew!

MAKES four 4-ounce jars

12 vanilla beans   **16 ounces 80-proof vodka**

1. Carefully cut a slit along each of the vanilla beans so the seeds are exposed. Place three vanilla beans into each of four 4-ounce jars. If they do not fit, you can slice them in half crosswise.

2. Pour the vodka over the top of the beans so they are fully submerged. Seal. Store in a cupboard at room temperature, shaking the bottle gently every other week.

3. The vanilla is ready to use in as little as 8 weeks, but for optimal results, wait 6 months and up to a year. As you use the vanilla, you can refill the bottles with more vodka for longer use. This extract can last several years, but the beans will eventually need to be replaced as the taste and scent become less intense.

Preserves, Powders, Ferments & Other Fun Stuff

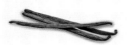

VANILLA BEANS

VODKA

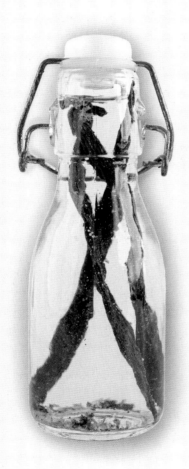

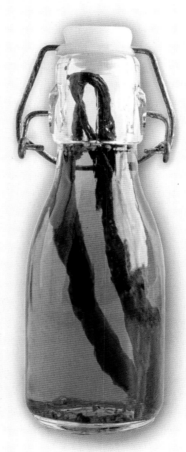

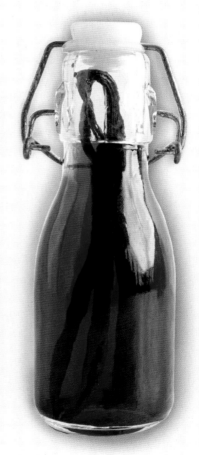

1 Day   1 Month   3 Months +

Perfect Preserved Lemons

You'll be feeling like a sourpuss if you miss out on these preserved lemons. Originating in Morocco, preserved lemons bring notes of citrus, tang, and sweetness to your cooking. They're excellent chopped into a salad, used in my Luscious Lemon Dressing (page 282), or on such side dishes as my Zucchini "Falafel" Fritters (page 186)—or as the perfect palate cleanser.

MAKES 5 to 7 lemons

5 to 7 Meyer lemons, organic if possible   **½ cup kosher salt, plus more as needed**

1. Scrub the lemons thoroughly.

2. With a sharp knife, carefully slice an X into four of the lemons, coming within ½ inch of their bottom. This should split them open, almost like an orange.

3. Transfer to a bowl and add 3 tablespoons of the kosher salt, packing it into the crevices of each lemon.

4. In a sterilized glass jar (I used a 16-ounce jar), put 2 tablespoons of the kosher salt, followed by one of the lemons. Using the back of a wooden spoon, press down the lemon to pack it in. Add an additional 2 tablespoons of salt, followed by another lemon. Repeat until the four lemons are packed into the jar, adding more split lemons and salt as needed if there is a lot of space in the jar.

5. Juice the final lemon into the jar, then pack it on top.

6. Add the lid, give it a shake, and place in a cool spot in your pantry for at least 1 week, shaking and flipping it every couple of days to make sure the lemon juice is evenly distributed.

7. After 1 week, transfer the jar of lemons to your refrigerator. When the peels become slightly translucent, after about 2 more weeks, they are ready to use.

8. Compost and try again if you see any signs of mold. When you are ready to use a lemon, remove it from the jar and rinse away any excess salt and seeds. Prepare according to recipes, or chop on top of salads or bowls for garnish.

Storage: Once the jar is open, store the preserved lemons in the fridge for up to 2 months.

LEMONS

SALT

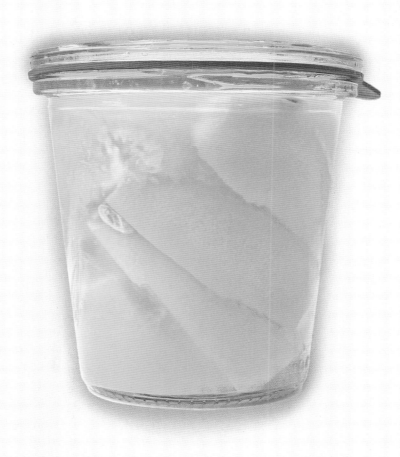

Sun-Dried Tomatoes

Time to let those cherry tomatoes soak up some rays and become the star of the show! Making your own sun-dried tomatoes is really easy. You can dry them in the sun, depending on your climate, or in the oven. They make a great addition to just about any dish, but you absolutely must try my Tuscan Sweet Potato Gnocchi with Sunflower Cream Sauce (pages 142 and 272).

MAKES about 1 cup ✦ **START TO FINISH:** 3 to 4 hours

1 pound cherry tomatoes (25 to 30 tomatoes)   Salt

1. If you live somewhere warm and sunny, place the tomatoes on a raised screen or rack outdoors to dry, bringing them in at night to avoid critters.

2. Alternatively, preheat the oven to 200°F and line a baking sheet with a reusable baking mat or parchment paper.

3. Slice the tomatoes in half. Place the tomatoes, cut side up, on the prepared baking sheet and sprinkle lightly with salt.

4. Roast for 2½ hours. Remove from the oven, and using the bottom of a glass, press down to express any juices.

5. Continue to bake until the tomatoes are your desired dryness.

   Storage: If completely dry, store in an airtight container in your pantry for up to 1 month.

CHERRY TOMATOES

SALT

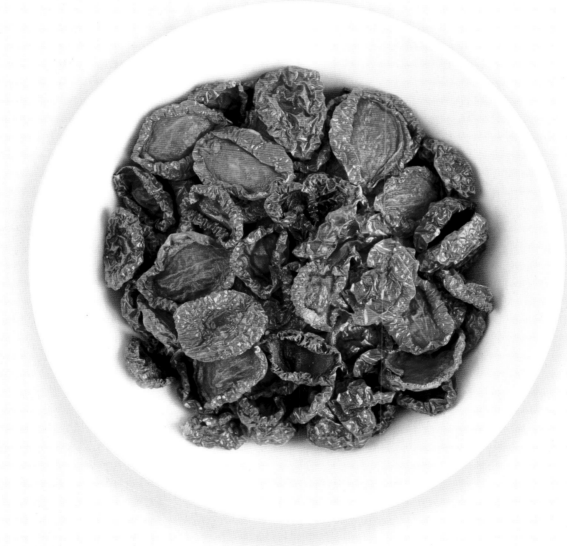

Herbed Bread Crumbs

Never let those stale bread slices go to waste again. Transform them into a flavorful versatile ingredient with these herbed bread crumbs. Like dashing pizzazz to a dish, these bread crumbs can take any meal from meh to magnificent. Try them out on my Bang-Bang Broccolicious Steaks (page 206).

MAKES 2½ cups ✦ **START TO FINISH:** 25 minutes

4 cups stale vegan bread, torn into chunks

1 tablespoon nutritional yeast

1 teaspoon garlic powder

2 teaspoons dried parsley

1 small shallot, diced

1. Preheat the oven to 350°F, and line a baking sheet with a reusable baking mat or parchment.

2. In a food processor or blender, combine the stale bread, nutritional yeast, garlic powder, and parsley. Process until bread crumbs are achieved. Mix with the diced shallot and pour onto the prepared baking sheet.

3. Bake the bread crumbs for 10 to 15 minutes, or until browned, mixing halfway through. Remove from the oven and transfer to an airtight jar when cool.

Storage: Store in an airtight container in the pantry for up to 5 days.

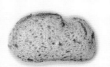

SOURDOUGH BREAD

NUTRITIONAL YEAST

GARLIC POWDER

DRIED PARSLEY

SHALLOTS

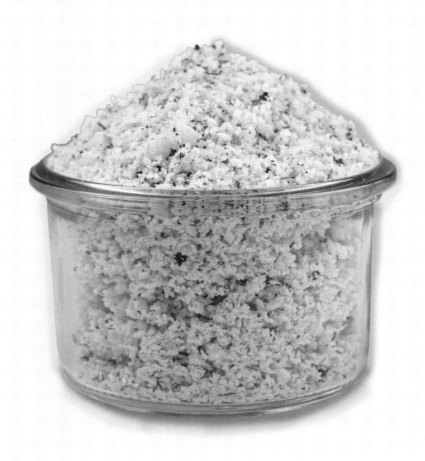

Citrus Peel Powder

Time to zest up your life! Instead of discarding those orange and lemon peels, put them to good use with sunshine in a jar. Collect your citrus peels and store them in a sealed container in your freezer. Then simply dehydrate and grind them to make an amazing bright powder, perfect to add a zesty note to such recipes as my "Death by Chocolate" Flapjacks (page 38) or desserts, or sprinkled on stir-fries.

MAKES ¼ cup ✦ START TO FINISH: 6 to 24 hours

10 orange or lemon peels, pith removed

1. Dehydrate the peels in the sun for 24 to 48 hours, bringing them in at night to avoid critters. Alternatively, line a baking sheet with a reusable baking mat or parchment paper, arrange the peels in a single layer on the prepared baking sheet, and dehydrate in the oven, at its lowest heat setting, for 6 hours.

2. Once they are dried, transfer the peels to a blender or coffee grinder. Blend until a powder is achieved.

Tomato Peel Powder

So, you just whipped up a batch of Scratch Tomato Sauce (page 164), and need a way to use up those tomato peels? I've got you covered. Tomato peels pack in a punch of tomato-y flavor and, when dehydrated, make an amazing spice reminiscent of paprika. The Canadian in me likes it sprinkled over popcorn for a ketchup-chip flair.

MAKES ¼ cup ✦ START TO FINISH: 12 hours

Peels from 8 to 20 tomatoes

1. Set the oven to its lowest temperature, and line a baking sheet with parchment paper or a reusable baking mat. Arrange the tomato skins in a single layer on the prepared baking sheet, and dehydrate in the oven for 4 to 6 hours, or until completely dried.

2. Alternatively, if you live somewhere warm and sunny, place the tomato peels on a raised screen or rack outdoors to dry, bringing them in at night to avoid critters.

3. Once dried, place the tomato peels in a coffee grinder or blender, and grind until a fine powder is achieved. Use on top of soups, stir-fries, and more for a subtle tomato kick or rehydrate with some water for a tomato paste alternative.

CITRUS PEEL POWDER

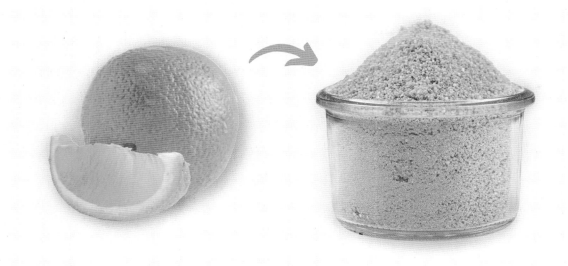

TOMATO PEEL POWDER

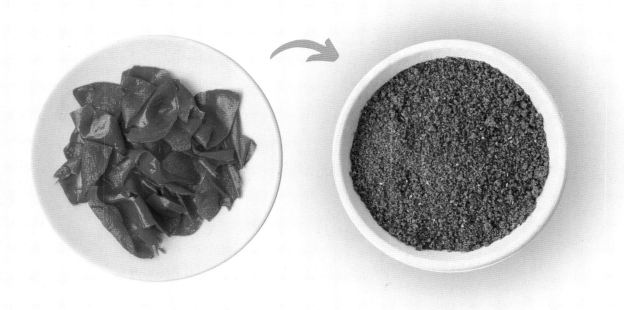

Storage: Store in a sealed jar in your pantry for up to 1 month.

Beet Powder

Did you know beet powder can act as a natural preworkout? One of the key ingredients in beet is dietary nitrates, which your body then converts to nitric acid, helping to more effectively increase oxygen in the blood. Stir it into water or your morning smoothie.

MAKES ¼ cup ✦ **START TO FINISH:** 2 to 3 hours

4 small beets, unpeeled

1. Thoroughly wash the beets. Grate and place on a baking sheet lined with parchment or a reusable baking mat.

2. Set the oven to its lowest temperature and dehydrate the beets for 40 minutes to 3 hours. The time can vary greatly depending on the moisture content of the beets.

3. Alternatively, if you live somewhere warm and sunny, place the beets on a raised screen or rack outdoors to dry, bringing them in at night to avoid critters.

4. Transfer the dried beets to a coffee grinder or blender and grind until a powder is achieved. Add 1 teaspoon to water or a smoothie an hour before a workout for a natural preworkout.

Pomegranate Peel Powder

Who says you can't have your pomegranate seeds and eat the peel too? Pomegranate peels have been used as a natural remedy for constipation for centuries, in the form of pomegranate peel tea.

MAKES ⅓ cup ✦ **START TO FINISH:** 2 to 3 days

3 organic pomegranate peels with rind

1. Wash the peels thoroughly by scrubbing with a sponge or brush with vegetable wash if possible. Chop into 1-inch chunks.

2. Set the oven to its lowest temperature, and line a baking sheet with parchment paper or a reusable baking mat. Arrange the pomegranate peels in a single layer on the prepared baking sheet, and dehydrate for 4 to 6 hours, or until completely dried.

3. Alternatively, if you live somewhere warm and sunny, place the pomegranate peels on a raised screen or rack outdoors to dry, bringing them in at night to avoid critters.

4. To make pomegranate peel tea, add 1 to 2 teaspoons of the pomegranate peel powder to a tea bag, and steep in hot water, as desired.

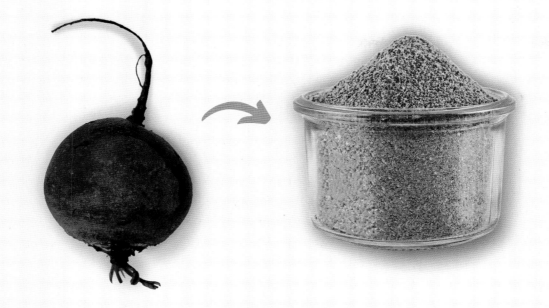

POMEGRANATE PEEL POWDER

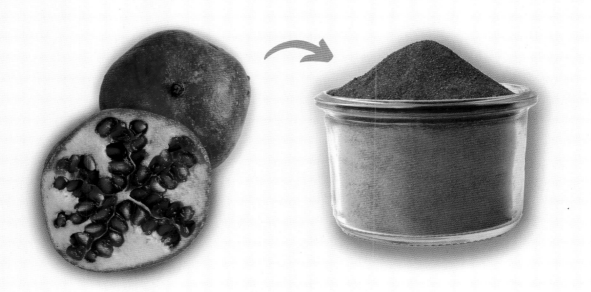

Storage: Store in a sealed jar in your pantry for up to 1 month.

Note: Do not consume more than one cup of pomegranate peel tea at a time, as it can speed up digestion.

Onion Peel Powder

Don't let those onion peels make you cry! Transform them into a delicious and versatile ingredient with this onion peel powder recipe. This sneaky zero-waste ingredient can act as a one-to-one replacement for onion powder in any dish, adding a kick of flavor to soups, stews, and stir-fries. Alternatively, you can powder garlic peels by using this method.

MAKES ⅓ cup ✦ START TO FINISH: 3 hours to 1 day

4 cups organic onion peels rinsed (dirty ones removed and discarded)

1. Soak your onion peels in water for 30 minutes, then drain and rinse. Dry with a clean cloth and make sure to discard any peels with dirt or residue.

2. Place on a dehydrator sheet to dry in the sun for 24 hours, bringing it in at night to avoid critters. Alternatively, arrange in a single layer on a parchment-lined baking sheet and leave in your oven at the lowest setting for 3 hours.

3. Using a blender or coffee grinder, grind the onion peels until a powder is formed. Use in recipes as you would onion powder.

Bouilliant Bouillon Powder

Who needs store-bought bouillon cubes when you can create your own delicious and zero-waste broth powder at home? This recipe utilizes common vegetable scraps, such as carrot peels, leek tops, and wilted herbs, to create a fragrant and flavorful bouillon that transforms soups, stews, and sauces from boring to bouilliant!

MAKES about 1½ cups bouillon powder

4 cups vegetable scraps—carrot peels, celery leaves, onion peels, garlic peels, leftover onions, herbs, and leek tops work best

¼ cup nutritional yeast

1 tablespoon salt

½ teaspoon ground turmeric

½ teaspoon freshly ground black pepper

½ teaspoon dried thyme

1. Finely chop the vegetables in a food processor. Transfer to a dehydrator sheet or lined baking sheet. You can dehydrate the vegetables in the sun, or on the lowest heat setting in the oven (typically 175°F) until completely dry, about 3 hours.

2. In a coffee grinder or blender, combine the dried vegetable scraps with the nutritional yeast, salt, turmeric, pepper, and thyme and blitz until a powder is formed.

3. One tablespoon of bouillon mixed with 1 cup of boiling water makes 1 cup of broth.

ONION PEEL POWDER

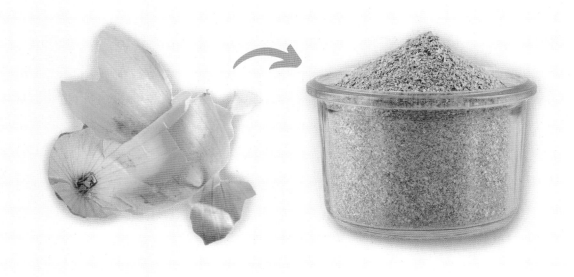

BOUILLIANT BOUILLON POWDER

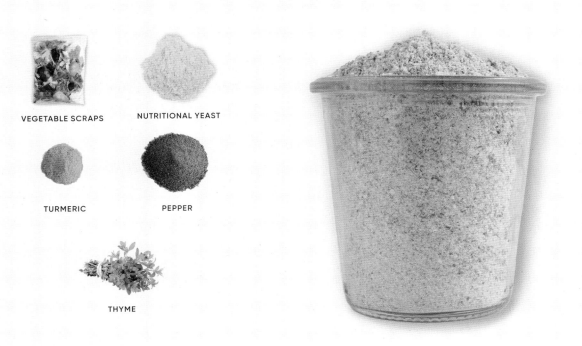

VEGETABLE SCRAPS

NUTRITIONAL YEAST

TURMERIC

PEPPER

THYME

Storage: Store in a sealed jar in your pantry for up to 1 month.

Lentil Sprouts

It's time to let lentils live their best life. I first learned about the magical power of sprouts from the sprout king himself, Doug Evans (*seriously, check this guy out if you want to dive into the wonderful world of sprouting*). Like a miracle in a jar, these lentil sprouts are a nutrient- and protein-packed superfood that costs cents on the dollar to make in your own kitchen. Sprouting lentils make such nutrients as vitamins B and C more bioavailable. Better yet, they taste amazing, adding a refreshing crunch to salads, wraps (check out my Sproutichoke Wrap, page 112), and sandwiches.

MAKES 1 jar of lentil sprouts

1 cup dried green or brown lentils, preferably organic

1. Before we begin, first rinse the lentils, then pick over and remove any small stones.

2. Place the lentils in a jar (I use a quart-size glass jar) and fill three-quarters of the way full with water. Close with the jar's perforated lid or a piece of cheesecloth, and allow the lentils to soak overnight on a countertop for 8 to 16 hours.

3. In the morning, drain the water from the jar and rinse the lentils well, either using the perforated lid or a fine-mesh strainer. Place the lentils back in the jar without the water, and either cover with the perforated lid or the cheesecloth held by a rubber band. Invert the jar so it is tilted on a diagonal with the lid end in a bowl.

4. Rinse the lentils twice a day for up to 4 days until sprouts begin to grow. Once the tails reach about ¼ inch in length, the lentil sprouts are ready to eat. Remove them from the jar and place on a clean cloth. Dry the lentil sprouts as much as possible. They should have no off-putting smell or signs of spoilage; if they do, you will want to discard them and try again.

   Storage: Store the sprouts in a sealed container in your fridge for up to 4 days.

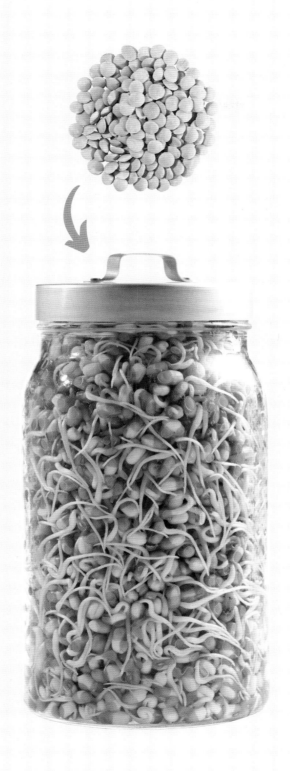

Turmeric Sauerkraut

Turmeric sauerkraut is the perfect way to use up that cabbage that's been sitting in your fridge. Finely shredded cabbage is fermented by lactic acid bacteria, resulting in a sour-and-savory accompaniment to such dishes as my Celeriac Corned "Beef" Sandwich (page 216). The essence of this dish is reflected in its name. The literal translation from German *sauerkraut* is "sour cabbage."

MAKES 1 to 2 jars ✦ **START TO FINISH:** 5 days

1 small green or red cabbage, around 3 pounds, cored and shredded finely

2 carrots, sliced or julienned

1½ tablespoons salt

1 teaspoon ground turmeric

1 teaspoon caraway seeds (optional)

1. In a bowl, combine the cabbage, carrots, and salt. Use your hands to mix everything thoroughly. Try to rub the salt into the cabbage.

2. Use a plate that fits just inside the bowl to cover the cabbage mixture. Weigh it down with canned food, jars, or something similar. As the cabbage begins to release moisture (which contains lactic acid), you want the cabbage to be submerged in the liquid. Leave the mixture at room temperature for 24 hours.

3. The next day, stir in the turmeric and caraway (if using). Divide the cabbage mixture, including its liquid, between two quart-size mason jars. Make sure the cabbage is tightly packed into the jar and submerged in its own brine. The jars should each be around three-quarters of the way full.

4. Once the cabbage is evenly dispersed in each jar, use either jar weights, pickle pebbles, or a smaller mason jar filled with dried beans to press the cabbage down and keep it submerged in the liquid. Cover the open mouth of each jar with a piece of cheesecloth held with a rubber band.

5. Leave the sauerkraut to ferment at a cool temperature (about 65°F) for at least 5 days. After the first 24 hours, lift the cheesecloth and press the cabbage down to ensure it stays submerged in the liquid, then cover the jar again.

6. It's up to you how sour you prefer the cabbage. You can ferment it anywhere between 5 and 10 days, with peak nutrition typically around 1 week. Once fermented, remove the weights and store in the fridge with a regular mason jar lid for up to 1 month.

Storage: Store in a jar in the fridge for up to 1 month.

GREEN CABBAGE

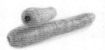

CARROT

TURMERIC

CARAWAY SEEDS

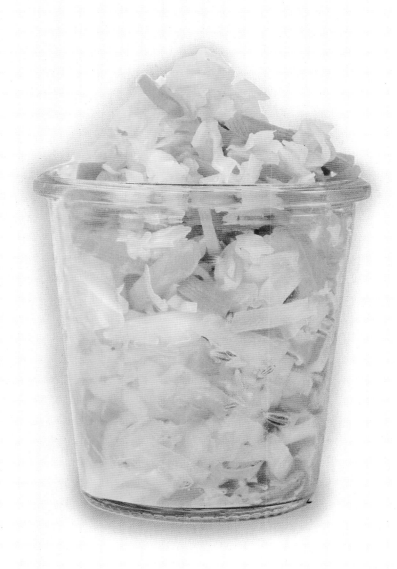

Preserves, Powders, Ferments & Other Fun Stuff

Spicy Pickled Red Onions

If you're looking to spice up your life (*and sandwiches*), these quick pickled red onions are the solution. They lend a perfect combo of heat, tang, and crunch to just about any dish. Plus, they're a great way to reduce food waste by making use of those onions that are starting to sprout! Best served with my Cuppa Joe Chili (page 218) or any dish where you want some extra kick.

MAKES one 20-ounce jar ✦ **START TO FINISH:** 1 hour

1 red onion, sliced thinly from the bottom to the root, with a mandoline, if possible

½ jalapeño pepper, deseed if you don't like heat, and sliced

1 tablespoon peppercorns

1 tablespoon vegan granulated sugar

1 cup hot water

1 cup Apple Scrap Vinegar (page 350) or store-bought apple cider vinegar

1. In a jar (I use a 20-ounce glass jar), combine the red onion and jalapeño slices with the peppercorns and sugar. Carefully pour in the hot water and Apple Scrap Vinegar until the onion and jalapeño are covered by the liquid. Stir and place a clean towel or cheesecloth over the top.

2. The pickled onions will be ready an hour later when they are vibrant in color and have a bold pickled taste. Seal with a lid, and enjoy as a garnish or in your favorite sandwiches.

Storage: Refrigerate in a sealed container for up to 1 week.

RED ONION

JALAPEÑO

BLACK PEPPERCORNS

WHITE SUGAR

APPLE CIDER VINEGAR

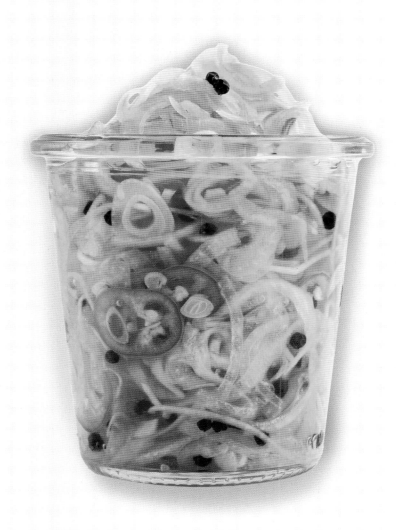

Preserves, Powders, Ferments & Other Fun Stuff

Quick 'n' Easy Homemade Pickles

Stuck in a pickle about what to do with all those cucumbers? Fear not, because this easy homemade pickle recipe is here to save the day. Pickles are actually one of the simplest recipes to make at home. The result is a tangy, crunchy snack or the perfect flavor enhancer for such recipes as my Dilly Orzo Soup (page 100), or any burger or sandwich.

MAKES 24 to 28 pickle spears ✦ **START TO FINISH:** 24 hours

1 pound pickling cucumbers, gherkins if possible

1 teaspoon black peppercorns

1 teaspoon mustard seeds

4 to 6 garlic cloves

Oak leaves (optional)

Dill flowers (optional)

1 cup water

1½ tablespoons salt

1 tablespoon vegan granulated sugar

½ cup distilled vinegar (5% acidity)

1. If you prefer whole pickles, soak them in water overnight. This will prevent them from being hollow inside. Otherwise, cut your cucumbers into spears!

2. At the bottom of two sterilized 16-ounce jars, combine the peppercorns, mustard seeds, garlic cloves, oak leaves (if using), and dill flowers (if using). Stuff in the cucumbers on top. Try to pack as many as you can into the jars.

3. In a small saucepan, combine the water with the salt and sugar. Bring to a simmer and whisk until the salt and sugar fully dissolve. Next, add the vinegar and bring the mixture back to a simmer for 2 to 3 minutes before removing from the heat.

4. Allow the mixture to cool for 7 to 10 minutes, then pour the brine into the jars, making sure the cucumbers are fully submerged in the liquid. Allow to cool completely before adding a lid.

5. Place the jars in the fridge and wait at least 24 hours before enjoying your pickles.

Storage: These pickles must be stored in the fridge and consumed within 3 weeks.

PICKLING CUCUMBERS

BLACK PEPPERCORNS

MUSTARD SEEDS

GARLIC CLOVES

VEGAN SUGAR

DISTILLED VINEGAR

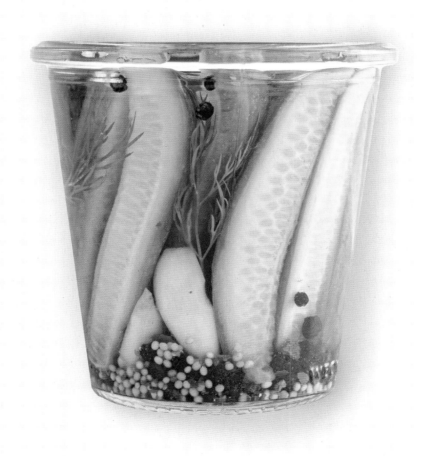

345

Preserves, Powders, Ferments & Other Fun Stuff

Pickled Watermelon Spears

Watermelon is my favorite summer fruit. There's just one problem . . . what to do with all the leftover rinds? Just when you think you've tried every type of pickle, here come these watermelon rind beauties. A little bit salty and a little bit sweet, these pickled watermelon spears make an amazing summer snack.

MAKES about two 16-ounce jars ✦ **START TO FINISH:** 24 hours

2 cups organic watermelon rind, green outer skin peeled and sliced into 2-inch spears

1 tablespoon sugar

1½ tablespoons salt

1 teaspoon black peppercorns

1 teaspoon mustard seeds

1 (1-inch) slice fresh ginger

½ cup Apple Scrap Vinegar (page 350) or store-bought apple cider vinegar

1. Bring a pot of salted water to a boil. Add the rind pieces and boil until tender, about 5 minutes. Drain, reserving 1 cup of the liquid and the rinds separately.

2. In a small saucepan, combine the reserved liquid with the sugar, salt, black peppercorns, mustard seeds, and ginger. Bring to a simmer and whisk until the salt and sugar fully dissolve. Next, add the Apple Scrap Vinegar and bring the mixture back to a simmer.

3. Stuff the rinds into two 16-ounce jars, fitting in as many spears as you possibly can. Allow the mixture to cool slightly so it is safe to handle, then pour the brine into the jars stuffed with watermelon, making sure the spears are fully submerged in the liquid.

4. Let cool completely before adding each lid. Place the jars in the fridge and wait at least 24 hours before enjoying the watermelon rind pickles.

Storage: These pickles must be refrigerated and consumed within 1 month.

WATERMELON

VEGAN SUGAR

BLACK PEPPERCORNS

MUSTARD SEEDS

GINGER ROOT

APPLE CIDER VINEGAR

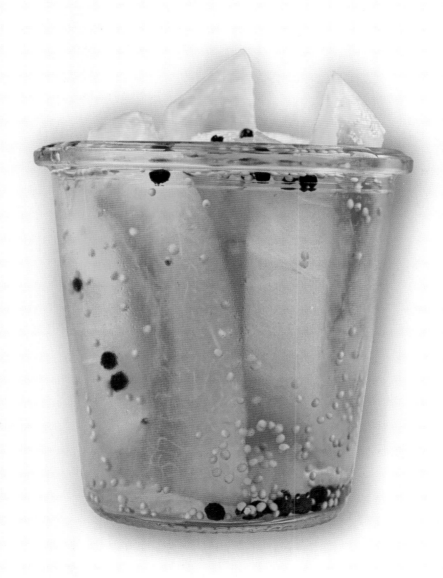

Preserves, Powders, Ferments & Other Fun Stuff

Strawberry Top Vinegar

Stop tossing those strawberry tops! Make this gorgeous strawberry top vinegar recipe instead. Steeping the tops transforms white wine vinegar into a red potion that has a subtle strawberry flavor, perfect as the base for my Strawberry Top Vinaigrette (page 280), for strawberry-infused cocktails, or even drizzled on ice cream.

MAKES 2 cups ✦ **START TO FINISH:** 2 days

½ cup strawberry tops **1½ cups white wine vinegar**

1. In a sealable jar, combine the vinegar and strawberry tops. Allow to rest at room temperature for at least 2 days.

2. Transfer the mixture to sealable bottles, discarding the tops for compost. Use as you would regular vinegar.

   Storage: Store in the pantry for up to 12 months.

STRAWBERRY TOPS

WHITE WINE VINEGAR

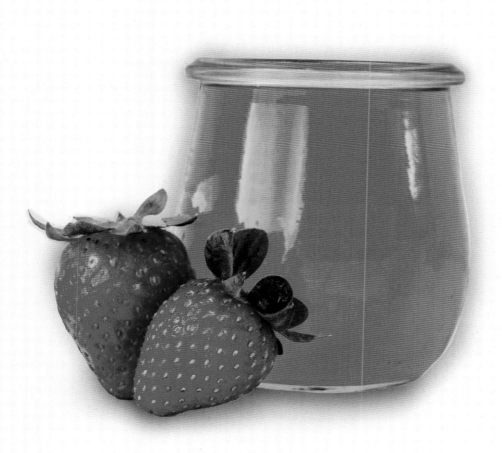

Preserves, Powders, Ferments & Other Fun Stuff

Apple Scrap Vinegar

Don't toss those apple scraps in the trash just yet. You can transform them into a delicious and sustainable ingredient with this simple recipe. This makes the perfect base for salad dressing, marinades, and more. Use as a one-to-one replacement in any recipe that calls for apple cider vinegar.

MAKES about 2 cups vinegar ✦ **START TO FINISH:** 4 weeks

2 cups warm water

3½ tablespoons vegan granulated sugar

Sliced cores and skins from 3 to 4 apples

1. In a bowl, combine the warm water and sugar. Stir until the sugar is dissolved.

2. Place the apple cores and skins in a sterilized wide-mouthed 32-ounce jar. Pour the sugar mixture over them, ensuring that the apple scraps are submerged and there are a few inches of airspace at the top.

3. Give it a stir and create a lid with either cheesecloth or an unused coffee filter on top. You should begin to see bubbles forming on the surface of the mixture within a couple of days. When this begins to happen, stir the mixture daily to prevent mold from forming.

4. Continue to ferment for 2 weeks, or until you no longer see bubbles forming in the liquid. Strain the mixture into a new, clean jar, composting the apple scraps at this time. Allow the vinegar mixture to ferment for an additional 2 weeks, stirring every couple of days, until it has the flavor and tang of vinegar to your liking.

Storage: Store lidded in the fridge for up to 3 months.

VEGAN SUGAR

APPLE SCRAPS

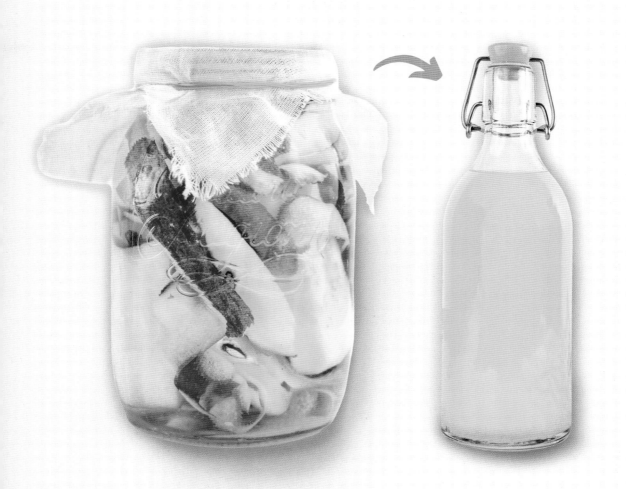

Preserves, Powders, Ferments & Other Fun Stuff

GROW YOUR OWN VEGETABLES FROM FOOD SCRAPS

Save money, reduce waste, and impress all your friends with your green thumb by regrowing vegetables from your food scraps! It's like having your own personal farm in your kitchen (minus the barnyard smell).

- **Green Onion:** When slicing green onions, leave 2 inches of the white bulbs and roots intact at the bottom. Reserve the bulbs and place them in a small jar, up to five per jar. Pour water into the jar, leaving around ½ inch of the green onions sticking out of the water. Refresh the water every 2 to 3 days, and you will have new green onions growing within 2 weeks. You can do this for up to three cycles with the same bulbs until they will stop producing as much green onion.

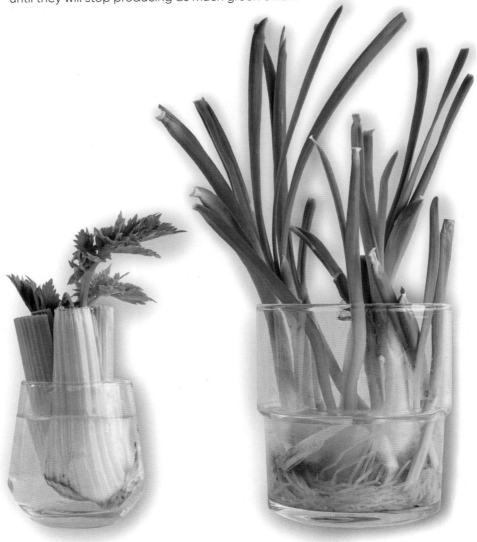

- **Lettuce:** Cut a head of romaine lettuce 1 to 2 inches from the bottom. Reserve the stem end and place it in a shallow dish. Add enough water to submerge the stem by about ½ inch. Place in a warm, sunny spot on a countertop, and change the water every 2 to 3 days. The lettuce will begin growing in a couple of days, and will be at full harvest at 10 to 12 days. This won't be as significant as the original romaine, but will provide you with enough lettuce for a small salad. You can also repot the stem at this point to continue growth.

- **Carrot Tops:** Using a knife, slice around ½ inch down from the carrot top. Also slice off the carrot tops, so they are about an inch long. Place the carrot tops, stump down, in a shallow bowl filled with about ⅜ inch of lukewarm water. Set this bowl by a window in direct sunlight. Change the water every 2 to 3 days. After 10 days, you will have carrot tops to harvest.

- **Celery:** Cut a bunch of celery 1 to 2 inches from the bottom. Reserve the stem end and place it in a shallow dish. Add enough water, about ½ inch, to submerge the stem. Place in a warm, sunny spot on a countertop, and change the water every 2 to 3 days. The leaves will begin growing in a couple of days, and will be at full harvest at 10 to 12 days.

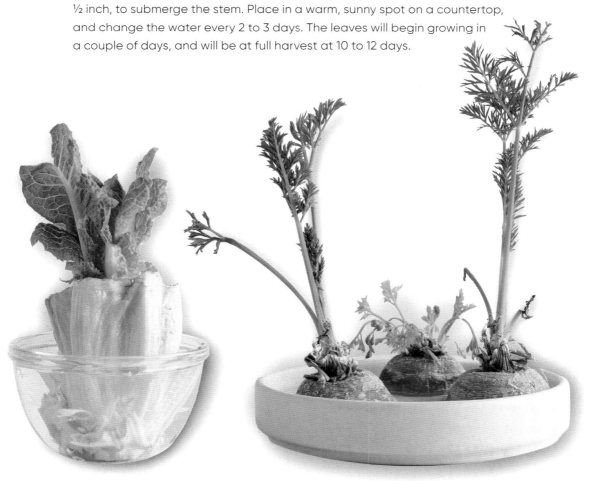

FREEZE YOUR SCRAPS

Leftover coffee, tomato paste, or red wine? Freeze these in ice cube trays for up to 3 months, and use in preportioned sizes as needed!

Preserves, Powders, Ferments & Other Fun Stuff

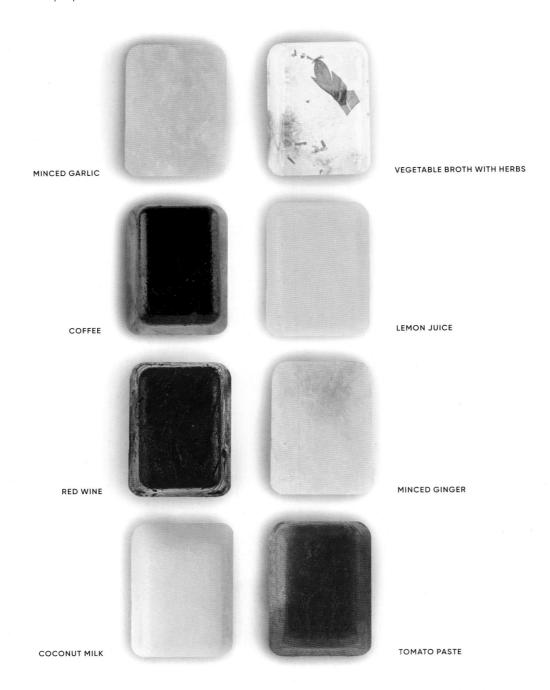

MINCED GARLIC

VEGETABLE BROTH WITH HERBS

COFFEE

LEMON JUICE

RED WINE

MINCED GINGER

COCONUT MILK

TOMATO PASTE

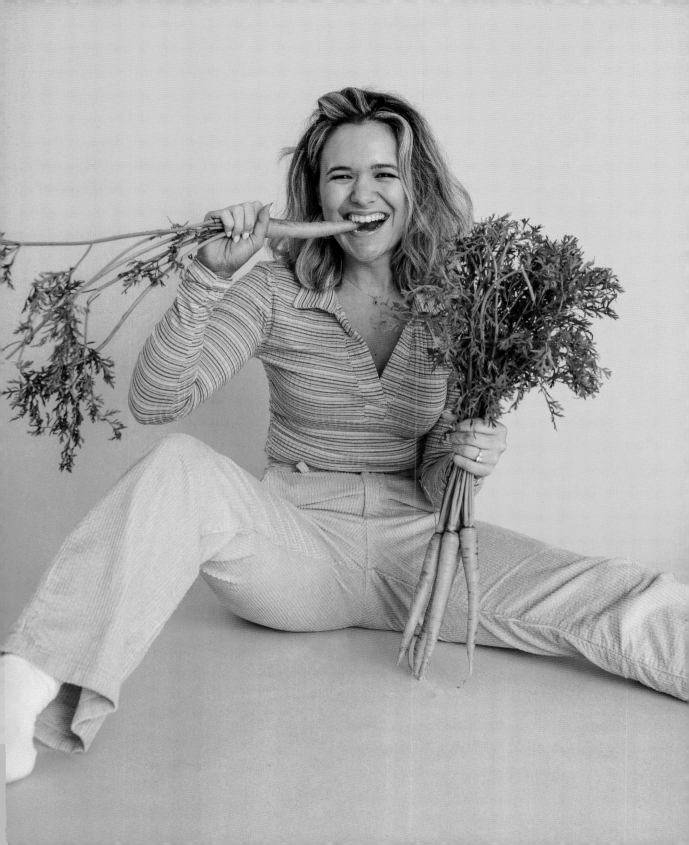

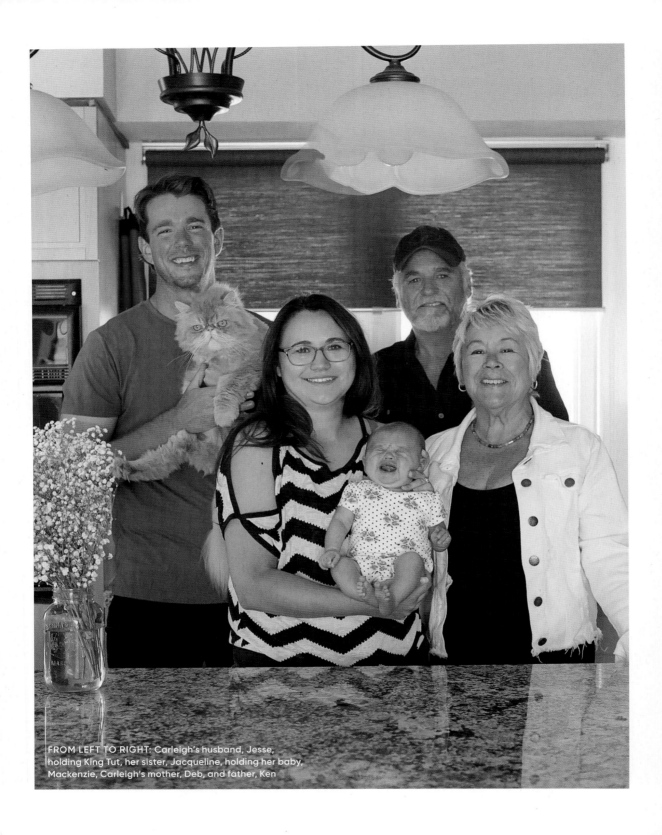

FROM LEFT TO RIGHT: Carleigh's husband, Jesse, holding King Tut, her sister, Jacqueline, holding her baby, Mackenzie, Carleigh's mother, Deb, and father, Ken

Acknowledgments

For me, the most challenging part of writing any cookbook comes down to the acknowledgments. It feels like an impossible task to capture in words the gratitude I have for the village of people who brought this massive project to fruition.

At the start of my *Scrappy* cookbook journey, one of my immediate family members fell very ill, and I didn't know if any of this would be possible. Then my sister, Jacqueline, quickly left her job as a veterinary technician to assist me in the recipe development, and I can truly say this book would not be half of what it is without her help and dedication. Thank you, Jake, for scraping me off the floor on the hard days, and for having me in stitches on the good ones.

Thank you to the rest of my family. My partner, Jesse, for being an unwavering support system, my biggest cheerleader, and my very favorite dishwasher. My mom and dad, for being the most supportive parents on the planet, and for always humbling me during the taste-testing phase of this project with your honest opinions.

My literary agent, Wendy. I am eternally grateful for the day we met, and for your ongoing support as a friend, agent, and confidant. You have made the process of publishing a book a dream come true.

To my editor, Renée. Thank you for believing in the vision of this book from day one, and for making it infinitely better with your genius mind. I feel so lucky to have an editor who truly understands the *why* behind these books and pushes them to be better. Every writer would be so lucky to have a Renée.

The entire Hachette team. I feel like I hit a jackpot being matched with the best publishing team in the world with members who are supportive, compassionate, and the hardest workers I've ever come across! Amanda, thank you for bringing the cover vision to life. Cisca, Nzinga, and Iris for your eagle eyes in editing the manuscript. To Michael and Ashley for the magical work you do in bringing this book to market, and to Michelle and Lauren for organizing amazing publicity opportunities for the launch. And finally to Laura, for your incredible talent in making each page as gorgeous as the next.

Shahad Odah and her simply awesome team at Foodie's Flare for shooting all the interior photos of this book. It was such a gift to be able to focus on recipe creation and have gorgeous photos being taken behind the scenes. I couldn't imagine a more professional and diligent team that made every single dish look spectacular. Cat Gavriusova for helping me with the perfect sourdough and fermenting recipes in this book. I don't know what I'd do without you. Alee LaPlaca of Alpaca Bakes for assisting me in developing a killer cake recipe.

Mandy, Linda, Victoria, Paige, Toni, Louis, Brian, and team for making a cover more whimsical than I could ever imagine. You made me feel like a movie star and the entire shoot was a dream come true!

Trish Sebben, my recipe tester. Your honest feedback made every recipe so much better, and as I told you with every batch, investing in you was one of the single best decisions I made for *Scrappy*.

Stephanie McKnight of Tidal Design and Shannon Bellisle of SB Creative Studio, for shooting the interior photos of me for this book with such care!

The PlantYou team, for keeping us afloat. Pam, my incredible online business manager extraordinaire. I'm so lucky to have you in my life and by my side for the highs and lows of entrepreneurship. Angee and Chelf—thank you for your incredible work to keep the cogs moving behind the scenes. You make it seem effortless, but I know the tireless effort that goes into the work we do every day.

And last, but certainly not least, YOU. For believing in *Scrappy Cooking*. Watching my videos. And most of all, for picking up this book. My absolute favorite part of this job is putting these recipes to paper, with a small hope that it can inspire you to eat more plants. THANK YOU for making that dream come true.

Love,
Carleigh

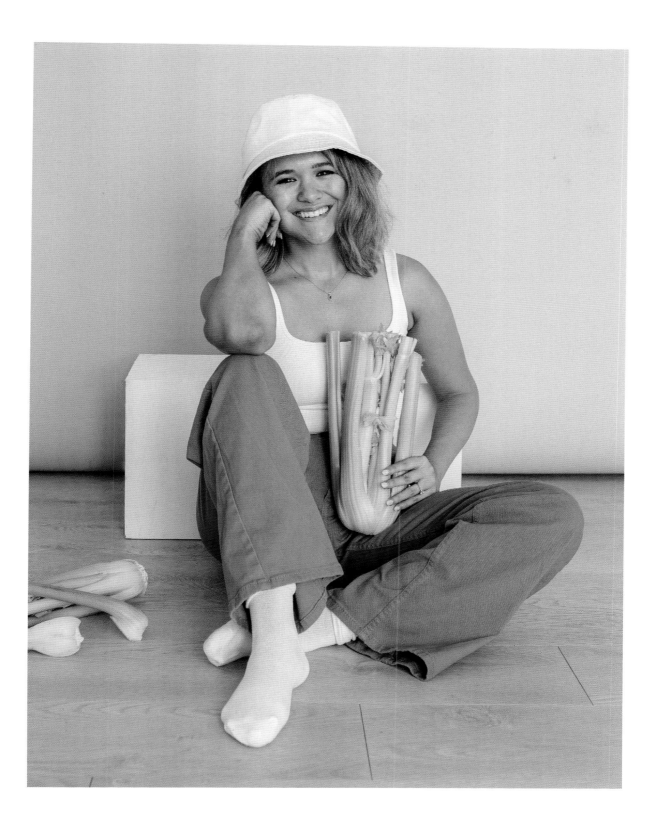

Nutritional Information

These nutritional calculations are an estimate and should be treated as such. The amounts will vary greatly, based on the ingredients you use. For example, some brands of almond milk have double the caloric amount than others. The nutritional information for these recipes is per individual serving, based on the lowest serving suggested. For example, in a recipe with 4 to 6 servings, the nutritional information is based on 4 servings. If there is an optional sauce or garnish with a recipe, it is not included in the calculations.

Scrappy Sunrises

Common Ground Granola
Calories: 234
Carbohydrates: 33 g
Protein: 7 g
Fat: 10 g
Fiber: 4 g

Chia Pudding Parfaits
Calories: 301
Carbohydrates: 29 g
Protein: 10 g
Fat: 7 g
Fiber: 8 g

Overnight Oat Fruity Parfaits
Calories: 373
Carbohydrates: 61 g
Protein: 11 g
Fat: 10 g
Fiber: 12 g

Berry Baked Oatmeal
Calories: 305
Carbohydrates: 47 g
Protein: 10 g
Fat: 10 g
Fiber: 8 g

Super Seedy Granola Bars
Calories: 238
Carbohydrates: 27 g
Protein: 8 g
Fat: 15 g
Fiber: 4 g

Brown Banana Muffins
Calories: 168
Carbohydrates: 34 g
Protein: 3 g
Fat: 3 g
Fiber: 3 g

"Death by Chocolate" Flapjacks
Calories: 119
Carbohydrates: 22 g
Protein: 4 g
Fat: 3 g
Fiber: 3 g

Optional Chocolate Sauce
Calories: 116
Carbohydrates: 11 g
Protein: 2 g
Fat: 9 g
Fiber: 1 g

Fritzy Fritters
Calories: 75
Carbohydrates: 14 g
Protein: 3 g
Fat: 1 g
Fiber: 7 g

Last Week's Loaf Breakfast Casserole
Calories: 502
Carbohydrates: 87 g
Protein: 17 g
Fat: 10 g
Fiber: 8 g

Eggless Omelet
Calories: 310
Carbohydrates: 52 g
Protein: 22 g
Fat: 5 g
Fiber: 17 g

Grab & Glow BurritOH
Calories: 468
Carbohydrates: 65 g
Protein: 34 g
Fat: 11 g
Fiber: 19 g

Cultured Vegan Yogurt
Calories: 388
Carbohydrates: 22 g
Protein: 9 g
Fat: 31 g
Fiber: 3 g

Two-Way "Bacon" Street
Calories: 128
Carbohydrates: 12 g
Protein: 6 g
Fat: 7 g
Fiber: 4 g

Juicer-Free Green Juice
Calories: 81
Carbohydrates: 18 g
Protein: 4 g
Fat: 0 g
Fiber: 1 g

Smoothie Bombs

Greens Bombs
Calories: 4
Carbohydrates: 1 g
Protein: 0 g
Fat: 0 g
Fiber: 0 g

Fruity, Spicy Anti-inflammatory Bombs
Calories: 17
Carbohydrates: 3 g
Protein: 0 g
Fat: 0 g
Fiber: 0 g

Fiber-Filled Chocolate Bombs
Calories: 84
Carbohydrates: 7 g
Protein: 4 g
Fat: 5 g
Fiber: 2 g

Very Berry Bombs
Calories: 28
Carbohydrates: 5 g
Protein: 1 g
Fat: 1 g
Fiber: 1 g

Scrappetizers & Sides

Fiesta Fries
Calories: 523
Carbohydrates: 92 g
Protein: 29 g
Fat: 8 g
Fiber: 18 g

We-Got-the-Beet Chips
Calories: 98
Carbohydrates: 14 g
Protein: 12 g
Fat: 1 g
Fiber: 9 g

Crispy Crunches
Calories: 67
Carbohydrates: 13 g
Protein: 4 g
Fat: 0 g
Fiber: 3 g

Dill Pickle Chips
Calories: 291
Carbohydrates: 58 g
Protein: 8 g
Fat: 3 g
Fiber: 11 g

The Knead for Flatbread
Calories: 138
Carbohydrates: 27 g
Protein: 5 g
Fat: 1 g
Fiber: 1 g

It's a (Flax) Wrap
Calories: 233
Carbohydrates: 16 g
Protein: 9 g
Fat: 13 g
Fiber: 12 g

Save the Seeds
Calories: 235
Carbohydrates: 16 g
Protein: 9 g
Fat: 12 g
Fiber: 3 g

Cornmeal Biscuits
Calories: 197
Carbohydrates: 28 g
Protein: 5 g
Fat: 8 g
Fiber: 3 g

Sweet & Spicy Carrot Showstopper
Calories: 321
Carbohydrates: 27 g
Protein: 6 g
Fat: 18 g
Fiber: 5 g

Greek Lemon Smashed Potatoes
Calories: 181
Protein: 3 g
Carbohydrates: 27 g
Fiber: 4.3 g
Fat: 7.2 g
Saturated Fat: 1 g

Scrappacia
Calories: 65
Carbohydrates: 13 g
Protein: 3 g
Fat: 0 g
Fiber: 2 g

Souperb Soups

Whatever Sheet-Pan Soup
Calories: 238
Carbohydrates: 25 g
Protein: 6 g
Fat: 15 g
Fiber: 6 g

Green Goddess Soup
Calories: 117
Carbohydrates: 11 g
Protein: 7 g
Fat: 6 g
Fiber: 3 g

Raid-the-Fridge Noodle Soup
Calories: 466
Carbohydrates: 74 g
Protein: 27 g
Fat: 9 g
Fiber: 9 g

Roasted Tomato Soup with Crispy Quinoa
Calories: 307
Carbohydrates: 56 g
Protein: 16 g
Fat: 4 g
Fiber: 13 g

Leeky Tuscan Minestrone
Calories: 229
Carbohydrates: 37 g
Protein: 15 g
Fat: 4 g
Fiber: 8 g

Cobby Chick'n Broth
Calories: 45
Carbohydrates: 7 g
Protein: 2 g
Fat: 0 g
Fiber: 0 g

Smoky Corncob Chowder
Calories: 296
Carbohydrates: 55 g
Protein: 15 g
Fat: 5 g
Fiber: 7 g

Caramelized French Onion Soup
Calories: 494
Carbohydrates: 65 g
Protein: 20 g
Fat: 19 g
Fiber: 6 g

Dilly Orzo Soup
Calories: 361
Carbohydrates: 49 g
Protein: 18 g
Fat: 11 g
Fiber: 7 g

Scrappy Broth
Calories: 17
Carbohydrates: 3 g
Protein: 0 g
Fat: 0 g
Fiber: 1 g

Sustainable Sammies, Wraps & Salads

Celery Leaf "Tabbouleh"
Calories: 69
Carbohydrates: 14 g
Protein: 3 g
Fat: 1 g
Fiber: 3 g

Broccoli Stem Summer Rolls
Calories: 474
Carbohydrates: 82 g
Protein: 15 g
Fat: 9 g
Fiber: 6 g

Life-Altering Mediterranean Wraps
Calories: 304
Carbohydrates: 45 g
Protein: 9 g
Fat: 11 g
Fiber: 7 g

Sproutichoke Wrap
Calories: 393
Carbohydrates: 59 g
Protein: 22 g
Fat: 9 g
Fiber: 10 g

A-Better-Burger Wrap
Calories: 294
Carbohydrates: 39 g
Protein: 13 g
Fat: 9 g
Fiber: 4 g

Stacked Veggie Sandwich
Calories: 447
Carbohydrates: 52 g
Protein: 15 g
Fat: 8 g
Fiber: 8 g

White Bean "Tuna" Sandwich (Filling)
Calories: 150
Carbohydrates: 27 g
Protein: 10 g
Fat: 2 g
Fiber: 8 g

Buffalo Chickpea Lettuce Cups
Calories: 312
Carbohydrates: 33 g
Protein: 11 g
Fat: 17 g
Fiber: 8 g

Citrus Cabbage Slaw
Calories: 136
Carbohydrates: 29 g
Protein: 5 g
Fat: 2 g
Fiber: 6 g

Grilled Romaine Salad
Calories: 161
Carbohydrates: 19 g
Protein: 3 g
Fat: 6 g
Fiber: 3 g

That's-a-Panzanella
Calories: 208
Carbohydrates: 27 g
Protein: 9 g
Fat: 8 g
Fiber: 4 g

The Saucy Kale
Calories: 453
Carbohydrates: 32 g
Protein: 19 g
Fat: 29 g
Fiber: 14 g

Brussels Sprouts Caesar Salad (with Garlic Croutons)
Calories: 279
Carbohydrates: 44 g
Protein: 11 g
Fat: 9 g
Fiber: 10 g

Street Corn Pasta Salad
Calories: 301
Carbohydrates: 41 g
Protein: 13 g
Fat: 12 g
Fiber: 6 g

Pantry Bean Salad
Calories: 200
Carbohydrates: 35 g
Protein: 11 g
Fat: 5 g
Fiber: 9 g

Strawberry Farro Salad
Calories: 345
Carbohydrates: 50 g
Protein: 10 g
Fat: 13 g
Fiber: 9 g

Beaming Lentil Lemon Salad
Calories: 411
Carbohydrates: 58 g
Protein: 13 g
Fat: 14 g
Fiber: 6 g

No-Waste Noodles

Tuscan Sweet Potato Gnocchi (2 servings)
Calories: 300
Carbohydrates: 61 g
Protein: 9 g
Fat: 3 g
Fiber: 10 g

Hot-Pink Pasta (4 servings)
Calories: 523
Carbohydrates: 78 g
Protein: 20 g
Fat: 15 g
Fiber: 3 g

The Whole Darn Squash Pasta (4 servings)
Calories: 597
Carbohydrates: 97 g
Protein: 23 g
Fat: 11 g
Fiber: 9 g

Skillet Lasagna (4 servings)
Calories: 489
Carbohydrates: 66 g
Protein: 23 g
Fat: 15 g
Fiber: 11 g

One-Pan Orzo Casserole (4 servings)
Calories: 574
Carbohydrates: 98 g
Protein: 24 g
Fat: 10 g
Fiber: 15 g

Vodka Penne with Broccolini (4 servings)
Calories: 644
Carbohydrates: 117 g
Protein: 14 g
Fat: 9 g
Fiber: 10 g

15-Minute Lemon Pepper Alfredo (4 servings)
Calories: 568
Carbohydrates: 104 g
Protein: 24 g
Fat: 8 g
Fiber: 8 g

Rock-Your-Broc Mac & Cheez (4 servings)
Calories: 653
Carbohydrates: 114 g
Protein: 32 g
Fat: 13 g
Fiber: 17 g

Instant Mac 'n' Cheez Powder (4 servings)
Calories: 140
Carbohydrates: 20 g
Protein: 15 g
Fat: 2 g
Fiber: 8 g

Mac 'n' Cheez Using the Powder (4 servings)
Calories: 535
Carbohydrates: 104 g
Protein: 32 g
Fat: 4 g
Fiber: 18 g

Green with Envy Spaghetti (4 servings)
Calories: 637
Carbohydrates: 113 g
Protein: 31 g
Fat: 7 g
Fiber: 4 g

Sunday Sauce (8 servings)
Calories: 359
Carbohydrates: 63 g
Protein: 66 g
Fat: 7 g
Fiber: 10 g

Scratch Tomato Sauce (4 servings)
Calories: 88
Carbohydrates: 19 g
Protein: 4 g
Fat: 1 g
Fiber: 4 g

Lemon Peel Pesto
Calories: 651
Carbohydrates: 83 g
Protein: 24.3 g
Fat: 27 g
Fiber: 3.5 g

The Main Bowl

Super Loaded Harvest Bowl
Calories: 380
Carbohydrates: 45 g
Protein: 12 g
Fat: 18 g
Fiber: 8 g

Microbiome Bowl
Calories: 435
Carbohydrates: 65 g
Protein: 21 g
Fat: 11 g
Fiber: 7 g

Pesto & Herb Vitality Bowl (4 servings)
Calories: 495
Carbohydrates: 99 g
Protein: 26 g
Fat: 3 g
Fiber: 19 g

Sea-Saving "Salmon" Bowl
Calories: 481
Carbohydrates: 69 g
Protein: 24 g
Fat: 13 g
Fiber: 5 g

Loaded Tortilla Bowls
Calories: 564
Carbohydrates: 80 g
Protein: 26 g
Fat: 20 g
Fiber: 19 g

Nutty Noodle Bowl
Calories: 517
Carbohydrates: 59 g
Protein: 20 g
Fat: 24 g
Fiber: 8 g

Eco Entrées

Firecracker Tofu with Coconut Rice
Calories: 536
Carbohydrates: 66 g
Protein: 30 g
Fat: 17 g
Fiber: 10 g

Zucchini "Falafel" Fritters
Calories: 95
Carbohydrates: 14 g
Protein: 6 g
Fat: 3 g
Fiber: 5 g

Any Vegetable Curry
Calories: 415
Carbohydrates: 71 g
Protein: 11 g
Fat: 8 g
Fiber: 9 g

Perfect Peanut Butter Curry
Calories: 354
Carbohydrates: 45 g
Protein: 16 g
Fat: 13 g
Fiber: 12 g

Palak "Paneer"
Calories: 193
Carbohydrates: 16 g
Protein: 11 g
Fat: 12 g
Fiber: 4 g

Golden Immunity Stew
Calories: 448
Carbohydrates: 55 g
Protein: 15 g
Fat: 7 g
Fiber: 10 g

Spicy Eggplant & White Bean Stew
Calories: 364
Carbohydrates: 67 g
Protein: 23 g
Fat: 3 g
Fiber: 18 g

What a Dahl!
Calories: 323
Carbohydrates: 58 g
Protein: 20 g
Fat: 2 g
Fiber: 20 g

Jackfruit Bourguignon
Calories: 228
Carbohydrates: 39 g
Protein: 10 g
Fat: 2 g
Fiber: 5 g

Stuffed Cabbage Dumplings
Calories: 257
Carbohydrates: 47 g
Protein: 11 g
Fat: 3 g
Fiber: 3 g

Can't-Miss Miso Cabbage Steaks
Calories: 297
Carbohydrates: 38 g
Protein: 12 g
Fat: 12 g
Fiber: 7 g

Bang-Bang Broccoli-cious Steaks
Calories: 329
Carbohydrates: 35 g
Protein: 12 g
Fat: 18 g
Fiber: 7 g

Bang-Bang Sauce
Calories: 206
Carbohydrates: 12 g
Protein: 6 g
Fat: 17 g
Fiber: 3 g

Whole Roasted Cauliflower, served with Roasted Red Pepper Sauce
Calories: 620
Carbohydrates: 84.7 g
Protein: 23 g
Fat: 23 g
Fiber: 11 g

Confetti Sheet-Pan Tacos (per taco, including taco shell)
Calories: 171
Carbohydrates: 28 g
Protein: 4 g
Fat: 6 g
Fiber: 4 g

Chickpea Potpie
Calories: 350
Carbohydrates: 64 g
Protein: 15 g
Fat: 5 g
Fiber: 9 g

Orange Peel Chick'n
Calories: 131
Carbohydrates: 16 g
Protein: 9 g
Fat: 4 g
Fiber: 1 g

Celeriac Corned "Beef" Sandwich
Calories: 267
Carbohydrates: 38 g
Protein: 9 g
Fat: 8 g
Fiber: 6 g

Cuppa Joe Chili
Calories: 324
Carbohydrates: 51 g
Protein: 24 g
Fat: 6 g
Fiber: 17 g

PlantYou Pizza Party
Calories: 425
Carbohydrates: 76 g
Protein: 14 g
Fat: 8 g
Fiber: 7 g

Vegan Ground Beef
Calories: 107
Carbohydrates: 14 g
Protein: 4 g
Fat: 5 g
Fiber: 4 g

Vegan Sticky "Ribs" & Seitan Chick'n
Calories: 110
Carbohydrates: 9 g
Protein: 13 g
Fat: 3 g
Fiber: 1 g

Pickled Tennessee Tenders
Calories: 259
Carbohydrates: 29 g
Protein: 19 g
Fat: 9 g
Fiber: 5 g

Broccoli 'n' "Beef" Stir-Fry
Calories: 417
Carbohydrates: 64 g
Protein: 17 g
Fat: 11 g
Fiber: 6 g

Second Chance Sheet-Pan "Fried" Rice
Calories: 390
Carbohydrates: 56 g
Protein: 14 g
Fat: 13 g
Fiber: 8 g

Veggie Masala Burgers
Calories: 208
Carbohydrates: 39 g
Protein: 7 g
Fat: 3 g
Fiber: 4 g

Vegan Meaty Hand Pies
Calories: 340
Carbohydrates: 48 g
Protein: 18 g
Fat: 8 g
Fiber: 17 g

Soy-Free Tofu
Calories: 64
Carbohydrates: 12 g
Protein: 5 g
Fat: 0 g
Fiber: 3 g

Sustainable Sweets

Wacky Cake
Calories: 343
Carbohydrates: 55 g
Protein: 3.7 g
Fat: 9 g
Fiber: 3 g

The Scrappy Cookie
Calories: 159
Carbohydrates: 18 g
Protein: 5 g
Fat: 8 g
Fiber: 1 g

Hot-Chocolate Cookies
Calories: 246
Carbohydrates: 31 g
Protein: 5 g
Fat: 13 g
Fiber: 4 g

Not-Picky Fruit Crisp
Calories: 319
Carbohydrates: 56 g
Protein: 7 g
Fat: 7 g
Fiber: 8 g

Leftover Quinoa Truffles
Calories: 135
Carbohydrates: 17 g
Protein: 4 g
Fat: 6 g
Fiber: 4 g

PB&J Chickpea Blondies
Calories: 293
Carbohydrates: 44 g
Protein: 9 g
Fat: 10 g
Fiber: 6 g

Mushy Berry Jam (per tbsp)
Calories: 7
Carbohydrates: 2 g
Protein: 0 g
Fat: 0 g
Fiber: 1 g

Candied Citrus Peels
Calories: 387
Carbohydrates: 101 g
Protein: 0 g
Fat: 0 g
Fiber: 0 g

Apple Scrap Honey (per tbsp)
Calories: 41
Carbohydrates: 11 g
Protein: 0 g
Fat: 0 g
Fiber: 0 g

Berry Fruit Leather
Calories: 49
Carbohydrates: 10 g
Protein: 1 g
Fat: 1 g
Fiber: 2 g

Coo-Coo for Coconut Caramel (Sauce)
Calories: 175
Carbohydrates: 20 g
Protein: 1 g
Fat: 11 g
Fiber: 1 g

Sticky Date Pudding
Calories: 394
Carbohydrates: 78 g
Protein: 6 g
Fat: 8 g
Fiber: 4 g

Nutritional Information

Mousse on the Loose
Calories: 240
Carbohydrates: 20 g
Protein: 1 g
Fat: 13 g
Fiber: 0 g

Mini Aquafaba Pavlovas
Calories: 11
Carbohydrates: 2 g
Protein: 0 g
Fat: 0 g
Fiber: 0 g

All the Earl Grey Tea Cake
Calories: 294
Carbohydrates: 56 g
Protein: 6 g
Fat: 6 g
Fiber: 3 g

Dressings, Dips & Saucy Things

Sunflower Cream Sauce
Calories: 28
Carbohydrates: 2 g
Protein: 1 g
Fat: 2 g
Fiber: 0 g

Carrot Top Chimichurri
Calories: 13
Carbohydrates: 2 g
Protein: 0 g
Fat: 0 g
Fiber: 1 g

Scrappy Pesto (4 servings)
Calories: 61
Carbohydrates: 4 g
Protein: 3 g
Fat: 4 g
Fiber: 1 g

Mango Peanut Sauce
Calories: 135
Carbohydrates: 18 g
Protein: 4 g
Fat: 6 g
Fiber: 2 g

Roasted Red Pepper Sauce
Calories: 201
Carbohydrates: 16 g
Protein: 8 g
Fat: 10 g
Fiber: 1 g

Creamy Vegan Tzatziki
Calories: 45
Carbohydrates: 7 g
Protein: 2 g
Fat: 1 g
Fiber: 1 g

Everything Tahini Dressing
Calories: 138
Carbohydrates: 9 g
Protein: 4 g
Fat: 11 g
Fiber: 2 g

Creamy Hummus Caesar
Calories: 63
Carbohydrates: 6 g
Protein: 3 g
Fat: 3 g
Fiber: 2 g

Strawberry Top Vinaigrette
Calories: 43
Carbohydrates: 6 g
Protein: 1 g
Fat: 2 g
Fiber: 1 g

Green Goddess Dressing
Calories: 109
Carbohydrates: 7 g
Protein: 3 g
Fat: 9 g
Fiber: 2 g

Luscious Lemon Dressing
Calories: 57
Carbohydrates: 6 g
Protein: 0 g
Fat: 4 g
Fiber: 1 g

(Almost) the Whole Can Hummus
Calories: 169
Carbohydrates: 24 g
Protein: 9 g
Fat: 5 g
Fiber: 7 g

High-Protein Kale, Asparagus & Edamame Spread
Calories: 174
Carbohydrates: 15 g
Protein: 14 g
Fat: 8 g
Fiber: 5 g

Whipped Feta Dip with Roasted Tomatoes
Calories: 196
Carbohydrates: 20 g
Protein: 9 g
Fat: 11 g
Fiber: 4 g

Tofu Feta
Calories: 48
Carbohydrates: 1 g
Protein: 2 g
Fat: 4 g
Fiber: 0 g

Vegan Nutty "Parm"
Calories: 70
Carbohydrates: 7 g
Protein: 8 g
Fat: 2 g
Fiber: 4 g

Balsamic Glaze
Calories: 73
Carbohydrates: 18 g
Protein: 0 g
Fat: 0 g
Fiber: 0 g

Sip & Save

Peanut Butter Jar Latte
Calories: 267
Carbohydrates: 31 g
Protein: 11 g
Fat: 12 g
Fiber: 3 g

Rose Water
Calories: 0
Carbohydrates: 0 g
Protein: 0 g
Fat: 0 g
Fiber: 0 g

Rose-Water Latte
Calories: 113
Carbohydrates: 14 g
Protein: 6 g
Fat: 3 g
Fiber: 1 g

Date Seed Coffee
Calories: 0
Carbohydrates: 0 g
Protein: 0 g
Fat: 0 g
Fiber: 0 g

Pineapple Skin Tea
Calories: 24
Carbohydrates: 6 g
Protein: 0 g
Fat: 0 g
Fiber: 0 g

Tangy Tepache
Calories: 72
Carbohydrates: 16 g
Protein: 0 g
Fat: 0 g
Fiber: 0 g

Ginger Turmeric Immunity Shots
Calories: 51
Carbohydrates: 13 g
Protein: 1 g
Fat: 0 g
Fiber: 3 g

Tummy-Soothing Lemon, Ginger & Mint Ice Cubes
Calories: 2
Carbohydrates: 0 g
Protein: 0 g
Fat: 0 g
Fiber: 0 g

DIY Ginger Ale
Calories: 10
Carbohydrates: 3 g
Protein: 0 g
Fat: 0 g
Fiber: 0 g

No-Waste Nut Milk
Calories: 94
Carbohydrates: 3 g
Protein: 4 g
Fat: 8 g
Fiber: 1 g

Strawberry Milk (4 cups)
Calories: 132
Carbohydrates: 13 g
Protein: 4 g
Fat: 8 g
Fiber: 2 g

Chocolate Nut Milk (4 cups)
Calories: 157
Carbohydrates: 19 g
Protein: 5 g
Fat: 8 g
Fiber: 3 g

Homemade Oat Milk
Calories: 77
Carbohydrates: 14 g
Protein: 3 g
Fat: 1 g
Fiber: 2 g

Preserves, Powders, Ferments & Other Fun Stuff

Small Sourdough Loaf (10 slices)
Calories: 134
Carbohydrates: 28 g
Protein: 4 g
Fat: 0 g
Fiber: 1 g

Sourdough Discard Crackers (largish crackers, 30 servings)
Calories: 31
Carbohydrates: 4 g
Protein: 1 g
Fat: 1 g
Fiber: 1 g

Homemade Vanilla Extract (per tsp)
Calories: 12
Carbohydrates: 0 g
Protein: 0 g
Fat: 0 g
Fiber: 2 g

Perfect Preserved Lemons
Calories: 21
Carbohydrates: 7 g
Protein: 1 g
Fat: 0 g
Fiber: 2 g

Sun-Dried Tomatoes (per ¼ cup)
Calories: 20
Carbohydrates: 4 g
Protein: 1 g
Fat: 0 g
Fiber: 1 g

Herbed Bread Crumbs (per ¼ cup)
Calories: 37
Carbohydrates: 7 g
Protein: 1 g
Fat: 1 g
Fiber: 1 g

Citrus Peel Powder (per tsp)
Calories: 8
Carbohydrates: 2 g
Protein: 0 g
Fat: 0 g
Fiber: 1 g

Tomato Peel Powder (per tsp)
Calories: 11
Carbohydrates: 2 g
Protein: 0 g
Fat: 0 g
Fiber: 1 g

Beet Powder (per tsp)
Calories: 15
Carbohydrates: 3 g
Protein: 1 g
Fat: 0 g
Fiber: 0 g

Pomegranate Peel Powder (per tsp)
Calories: 33
Carbohydrates: 4 g
Protein: 0 g
Fat: 0 g
Fiber: 0 g

Onion Peel Powder (per tsp)
Calories: 8
Carbohydrates: 2 g
Protein: 0 g
Fat: 0 g
Fiber: 0 g

Bouilliant Bouillon Powder (per tbsp)
Calories: 15
Carbohydrates: 3 g
Protein: 1 g
Fat: 0 g
Fiber: 1 g

Lentil Sprouts (per cup)
Calories: 82
Carbohydrates: 17 g
Protein: 7 g
Fat: 0 g
Fiber: 0 g

Turmeric Sauerkraut (per cup)
Calories: 61
Carbohydrates: 14 g
Protein: 3 g
Fat: 0 g
Fiber: 6 g

Spicy Pickled Red Onions (per tbsp)
Calories: 14
Carbohydrates: 3 g
Protein: 0 g
Fat: 0 g
Fiber: 0 g

Quick 'n' Easy Homemade Pickles (per gherkin/4 spears)
Calories: 23
Carbohydrates: 1 g
Protein: 0 g
Fat: 0 g
Fiber: 1 g

Pickled Watermelon Spears (per ¼ cup)
Calories: 23
Carbohydrates: 5 g
Protein: 0 g
Fat: 0 g
Fiber: 0 g

Strawberry Top Vinegar (per tbsp)
Calories: 4
Carbohydrates: 0 g
Protein: 0 g
Fat: 0 g
Fiber: 0 g

Apple Scrap Vinegar (per tbsp)
Calories: 9
Carbohydrates: 0 g
Protein: 0 g
Fat: 0 g
Fiber: 0 g

Metric Conversion Charts

The recipes in this book have not been tested with metric measurements, so some variations might occur.

Remember that the weight of dry ingredients varies according to the volume or density factor: 1 cup of flour weighs far less than 1 cup of sugar, and 1 tablespoon doesn't necessarily hold 3 teaspoons.

General Formula for Metric Conversion

Ounces to grams	multiply ounces by 28.35
Grams to ounces	multiply ounces by 0.035
Pounds to grams	multiply pounds by 453.5
Pounds to kilograms	multiply pounds by 0.45
Cups to liters	multiply cups by 0.24
Fahrenheit to Celsius	subtract 32 from Fahrenheit temperature, multiply by 5, divide by 9
Celsius to Fahrenheit	multiply Celsius temperature by 9, divide by 5, add 32

Volume (Liquid) Measurements

1 teaspoon = ⅙ fluid ounce = 5 milliliters

1 tablespoon = ½ fluid ounce = 15 milliliters

2 tablespoons = 1 fluid ounce = 30 milliliters

¼ cup = 2 fluid ounces = 60 milliliters

⅓ cup = 2⅔ fluid ounces = 79 milliliters

½ cup = 4 fluid ounces = 118 milliliters

1 cup or ½ pint = 8 fluid ounces = 250 milliliters

2 cups or 1 pint = 16 fluid ounces = 500 milliliters

4 cups or 1 quart = 32 fluid ounces = 1,000 milliliters

1 gallon = 4 liters

Volume (Dry) Measurements

¼ teaspoon = 1 milliliter

½ teaspoon = 2 milliliters

¾ teaspoon = 4 milliliters

1 teaspoon = 5 milliliters

1 tablespoon = 15 milliliters

¼ cup = 59 milliliters

⅓ cup = 79 milliliters

½ cup = 118 milliliters

⅔ cup = 158 milliliters

¾ cup = 177 milliliters

1 cup = 225 milliliters

4 cups or 1 quart = 1 liter

½ gallon = 2 liters

1 gallon = 4 liters

Weight (Mass) Measurements

1 ounce = 30 grams

2 ounces = 55 grams

3 ounces = 85 grams

4 ounces = ¼ pound = 125 grams

8 ounces = ½ pound = 240 grams

12 ounces = ¾ pound = 375 grams

16 ounces = 1 pound = 454 grams

Linear Measurements

½ in = 1 ½ cm

1 inch = 2 ½ cm

6 inches = 15 cm

8 inches = 20 cm

10 inches = 25 cm

12 inches = 30 cm

20 inches = 50 cm

Oven Temperature Equivalents

Fahrenheit (F) and Celsius (C)

100°F = 38°C

200°F = 95°C

250°F = 120°C

300°F = 150°C

350°F = 180°C

400°F = 205°C

450°F = 230° C

Index

Stuffed Cabbage Dumplings, 202
    Whole Roasted Cauliflower, 208–209
Rose Water, 294
Rose-Water Latte, 298

S